A Guide to Quick and Easy Access to Information in this Book

This book has 5 major sections. Select the topic of interest by the table of contents or the index.

* If you want to learn about tumor growth principles, epidemiology information, prevention/screening/detection guidelines, and/or diagnosis and staging classifications, refer to Section I.

* To locate cancer disease management with oncologic complications, site-specific cancers are listed in alphabetical order in Section II.

* If you want information about cancer disease treatment, refer to Section III. The 5 major treatments (surgery, radiation therapy, chemotherapy, biotherapy, and bone marrow transplantation) and cancer clinical trials contain the who, what, where, when, why, and how aspects of care.

* To learn about cancer supportive care interventions, refer to Section IV. Relevant clinical guidelines can be found for pain, nutrition, psychosocial, sexuality, and home care needs.

* To find clinical practice guidelines for multifaceted infusion therapies refer to Section V. The drugs/blood products, dose, route, and infusion principles with nursing management are listed alphabetically in a table format. Venous access devices can also be found in this section.

D0222454

Pocket Guide to
Oncology Nursing

Pocket Guide to
Oncology Nursing

Shirley E. Otto, MSN, RN, OCN, CRNI

Clinical Nurse Specialist
St. Francis Regional Medical Center
Wichita, Kansas

Illustrated

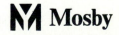 **Mosby**

St. Louis   Baltimore   Berlin   Boston   Carlsbad   Chicago   London   Madrid
Naples   New York   Philadelphia   Sydney   Tokyo   Toronto

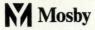

Mosby

Dedicated to Publishing Excellence

Publisher: Nancy L. Coon
Managing Editor: Jeff Burnham
Associate Developmental Editor: Linda Caldwell
Production: Page Two Associates
Cover Art: Catherine Chang

First Edition
Copyright© by Mosby-Year Book, Inc.

A NOTE TO THE READER
The author and publisher have made every attempt to check dosages and nursing
content for accuracy. Because the science of pharmacology is continually
advancing, the knowledge base continues to expand. Therefore, we recommend
that the reader always check product information for changes in dosage or
administration before administering any medication. This is particularly important
with new or rarely used drugs.

Printed in the United States of America
Composition by Page Two Associates
Printing/binding by R.R. Donnelly

Mosby-Year Book, Inc.
11830 Westline Industrial Drive, St. Louis, Missouri 63146

Library of Congress Cataloging in Publication Data
Oncology Nursing / Shirley E. Otto — 1st ed.
Includes bibliographical references and index.
ISBN 0-8015-6547-1
1. Cancer —Nursing. I. Otto, Shirley E.

DNLM/DLC
for Library of Congress
93 94 95 96 97 / 9 8 7 6 5 4 3 2 1

I would like to thank the contributors to
Oncology Nursing, 2nd edition, whose knowledge
and expertise has helped
form the basis of this pocket guide.

Joyce Alexander, MSN, RN, OCN
Cynthia Brogden, MSN, RN, OCN
Stephanie Chang, MN, RN, OCN
Jane C. Clark, MN, RN, OCN
Frances Cornelius, MSN, RN
Rebecca Crane, MN, RN, OCN
Betty Thomas Daniel, MS, RN, OCN
Marilyn Davis, MS, RN
Mary Gullatte, MN, RN, OCN
Ryan Iwamoto, ARNP, MN
Noella Devolder McCray, MN, RN, OCN
Linda Meili, BSN, RN, OCN
Jill Grodecki Moore, MSN, RN
Mary E. Murphy, MS, RN, OCN
Jeanne Parzuchowski, MS, RN, OCN
Karen Pfeifer, MSN, RN, CNA, OCN
Paula Trahan Rieger, MSN, RN, OCN
Sandra Lee Schafer, MN, RN, OCN
Susan L. Penny Schmidt, MS, RN, OCN
Lisa Schulmeister, MN, RN, CS, OCN
Suzanne Shaffer, MN, RN, OCN
Judith A. Shell, MS, RN, OCN
Carol J. Swenson, MS, RN, OCN
Sandra Szekely, RSN, RN

Shirley E. Otto, MSN, RN, OCN, CRNI

Preface

Health care in the 90's is in a constant state of transition. Competent, quality and cost-effective patient care is required by all health-care professionals. Patients with cancer are provided multi-option care in varied clinical settings: acute, ambulatory, home, and extended-care. The nurses working in these settings have many demands placed upon their skills and resources. Time, astute clinical observations, prudent nursing interventions and communication with other health-care professionals have become VERY IMPORTANT ISSUES to the nurse.

POCKET GUIDE TO ONCOLOGY NURSING was developed to keep pace with the many demands and changes placed upon the nurse. It contains the "necessary to know for oncology nursing practice" plus Infusion Therapies Guidelines for antibiotics, antifungals, antivirals; biotherapy; chemotherapy; blood component therapy; venous access; and ambulatory infusion pumps. Additional resources include: laboratory values, diagnostic tests and cancer resources.

To facilitate easy use of the text, multiple boxes, tables, and quick reference guides are used. Priorities of Patient Teaching, Geriatric Considerations, Disease and Treatment Complications have been incorporated into the disease and treatment chapters. The American Cancer Society Guidelines for prevention, screening, and detection are listed as well as the American Joint Committee for Diagnosis and Staging for all major cancer disease sites. The disease chapters [bone, brain, breast, colorectal, gastrointestinal, genitourinary, gynecological, head and neck, HIV and related cancers, leukemia, lung, lymphoma, myeloma, skin cancers] contain succinct clinical management issues. Cancer treatment modalities include surgery, radiation therapy, chemotherapy, biotherapy, bone marrow transplantation, and cancer clinical trials provide concise information on the treatment rationale, types of therapy, and nursing diagnoses/interventions.

Prudent clinical interventions for oncological complications, home care, pain management, nutrition, protective mechanisms, psychosocial and sexuality issues are provided in the last section of the text.

Brief Contents

Detailed Contents

Clinical Aspects

of the Cancer

Diagnosis

Pathophysiology

Medical researchers have identified approximately 100 different types of cancers. Each cancer cell within these various diseases has an altered morphology and biochemistry from the normal cell. Cancer is not a disorderly growth of immature cells, but, rather, a logical coordinated process in which a normal cell undergoes changes and acquires special capabilities.

The Normal Cell

The basic unit of structure and function in all living things is the *cell*. Approximately 60 trillion cells are in the adult human body, and, although there are many different types of cells, all of them have certain common characteristics. Whenever cells are destroyed, the remaining cells of the same type reproduce until the correct number has been replenished. This orderly replacement of cells is governed by a control mechanism that stops when the loss or damage has been corrected. Dynamic, active, and orderly, the healthy cell is a small powerhouse, laboratory, factory, and duplicating machine—perfectly copying itself over and over.[6] Figure 1-1 shows the phases and characteristics of *mitosis* (cell division).

Proliferative Growth Patterns

Cancer cells are not subject to the usual restrictions placed by the host on cell proliferation. Abnormal cellular growth is classified as *nonneoplastic* and *neoplastic growth*.[11,15]

Nonneoplastic Growth Patterns

The four common nonneoplastic growth patterns are hypertrophy, hyperplasia, metaplasia, and dysplasia.

- *Hypertrophy*—an increase in cell size. It commonly results from increased workload, hormonal stimulation, or compensation directly related to the functional loss of other tissue.

- *Hyperplasia*—a reversible increase in the number of cells of a certain tissue type, resulting in increased tissue mass. Hyperplasia commonly occurs as a normal physiological response at times of rapid growth and development (e.g., pregnancy and adolescence). It is abnormal when the volume of cells produced exceeds the normal physiological demand.

- *Metaplasia*—one adult cell type is substituted for another type not usually found in the involved tissue (e.g., glandular for squamous). The process is reversible if the stimulus is removed, or metaplasis may progress to dysplasia if the stimulus persists. Metaplasia can be induced by inflammation, vitamin deficiencies, irritation, and various chemical agents. A common area for metaplasia to occur is the uterine cervix.

- *Dysplasia*—characterized by alteration in normal adult cells in which the cell varies its normal size, shape, or organization, or one mature cell type is replaced with a less mature cell type. The common stimulus creating a dysplasia is usually an external one (e.g., radiation, inflammation, toxic chemicals, or chronic irritation). Dysplasia is possibly reversible if the stimulus is removed.

Neoplastic Growth Patterns

- *Anaplasia* means "without form" and is an irreversible change where the structure of adult cells regress to more primitive levels, e.g., cancer.

- *Neoplasia* means "new growth" and describes an abnormal tissue mass that extends beyond the boundaries of normal tissue, failing to fulfill the normal function of cells in that tissue. Neoplasms are characterized by uncontrolled functioning, unregulated division and growth, and abnormal motility. Neoplastic growths are referred to as *benign neoplasms* or *malignant neoplasms*. Benign neoplasms include papillomas or warts. Malignant neoplasms include solid tumors and leukemia. *Cancer* is the common term for all malignant neoplasms. Table 1-1 summarizes the difference between benign and malignant growths.[9,20]

Interphase
- Cell grows in size
- Chromosomes elongate
- DNA replicates

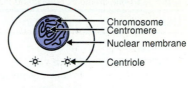

Chromosome
Centromere
Nuclear membrane
Centriole

Prophase
- DNA coils
- Centrioles move to opposite poles

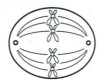

Metaphase
- Chromosomes align across cell equator
- Nucleoli and nuclear membrane disappear

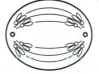

Anaphase
- Chromosomes divide
- Chromosomes move to opposite poles

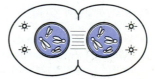

Telophase
- Chromosomes elongate
- Nuclear membranes reappear and enclose chromosomes
- Cytokinesis occurs
- Centrioles replicate

Figure 1-1. Mitosis: phases and characteristics. (From Griffiths M, Murray K, and Russo P: *Oncology nursing: pathophysiology, assessment, and intervention*, New York, 1984, Macmillan Publishing Co.)

Table 1-1 Comparison of Benign and Malignant Growths

Characteristic	Malignant Tumor	Benign Tumor
Encapsulated	Rarely	Usually
Differentiated	Poorly	Partially
Metastasis	Frequently present	Absent
Recurrence	Frequent	Rare
Vascularity	Moderate to marked	Slight
Mode of growth	Infiltrative and expansive	Expansive
Cell characteristics	Cells abnormal and become more unlike parent cells	Fairly normal and similar to parent cells

From Bender CM and Yasko JM: Problems with abnormal cell growth. In Lewis SM and Collier IC, editors: *Medical-surgical nursing: assessment and management of clinical problems,* ed 3, St Louis, 1992, Mosby. Characteristics of Cancer Cells.

Characteristics of Cancer Cells

Microscopic Properties

- *Pleomorphism*—cancer cells vary in size and shape. Some are unusually large, while others are too small. Multiple nuclei may be seen.
- *Hyperchromatism*—nuclear chromatin, the major component of genes, is more pronounced upon staining.
- *Polymorphism*—the nucleus is larger and varies in shape.
- *Aneuploidy*—unusual numbers of chromosones are seen.
- *Abnormal chromosome arrangements*—a variety of possibilities exists including *translocations*, the exchange of material between chromosomes, *deletions*, loss of chromosome sections, *additions*, extra chromosomes, and *fragile sites*, weak sections on chromosomes.[6,7,9,15]

Kinetic Properties

- *Loss of proliferate control*—cell renewal or replacement is the stimulus for cell proliferation.
- *Loss of capacity to differentiate*—differentiation refers to the extent to which cancer cells resemble comparable

normal cells. Cells that closely resemble the normal cell but form slow-growing, usually encapsulated tumors are *well-differentiated*. Cells that grow rapidly and do not have the original tissue's morphologic characteristics and specialized cell functions are called undifferentiated. The process by which cells lose characteristics of normal cells is called dedifferentiation. The more undifferentiated a malignant cell, the more virulent it is thought to be.

■ *Altered biochemical properties*—cells may acquire new properties because of enzyme pattern changes or alterations in DNA. Examples of these *altered biochemical properties* include production of tumor-associated antigens marking the cancer as "non-self;" continued reproduction despite diminished concentrations of growth hormones; higher rates of anaerobic glycolysis, making the cell less dependent on O_2; loss of cell-to-cell cohesiveness and adhesiveness; and abnormal production of hormones or hormone-like substances that induce paraneoplastic syndromes. (Table 1-2.)[7,16]

■ *Chromosomal instability*—chromosomal instability results in new, increasingly malignant mutants as cancer cells create a surviving subpopulation of advanced neoplasms with unique biologic and cytogenetic characteristics that are highly resistant to therapy.[15]

■ *Capacity to metastasize*—metastasis, the spread of cancer cells from a primary (parent) site to distant secondary sites, aided by the production of enzymes on the surface of the cancer cell. Cancer and cells become increasingly malignant with each mutation.

Cellular Kinetics

The field of cellular kinetics is the study of the quantitative growth and division of cells.[15]

Cell Cycle

The *cell cycle* is the sequence of events involved in replication and distribution of DNA to the daughter cells produced by cell division. All cells, nonmalignant and malignant, progress through the five phases of the cell cycle. These five phases are G_0, G_1, S, G_2, and M (Figure 1-2).

Table 1-2 Paraneoplastic Syndromes

Clinical Syndrome	Underlying Cancers	Causal Substance
Cushing's syndrome	Bronchogenic carcinoma (small cell) Pancreatic carcinoma Neural tumors	Adrenocortotropic hormone (ACTH) or ACTH-like substance
Hyponatremia	Bronchogenic carcinoma Intracranial neoplasms	Antidiuretic hormone (ADH) or ADH-like substance
Hypercalcemia	Bronchogenic carcinoma (squamous cell) Breast carcinoma Renal carcinoma Adult T-cell lymphoma	(?) Parathyroid hormone-like substance Transforming growth factor (TGF)-a
Hyperthyroidism	Blood dyscrasias Bronchogenic carcinoma Prostatic carcinoma	Thyroid-stimulating hormone (TSH) or TSH-like substance

Hypoglycemia	Fibrosarcoma Other mesenchymal sarcomas Hepatocellular carcinoma	Insulin or insulin-like substance
Carcinoid syndrome	Bronchial adenoma (carcinoid) Pancreatic carcinoma Gastric carcinoma	Serotonin, bradykinin, (?) histamine
Polycythemia	Renal Carcinoma Cerebellar hemangioma Hepatocellular carcinoma	Erythropoietin
Venous thrombosis	Pancreatic carcinoma Bronchogenic carcinoma Other cancers	(?) Hypercoagulability

From Volker DL: Pathophysiology of cancer. In Clark JC and McGee RF, editors: *Core curriculum for oncology nursing*, Philadelphia, 1992, WB Saunders. Modified from Cotran RS, Kumar V, and Robbins SL: *Robbins pathologic basis of disease*, ed 4, Philadelphia, 1989, WB Saunders.

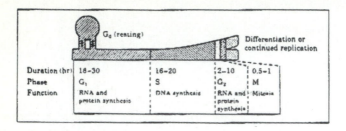

Figure 1-2. Cell cycle time.

- *G_0 Phase (postmitotic resting phase)*—encompasses that period of the cell cycle when normal renewable tissue is not actively proliferating; includes nondividing cells and resting cells.
- *G_1 Phase (growth or postmitotic presynthesis period)*—lasts from 18 to 30 hours, extends from the completion of the previous cell division to the beginning of chromosome replication; period of decreased metabolic activity; synthesizes proteins needed in the formation of ribonucleic acid (RNA).
- *S Phase (synthesis)*—lasts approximately 16 to 20 hours; RNA is synthesized, which is essential for the synthesis of deoxyribonucleic acid (DNA).
- *G_2 Phase (postsynthetic/premitotic phase)*—lasts from 2 to 10 hours, is one of relative hypoactivity, as the cells await entry into the mitotic phase; termination of DNA synthesis to the beginning of cell division.
- *M Phase (mitosis)*—lasts from 30 minutes to 1 hour, mitosis and cell division occur. Duplication of DNA must be complete before cells enter the mitotic cycle. This phase is further subdivided into four stages: *prophase, metaphase, anaphase,* and *telophase.* (Figure 1-1).

Cancer cells are able to complete the cell cycle quicker by decreasing the length of time spent in the G_1 phase, and are less likely to enter or remain in the G_0 phase of the cell cycle than are normal cells. Those cells in the late G_1 or early S phase of the cell cycle are the most vulnerable to dedifferentiation.[1,11,15,18]

Tumor Growth Properties

In general, cancer cells possess the following properties:

- *Immortality of transformed cells*—cancer cells are capable of passing through an infinite number of population doublings if insufficient nutrition and growth factors are available.
- *Decreased contact inhibition of movement*—normal cells adjust to the proximity of neighboring cells by halting growth. Cancer cells invade others without respect to these constraints.
- *Decreased contact inhibition of cell division*—cancer cells lack or exhibit decreased contact inhibition of growth, continuing to divide, even piling atop one another.
- *Decreased adhesiveness*—cancer cells are less adhesive, resulting in increased cell mobility.[14]
- *Loss of anchorage dependence*—cancer cells do not need a surface on which to attach and proliferate. This property affects cells' shape and adhesiveness.
- *Loss of restrictive point control*—cancer cells lose this stringent restriction point control and continue to proliferate in spite of suboptimal nutrition and high cell density.

Tumor Growth Concepts

Normal cells are divided into three major categories of cell growth: *static* (nondividing), *expanding* (resting), and *renewing* (continuously dividing). Static cells do not continue to divide after the postembryonic period. If these cells are damaged or destroyed, they cannot be replaced. Examples are nerve and brain cells. Expanding cells temporarily stop reproduction on reaching normal size, but they can reenter the cell cycle and divide during times of physiological need. Examples are liver, kidney, and endocrine gland cells. Renewing cells have the highest level of reproductive activity. These cells have a finite lifespan and continuously replicate to replace dying cells. Examples are germ cells, epithelial cells of the gastrointestinal mucosa, and blood cells. Tumors are composed of mixtures of nondividing, resting, and continuously dividing cells.[9,11]

The growth rate of tumors is expressed in doubling time. *Tumor volume-doubling time* (DT) is the time needed for a tumor mass to double its volume. Tumor cells undergo a series of doublings as the tumor increases in size. The average DT of most primary solid tumors is approximately 2 to 3 months, with a range of 11 to 90 weeks. In general, a tumor must progress through approximately 30 doublings before becoming palpable. The minimum clinically detectable body burden of tumor (*tumor volume*) is 10 billion cells (1 g). Tumor masses are usually 100 billion cells or 10 g at detection.

Because not all tumor cells divide simultaneously, *growth fraction* (GF) is an important concept in the determination of DT. GF is the ratio of the total number of cells to the number of proliferating cells. Tumors with larger GFs increase their tumor mass more quickly. As tumor volume increases, GF decreases. The rapid proliferation of tumor cells followed by continuous, but slowed, proliferation is called the *Gompertz function*. The Gompertz function can be expressed by the *Gompertz growth curve* (Figure 1-3). The growth curve illustrates the initial exponential growth of cancer cells, followed by the steady and progressive decrease in the GF due to a decrease in the fraction of proliferating cells and an increase in the rate of cell death.[9,15,19]

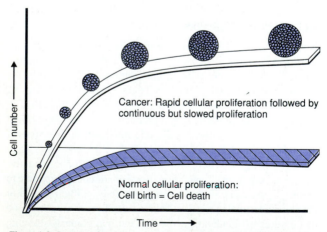

Figure 1-3. Gompertz function as viewed by growth curve. (From Goodman M: *Cancer: chemotherapy and care, part I,* 1990, Bristol Laboratories, Division of Bristol-Myers Co., Evansville, Inc.)

Carcinogenesis

Carcinogenesis is the process by which normal cells are transformed into cancer cells.

- *Initiating agent (carcinogen)*—a chemical, biologic, or physical agent capable of permanently, directly, and irreversibly changing the molecular structure of the genetic component (DNA) of a cell. Viral, environmental or lifestyle, and genetic factors have all been identified as initiators of carcinogenesis.[20]

- *Promoting agent (cocarcinogen)*—alters the expression of genetic information of the cell, thereby enhancing cellular transformation; includes hormones, plant products, and drugs. Promoting agents, themselves, do not cause cancer. The effects are temporary and reversible.[10]

- *Complete carcinogen*—possesses both initiating and promoting properties and is capable of inducing cancer on its own, e.g., radiation.

- *Reversing agent*—inhibits the effects of promoting agents by stimulating metabolic pathways in the cell that destroy carcinogens or by altering the initiating potency of chemical carcinogens, e.g., drugs, enzymes, and vitamins.[6]

- *Oncogene*—a gene that has evolved to control growth and repair of tissues; includes protooncogenes, the portion of DNA that regulates normal cell proliferation and repair, and antioncogenes, the portion of DNA that stops cell division.[18,20]

- *Progression*—the change in a tumor from a preneoplastic state, or low degree of malignancy, to a rapidly growing, virulent tumor, characterized by changes in growth rate, invasive potential, metastatic frequency, morphologic traits, and responsiveness to therapy.[9]

- *Heterogeneity*—refers to differences among individual cells within a tumor (e.g., genetic composition, growth rate, metastatic potential, hormone receptors, and susceptibility to antineoplastic therapy). The degree of heterogeneity increases as the tumor increases in size.[7]

- *Transformation*—transformation is a multistep process by which cells become progressively dedifferentiated after exposure to an initiating agent. Transformation results from a genetic alteration in the cell, which deregulates the control of cell proliferation.[6,18,20]

A Theory of Carcinogenesis

The *Berenblum theory* states that cancer occurs as the result of two distinct events: *initiation* and *promotion*. Initiation occurs first and is usually believed to be rapid and mutational. The change is brought about by an initiating agent (e.g., a chemical substance). The second event involves a promoting agent, and its effect is generally believed to include changes in cell growth, transport, and metabolism. Without promotion, initiation will not result in a truly transformed cell. Promotion may occur shortly after initiation or much later in an individual's life. Initiation produces a change in the cell, but cancer will not develop until the cell is affected by one or several promoting agents (Figure 1-4).[2]

Promoting Agents

Hormones

Hormones promote the carcinogenic process by sensitizing a cell to the carcinogenic insult or modifying the growth of an established tumor. Four main types of human cancer (i.e., cancer of the prostate, brain, breast, and endometrium) occur in hormone-responsive tissues (target tissues).[10]

Chemicals

Chemical carcinogens include compounds or elements that alter DNA. Environmental chemical carcinogens range from food preservatives to atmospheric pollution.

Viruses

Viruses are thought to contribute to human carcinogenesis by infecting the host DNA, resulting in proto-oncogenic changes and cell mutation. Viral carcinogens may be *slow-acting* (adenoviruses, herpes viruses) or *fast-acting* (human T-cell lymphomaleukemia virus or HTLV) and are *tissue specific*, infecting tissue selectively. Age and immunocompetence are believed to interact with and affect a person's vulnerability to viral carcinogens (Table 1-3).[18]

Table 1-3 Oncogenic Viruses

Family	Virus	Associated Tumors	Other Risk Factors
DNA VIRUSES			
Hepadenovirus	Hepatitis B group (HBV)	Liver cancer	Alcohol/Smoking Fungal toxins/Other viruses
Papovavirus	Human papilloma virus (HPV)	Genital, laryngeal, and skin warts Skin cancers in clients with epidermodysplasia verruciformis In situ and invasive cancers of the vulva and uterine cervix	Sunlight Genetic disorders possibly affecting immunity
Herpesvirus	Epstein-Barr virus (EBV)	Burkitt's lymphoma Immunoblastic lymphoma Nasopharyngeal carcinoma	Malaria Immune deficiency Histocompatibility antigen genotype
	Herpes simplex type 2 (HSV-2)	Cancer of uterine cervix	
	Cytomegalovirus (CMV)	Kaposi's sarcoma	Immune deficiency
RNA VIRUSES			
Type D	Human T-cell leukemia virus-1 (HTLV-1)	Adult T-cell leukemia/ lymphoma	Histocompatibility antigen genotype

From Fernoglio-Preiser CM et al: *New concepts in neoplasia as applied to diagnostic pathology*, Baltimore, 1986, Williams & Wilkins.

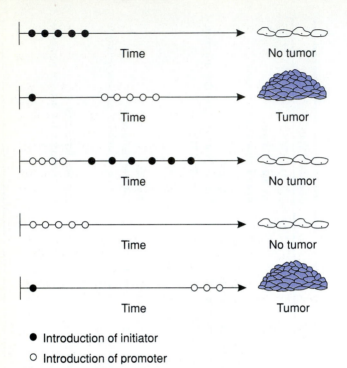

● Introduction of initiator
○ Introduction of promoter

Figure 1-4. The interactions of initiation and promotion.

Radiation

Radiation appears to initiate carcinogenesis by damaging susceptible DNA, producing changes in the DNA structure. Cell death may result, or the cells may become permanently altered and escape normal control mechanisms.

Both *ionizing* and *electromagnetic radiation* have been known to cause cancer in animals and humans. Sources of ionizing radiation exposure include: radioactive ground minerals, diagnostic or therapeutic x-rays, and synthetic radioactive materials. Factors that apparently influence the risk of carcinogens by ionizing radiation include the following:

- Host characteristics—genetic make-up, age, and degree of stress.
- Cell cycle phase—cells in G_2 are more sensitive than cells in S or G_1.
- Degree of differentiation—immature cells are most vulnerable.
- Cellular proliferation rate—cells with high mitotic rates are most vulnerable.
- Tissue type—gastrointestinal and hematopoietic tissues are extremely sensitive to radiation.
- Rate of dose and total dose—the higher the dose rate and total dose, the greater is the chance for mutation to occur.

Immune System

Human immunity to malignant disease is a function of *humoral factors* (tumor-specific antibodies) and *cellular factors* (sensitized *lymphocytes* and macrophages). Cancer cells often possess antigens and, therefore, are recognized as foreign cells by the immune system and are destroyed.

Tumor Nomenclature

Histogenetic Classification System

Tumors are grouped according to the tissue from which they originate and are described by the *histogenetic classification* system. (Table 1-4). Benign tumors also use the suffix *oma* to designate the presence of a tumor. However, malignant tumors of epithelial origin are designated by the root *carcin* (crablike) and those of connective tissue origin are designated by the root *sarc* (flesh). Mixed tumors contain more than one neoplastic cell type. Teratomas are a special type of mixed tumor and may be benign or malignant. These tumors arise from totipotential (germ) cells and may be composed of several differentiated tissue types. Teratomas arise from three germ layers: endoderm, ectoderm, and mesoderm.[9,11,18]

Table 1-4 Classification of Tumors

Site	Benign	Malignant
EPITHELIAL TISSUE TUMORS*	—OMA	—CARCINOMA
Surface epithelium	Papilloma	Carcinoma
Glandular epithelium	Adenoma	Adenocarcinoma
CONNECTIVE TISSUE TUMORS†	—OMA	—SARCOMA
Fibrous tissue	Fibroma	Fibrosarcoma
Cartilage	Chondroma	Chondrosarcoma
Striated muscle	Rhabdomyoma	Rhabdomyosarcoma
Bone	Osteoma	Osteosarcoma
NERVOUS TISSUE TUMORS‡	—OMA	—OMA
Astrocytes	—	Astrocytoma
Meninges	Meningioma	Meningeal sarcoma
Nerve cells	Ganglioneuroma	Neuroblastoma
HEMATOPOIETIC TISSUE TUMOR		
Lymphoid tissue		Hodgkin's disease, malignant lymphoma
Plasma cells		Multiple myeloma
Bone marrow		Lymphocytic and myelogeneous leukemia

* Body surfaces, lining of body cavities, and glandular structures.
† Supporting tissue, fibrotic tissues, and blood vessels.
‡ Brain nerves and retina.

From Bender CM and Yasko JM: Problems with abnormal cell growth. In Lewis SM and Collier IC, editors: *Medical-surgical nursing: assessment and management of clinical problems*, ed 3, St Louis, 1992, Mosby.

Nomenclature of Hematologic Malignancies

Leukemia is a cancer of the hematologic system and is a diffuse rather than a solid tumor, characterized by the abnormal proliferation and release of leukocyte precursors. These are classified as either *lymphoid* or *myeloid* according to the predominant cell type and as *acute* or *chronic* according to the level of maturity shown by the predominant cell. The prefix *lympho* describes a leukemia of lymphoid (lymphatic system) origin, and *myelo* or *granulo* describes a leukemia of myeloid (bone marrow) origin. The suffix *blastic* describes immature white blood cells, while the suffix *cystic* describes the presence of more mature cells.

Malignant lymphoma is a cancer of the lymphoid tissue. Both *non-Hodgkin's lymphoma* and *Hodgkin's disease* are classified according to four primary features: cell type, degree of differentiation, type of reaction elicited by tumor cells, and growth patterns, *nodular* or *diffuse*.[4,11]

Multiple myeloma is a cancerous proliferation of plasma cells (B lymphocytes), characterized by bone marrow involvement, bone destruction, and the presence of a homogeneous immunoglobulin in the urine or serum.

Routes of Tumor Spread

The spread of cancer cells from a primary tumor occurs by two major processes: *direct spread* to contiguous areas or *metastatic spread* to nonadjacent tissues.

Direct Spread

Direct invasion is the ability of a tumor to penetrate and destroy adjoining tissue.[4,12]

- *Tumor angiogenesis factor*—a substance secreted by cancer cells, stimulates new capillary formation, increases growth rate and local tissue invasion.
- *Mechanical pressure and rate of tumor growth*—uncontrolled replication produces densely packed and expanding tumor masses that exert pressure on adjacent tissues.
- *Cell motility and loss of cellular adhesiveness*—has a propensity for locomotion and promotes tumor cell dispersion.[14]

■ *Tumor-secreted enzymes*—causes destruction of normal tissue barriers, allowing invasion of cancer cells.

■ *Serosal seeding*—cells spread locally into tissue and penetrate body cavities. e.g., lung, ovarian, pleural, and peritoneal cavities.[8,12,13]

■ *Surgical instrumentation*—tumor cells may be seeded by needles as they are removed, or manipulation of the tumor during surgery may release cells into the circulation.[9,13]

Metastatic Spread

This process permits the release of cells from the primary site and subsequent spread and attachment to structures in distant sites (Figure 1-5).

The sequence of events in the metastatic process by hematogenous channels (dissemination of tumor cells through veins or arteries) is as follows:

■ Growth and progression of the primary tumor
■ Angiogenesis at the primary site
■ Detachment
■ Circulation of tumor cells
■ Arrest of tumor cells on vascular endothelium
■ Site predilection
■ Escape from the circulation (extravasution)
■ Angiogenesis of metastatic implant.

Lymphatic Spread

Lymphatic spread occurs when the cancer cells penetrate lymphatic channels draining the affected site. *Carcinomatosis*, the extensive dissemination of tumor cells by gravity, may also be a causal factor of metastasis.[19]

Host and Treatment Factors as Modifiers of Metastasis

Factors known to increase the likelihood of metastasis include a primary tumor of long duration; a high mitotic rate; trauma, including biopsy and tumor massage; heat; radiation; and chemotherapy. Factors known to decrease the likelihood of metastasis

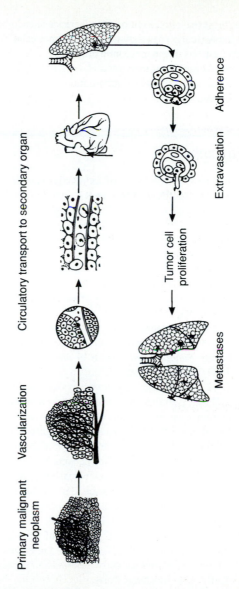

Figure 1-5. Lymphatic-hematogenic spread. (From Beare P and Meyers J: *Principles and practice of adult health nursing*, ed 1, St Louis, 1990, Mosby.)

include those that reduce tumor cell adherence to endothelial cells, retard intravascular coagulation, and kill tumor cells.[11]

Other aspects of the metastatic process:

- Metastases from metastasis
- Inhibitory effect of primary tumors
- Dormancy

Bibliography

1. Bender C: Implications of antineoplastic therapy for nursing. In Clark JC and McGee RF, editors: *Core curriculum for oncology nursing*, ed 2, Philadelphia, 1992, WB Saunders.

2. Berenblum I: *Established principles and unresolved problems in carcinogenesis,* J Natl Cancer Inst 60:723, 1978.

3. Bunn PA Jr and Ridgway EC: Paraneoplastic syndrome. In DeVita VT Jr, Hellman S, and Rosenberg SA, editors: *Cancer: principles and practice of oncology*, ed 4, Philadelphia, 1993, JB Lippincott.

4. Chew EC, Josephson RL, and Wallace AC: Morphologic aspects of the arrest of circulating cancer cells. In Weiss L, editor: *Fundamental aspects of metastasis,* Amsterdam, 1975, North-Holland.

5. Cook MB: *Multiple myeloma*. In Groenwald SL, Frogge MH, and Goodman M, editors: *Cancer nursing: principles and practice*, ed 3, Boston, 1993, Jones and Bartlett.

6. Donehower MG: The behavior of malignancies. In Johnson BL and Gross J, editors: *Handbook of oncology nursing*, New York, 1985, John Wiley & Sons.

7. Fidler IJ: The evolution of biological heterogeneity in metastatic neoplasms. In Nicolson GL and Miles L, editors: *Cancer invasion and metastasis: biologic and therapeutic aspects*, New York, 1984, Raven Press.

8. Folkman J and Cotran RS: Relation of vascular proliferation to tumor growth. In Richter GW and Epstein MA, editors: *International review of experimental pathology,* New York, 1976, Academic Press.

9. Goldfarb S: Pathology of neoplasia. In Kahn SB and others, editors: *Concepts in cancer medicine*, New York, 1983, Grune & Stratton.

10. Jordan VC: Hormones. In Kahn SB and others, editors: *Concepts in cancer medicine*, New York, 1983, Grune & Stratton.

11. Kupchella CE: Cellular biology of cancer. In Groenwald SL, Frogge MH, and Goodman M, editors: *Cancer nursing: principles and practice*, ed 3, Boston, 1993, Jones and Bartlett.

12. Kupchellas CE: The spread of cancer: invasion and metastasis. In Groenwald SL, Frogge MH, and Goodman M, editors: *Cancer nursing: principles and practice,* ed 3, Boston, 1993, Jones and Bartlett.

13. Luckmann J and Sorensen KC: *Medical-surgical nursing: a psychophysiologic approach,* ed 4, Philadelphia, 1991, WB Saunders.

14. Nicolson G: *Organ specificity of tumor metastasis: role of preferential adhesion, invasion and growth of malignant cells at specific secondary sites,* Cancer Metastasis Rev 7:143, 1988.

15. Potter VR: The cancer cell. In Kahn SB and others, editors: *Concepts in cancer medicine*, New York, 1983, Grune & Stratton.

16. Shields PG and Harris CC: Principles of carcinogenesis: chemical. In DeVita VT Jr, Hellman S, and Rosenberg SA, editors: *Cancer: principles and practice of oncology,* ed 4, Philadelphia, 1993, JB Lippincott.

17. Sirica AE: Classification of neoplasms. In Sirica AE, editor: *The pathobiology of neoplasia*, New York, 1989, Plenum Press.

18. Volker DL: Pathophysiology of cancer. In Clark JC and McGee RF, editors: *Core curriculum for oncology nursing*, ed 2, Philadelphia, 1992, WB Saunders.

19. Wolber WH: Metastasis. In Kahn SB and others, editors: *Concepts in cancer medicine*, New York, 1983, Grune & Stratton.

20. Yarbro JW: Carcinogenesis. In Groenwald SL, Frogge MH, and Goodman M, editors: *Cancer nursing: principles and practice*, ed 3, Boston, 1993, Jones and Bartlett.

Epidemiology

2

Terminology

Incidence

The number of newly diagnosed cases of cancer in a specified period of time (usually a calendar year) in a defined population is called the cancer *incidence*. For example, the incidence of breast cancer in the United States in 1994 was 183,000 newly diagnosed cases. Incidence is frequently expressed in the literature as a rate per 100,000 population at risk. Incidence data collection focuses on two specific areas: demographic and medical. Demographic information extrapolates age, sex, race, marital status, and place of residence. Medical data on the same individual reports onset of illness, location of tumor, stage, histology, treatment, and survival over time.[4,5,8]

Incidence rate = number of persons developing cancer
in a specified period of time

_____

total population living at that time

SEER Data

In 1973, the NCI established and funded the Surveillance, Epidemiology, and End-Results Program (SEER), consisting of 11 population-based registries to collect data on individual cancer sites. These registries continuously gather information on cancer incidence, mortality, and survival. In addition to SEER data, incidence information is also collected in individual hospital cancer registries.[7]

Prevalence

The measurement of all cancer cases, both old and new, at a *designated point in time,* is called cancer *prevalence*.

$$\text{Prevalence rate} = \frac{\text{number of persons with cancer at a given point in time}}{\text{total population living at that time}}$$

Prevalence information is used for healthcare planning including physical facilities, manpower, and the design and implementation of screening programs.

Mortality

The number of deaths attributed to cancer in a specified time period and in a defined population is the cancer mortality. The 1994 estimated cancer mortality rate in the United States is 538,000 persons or about 1,474 people a day.[1]

$$\text{Mortality rate} = \frac{\text{number of persons dying from cancer in a specified time period}}{\text{total population living at that time}}$$

Mortality data determines trends over time in the magnitude of cancer as a cause of death among members of our population.

Survival

The link between incidence and mortality data is *survival analysis,* the observation over time of persons with cancer and the calculation of their probability of dying over several time periods. Survival data are a useful measure of the end result of cancer treatment and can indicate improvements over time in the management of cancer. For most cancers, the chances of surviving the second 5 years are greater than surviving the first 5 years.

Identification of Trends

The trends found in monitoring cancer incidence and mortality statistics have significant implications for cancer education and prevention. Some examples of current trends in cancer incidence, mortality, and survival are listed in Box 2-1.

Box 2-1

Current Trends in Cancer Incidence, Mortality, and Survival

Incidence

There were over 1,208,000 newly diagnosed cases in the United
  States in 1994.

Higher rate of incidence is seen in males than females.

Overall incidence is highest in Hawaiians, lowest in American
  Indians.

Blacks have three times more esophageal cancer than whites.

The leading sites of incidence in males are: prostate, lung, colon.

The leading sites of incidence in females are: breast, colon, lung.

Cancers of the colon and rectum are the most frequently diagnosed malignancies.

Melanoma incidence has increased 1000% in the past 50 years.

Mortality

Over 538,000 cancer-related deaths in the United States in 1994.

Lung cancer accounts for 33% of male cancer deaths.

Lung cancer accounts for 23% of female cancer deaths.

Leading causes of male death are cancers of the lung, prostate,
  colon, pancreas, and leukemia.

Leading causes of female death are cancers of the lung, breast,
  colon, pancreas, and ovary.

Cancer is the leading cause of death in women from age 35 to
  74.

For all ages, cancer is the second most common cause of death,
  following heart disease.

Survival

Overall 5-year survival rate for all cancers is 50%.

Large survival increases seen in Hodgkin's disease, melanoma skin
  cancers, and cancer of the testis, prostate, and bladder.[1]

Survival depends on extent of disease at diagnosis.

Less favourable survival rates are seen in blacks.

Five-year survival for all types of childhood cancer increased from
  28% in the early 1960s to 63% in the early 1980s.[1]

Data from American Cancer Society: *Cancer facts and figures—1994*, Atlanta,
1994, American Cancer Society.

Types of Studies

The epidemiologic method is composed of an orderly progression of three types of studies: descriptive, analytic, and experimental.

Descriptive Studies

Descriptive studies are observational in nature and record the existing patterns of disease. Person, place, and time are epidemiologic variables that serve as a major source of clues to cancer etiology.

Person

Age, sex, and racial differences account for fundamental differences in cancer rates.

- *Age*—With a few exceptions, cancer becomes more prevalent in older people. The increased incidence reflects the importance of duration of carcinogen exposure and of long induction periods of some cancers. More than half of all cancers are diagnosed after the age of 65.
- *Sex*—Men tend to develop cancer more often the women, and they die more frequently from cancer than women.
- *Race*—The male incidence of cancer is highest in blacks, followed by whites, then Hawaiians. In females, Hawaiians have the highest incidence, followed by whites, then blacks. Whites have especially high rates of melanoma, Hodgkin's disease, non-Hodgkin's lymphomas, and leukemia. Blacks have elevated rates of multiple myeloma and cancers of the oral cavity, esophagus, and colon. Hispanics have especially high rates of cervical cancer, and American Indians have a remarkable prevalence of stomach cancer. Chinese people have more liver cancer diagnosed , and Japanese people have a high percentage of stomach cancers.[2,3,6]
- *Other Factors*—Host factors such as general health/wellness status—including nutritional status, cultural and socioeconomic variables, marital status, psychologic factors, and susceptibility factors—add to the body of information and may help define the hypothesis of a particular cancer cause.

Place

The category of place in descriptive studies involves physical and biologic environmental variables such as geologic structure, water sources, flora, weather, climate, plants, animals, urban versus rural, waste disposal systems, industrialization, and pollution.

Time

Evaluating the incidence of cancer over time may indicate significant trends, e.g., increases in melanoma and lung cancer deaths over the past several decades.

Analytical Studies

This type of study is observational in nature and its purpose is to elucidate which type of exposure causes which kind(s) of cancer.[9] The three types of analytical studies are cross-sectional studies, cohort design, and case-control design.[5,9]

Cross-Sectional Studies

Occur in the present and these studies may also be called prevalence surveys. The purpose is to canvass a population of subjects to ascertain a relationship between the disease and variables of interest as they exist in the group at a specific time.

Cohort Design

It examines populations who have been exposed to see if they develop the disease in the future. This type of study is a prospective investigation and may also be called a *concurrent study*.

A second type of cohort study is the *historical cohort design*, also called the *historical prospective study*. This design is frequently used in occupational studies as both the exposure and onset of cancer have already occurred.

It is important in a cohort or prospective study that the time the study begins is clearly identified, that all of the participants are free of cancer when enrolled in the study, and that all participants are followed the same way.

Case-Control Design

This method evaluates a case group of persons diagnosed with the cancer under study who have exposure to the suspected cancer-causing agent. This group is compared to a control group chosen from the general population. The case-control design is a retrospective study that evaluates the outcome of past events.

Study Analysis

The endpoint of an analytic study is the determination of risk. Risk refers to the likelihood that people who are without a disease, but who come in contact with certain factors thought to increase the disease risk, will acquire the disease.

Risk can be calculated as either relative or attributable. *Relative risk* estimates how much the risk of acquiring cancer increases with exposure to a risk factor or the ratio of the rate of cancer between exposed and unexposed individuals. The higher the relative risk, the stronger the association between the risk factor and the cancer.

Attributable risk describes the expected or normal number of unexposed people who acquire cancer, such as the number of nonsmokers expected to develop lung cancer in a year. Attributable risk is calculated by simply subtracting the rate of incidence in the exposed population from the rate of incidence in the nonexposed population.

Experimental Studies

Experimental studies are prospective and may be called intervention studies, clinical trials, or prophylactic studies.

Causes of Cancer

Descriptive epidemiology factors used to discover the causes of cancer are found in Box 2-2. Environmental causes and types of cancer are found in Table 2-1.

Box 2-2 Descriptive Epidemiology Factors

Frequency	Disease	Person	Place	Time
Incidence	Site	Age	Physical environment	Changes
Prevalence	Morphology	Sex	Biological environment	in frequency
Mortality	Grade	Race	Geographic location	patterns
	Stage	Marital status		over
		Nutritional status		specified
		Cultural differences		periods
		Socioeconomic variables		of time
		Psychological factors		
		Susceptibility factors		

Table 2-1 lists a number of environmental causes of cancer, the type of exposure, and the kind of resulting cancer. Some of these carcinogenic agents were identified by laboratory research; others were identified by the epidemiologic methods.

Table 2-1 Environmental Causes of Human Cancer

Agent	Type of Exposure	Site of Cancer
Alcoholic beverages	Drinking	Mouth, pharynx, esophagus, larynx, liver
Alkylating agents (melphalan, cyclophosphamide, chlorambucil, semustine)	Medication	Leukemia
Androgen-anabolic steroids	Medication	Liver
Aromatic amines (benzidine, 2-naphthylamine, 4-aminobiphenyl)	Manufacturing of dyes and other chemicals	Bladder
Arsenic (inorganic)	Mining and smelting of certain ores, pesticide manufacturing and use, medication, drinking water	Lung, skin, liver (angiosarcoma)
Asbestos	Manufacturing and use	Lung, pleura, peritoneum
Benzene	Leather, petroleum, and other industries	Leukemia
Bis(chloromethyl)ether	Manufacturing	Lung (small cell)
Chlornaphazine	Medication	Bladder

Chromium compounds	Manufacturing	Lung
Estrogens	Medication	Cervix, vagina (adenocarcinoma)
Synthetic (DES)		
Conjugated (Premarin)		Endometrium
Steroid contraceptives		Liver (benign)
Immunosupressants (azathioprine, cyclosporin)	Medication	Non-Hodgkin's lymphoma, skin (squamous carcinoma and melanoma), soft tissue tumors (including Kaposi's sarcoma)
Ionizing radiation	Atomic bomb explosions, treatment and diagnosis, radium dial painting, uranium and metal mining	Most sites
Isopropyl alcohol production	Manufacturing by strong acid process	Nasal sinuses
Leather industry	Manufacturing and repair (boot and shoe)	Nasal sinuses, bladder
Mustard gas	Manufacturing	Lung, larynx, nasal sinuses
Nickel dust	Refining	Lung, nasal sinuses
Parasites	Infection	
Schistosoma haematobium		Bladder (squamous carcinoma)
Clonorchis sinensis		Liver (cholangiocarcinoma)

Continued.

Agent	Type of Exposure	Site of Cancer
Phenacetin-containing analgesics	Medication	Renal pelvis
Polycyclic hydrocarbons	Coal carbonization products and some mineral oils	Lung, skin (squamous carcinoma)
Tobacco chews, including betel nut	Snuff dipping and chewing of tobacco, betel, lime	Mouth
Tobacco smoke	Smoking, especially cigarettes	Lung, larynx, mouth, pharynx, esophagus, bladder, pancreas, kidney
Ultraviolet radiation	Sunlight	Skin (including melanoma), lip
Viruses	Infection	
Epstein-Barr virus		Burkitt's lymphoma; nasopharyngeal carcinoma
Hepatitis-B virus		Hepatocellular carcinoma
Human T-lymphotrophic virus, type I		T-cell leukemia/lymphoma
Vinyl chloride	Manufacturing of polyvinyl chloride	Liver (angiosarcoma)
Wood dusts	Furniture manufacturing (hardwood)	Nasal sinuses (adenocarcinoma)

From Fraumeni JF and others: Epidemiology of cancer. In DeVita VT, Hellman S, and Rosenberg SA, editors: *Cancer principles and practice of oncology*, ed 4, Philadelphia, 1993, JB Lippincott.

Bibliography

1. American Cancer Society: *Cancer facts and figures— 1994*, Atlanta, 1994, American Cancer Society, Inc.
2. Boring CC, Squires TS, Tong T: *Cancer statistics, 1994*, Cancer 44(1):7, 1994
3. Feinstein AR, Sosin DM, and Wells CK: *The Will Rogers phenomenon: stage migration and new diagnostic techniques as a source of misleading statistics for survival in cancer*, N Engl J Med 312:1604, 1985.
4. Fraumeni JF and others: Epidemiology of cancer. In DeVita VT, Hellman S, and Rosenberg SA, editors: *Cancer: principles and practice of oncology*, ed 4, Philadelphia, 1993, JB Lippincott.
5. Hutchinson GB: The epidemiologic method. In Schottenfeld D and Fraumeni JF, editors: *Cancer epidemiology and prevention*, Philadelphia, 1982, WB Saunders.
6. Mettlin C: *Trends in years of life lost to cancer*, 1970-1985, CA 39(1):33, 1989.
7. Myers MH and Ries LG: *Cancer patient survival rates: SEER Program results for 10 years of follow-up*, CA 39(1):21, 1989.
8. Newell GR and others: Epidemiology of cancer. In DeVita VT, Hellman S, and Rosenberg SA, editors: *Cancer: principles and practice of oncology*, ed 4, Philadelphia, 1993, JB Lippincott.
9. Oleske DM: Epidemiologic principles for nursing practice: assessing the cancer problem and planning its control. In Baird SB, McCorkle R, and Grant M, editors: *Cancer nursing: a comprehensive textbook*, Philadelphia, 1991, WB Saunders.

Prevention, Screening, and Detection

3

Approximately 76 million Americans alive today will eventually have cancer; about one in three according to present rates, striking approximately three of four families. Cancer continues to be the second leading cause of death in the United States. The American Cancer Society (ACS) estimates that more than one million new cancer cases will be diagnosed in 1994.

Prevention, screening, and early detection are among the best strategies available in the quest to conquer cancer. The United States' goal in cancer control, as identified by the National Cancer Institute (NCI), is to reduce the cancer death rate by 50% for all Americans by the year 2000; saving some 230,000 lives each year. These reductions are to be achieved by smoking cessation, diet modification, and early detection through screening programs, state-of-the-art cancer treatments, elimination of occupational and environmental risks, and changes in lifestyle, focusing on healthy choices in diet and exercise.[3,9,20]

Cancer Prevention Guidelines

Cancer prevention, as discussed here, is two-dimensional: *primary prevention* aimed at measures to ensure that the cancer never develops and *secondary prevention* aimed at detecting and treating the cancer early while in its most curable stage.

The American Cancer Society estimates that 80% of all cancers may be associated with environmental exposures and are potentially preventable. Major factors placing humans at risk for developing cancer include: tobacco, diet, lifestyle, occupational and environmental exposures. Site specific guidelines related to cancer risk factors, signs and symptoms, screening, and early detection are presented in Table 3-1.[7,8,10,16,22]

Table 3-1 Site-Specific Cancer Risk, Screening, and Early Detection Guidelines [14,17,37]

Site	Associated Risk Factors	Signs and Symptoms	Screening and Detection
Biliary tract (Gallbladder and bile ducts)	Older Americans (age 60-70s) Female predominance Higher in white females than African American females Chronic infection with liver parasites (*Clonorchis sinensis*) Eating raw or pickled freshwater fish from Southeast Asia Chronic ulcerative colitis	Pruritus, jaundice, abdominal pain Nausea and vomiting Fever, malaise, enlarged liver Palpable mass upper right quadrant Lower extremity edema Ascites	Physical examination Ultrasound
Bladder	Occupational exposure (textile, rubber) Cigarette smoking Chronic bladder infections	Microscopic or gross hematuria Dysuria, bladder irritability Urinary urgency, frequency and/or hesitancy	Urinalysis Urine cytology Physical examination
Brain	Environmental exposures (vinyl chlorides) Epstein-Barr virus	Persistent generalized headache Vomiting, seizures Loss of fine motor control Unsteady gait, lethargy Change in personality Slurring of speech Loss of memory, impaired vision	Physical examination Prompt follow-up with onset of signs and symptoms

Breast	Previous history of cancer (colon, thyroid, endometrial, ovary, breast) Obesity High fat intake Family history of breast cancer Exposure to ionizing radiation before age 35 Early menarche Late menopause	Painless mass or thickening in breast or axilla Skin dimpling, puckering, or nipple retraction Nipple discharge or scaliness Edema (peau d'orange) Erythema, ulceration Change in size, contour, shape of breast	Consist of three modalities:[8] 1. *Breast self-examination* monthly at age 20 and older. 2. *Clinical examination* age 20–40: every 3 years over 40: every year 3. *Mammography* age 40–49: every 1–2 years age 50 & over: every year * Baseline mammogram at age 25 has been recommended for genetically predisposed women. Fine needle aspiration Ultrasound
	Nulliparity First pregnancy after age 30		
Central nervous system	Unknown etiology Speculation related to genetic disorders	Headache, nausea/vomiting Edema Loss of motor coordination	No effective screening measures Family history

Continued.

Table 3-1 Cont'd.

Site	Associated Risk Factors	Signs and Symptoms	Screening and Detection

Central nervous system cont'd		Unsteady gait, seizures
		Vision and speech problems
			CT scan of the brain, MRI
			Cerebrospinal fluid analysis
			Tumor markers
			  Alpha-fetoprotein
			  Beta human chrorionic-gonadotropin

Cervix	Early age at first intercourse (before age 20) Multiple sex partners Smoking, diet HPV infection (condyloma or warts) Herpes simplex virus II	Abnormal vaginal bleeding Persistent postcoital spotting	Pap test Pelvic examination

Colon and rectum	Colorectal polyp(s)
	Diets high in fat
	Diets low in fiber
	Genetic component:
	  Familial polyposis
	  Gardner's syndrome
	  Peutz-Jeghers syndrome
		Depend on the location of the tumor:
		Right colon
		Anemia
		GI bleeding
		Persistent lower abdominal pain
		Right lower quadrant mass
			Digital rectal examination
			Stool occult blood testing
			Flexible sigmoidoscopy (see Table 3-12 for frequency of these tests/procedures

Inflammatory bowel disease
Crohn's disease
Ulcerative colitis

Left colon
Gross blood in the stool
Decrease in stool caliber
Change in bowel habits,
  constipation, diarrhea
Rectum
Hematochezia; Tenesmus
Feeling of incomplete evacuation
Rectal pain (late sign)
Prolapse of tumor

Endometrium
Post menopause
High socioeconomic status
Nulliparity; Hypertension
Obesity >50 pounds over
  ideal body weight
Prolonged use of exogenous
  estrogen without supplemental
  progesterone
High fat intake; Diabetes
Stein-Leventhal syndrome (failure to
  ovulate/infertility—polycystic ovaries)
Menstrual aberration

Early sign
Abnormal vaginal bleeding
Late signs
Pain in pelvis, legs, or back
General weakness
Weight loss

Aspiration curettage

Continued.

Table 3-1 Cont'd.

Site	Associated Risk Factors	Signs and Symptoms	Screening and Detection
Esophagus	Elderly male (70-80 years old) Nitrosamines and ethanol consumption Cigarette smoking	*Early signs* Dysphagia Weight loss Regurgitation	Esophagoscopy with staining techniques Brush biopsy Radioisotopes in tumor scanning
	Precancerous lesions Achalasia (failure of the lower esophagus to relax with swallowing) Combined smoking and drinking Barrett's esophagus (chronic gastric reflux)	Aspiration Odynophagia (pain on swallowing) Gastroesophageal reflux *Advanced signs* Cervical adenopathy Chronic cough; Hoarseness Choking after eating Massive hemoptysis Hematemesis	
Head and neck	Tobacco (inhaled or chewed) Ethyl alcohol Combination of tobacco and alcohol Poor oral hygiene Wood dust inhalation	*Mouth and oral cavity* Swelling Ulcer that does not heal *Nose and Sinuses* Pain; Swelling	Semiannual dental oral examination Awareness of signs and symptoms (cancer's seven warning signs)

Type	Risk factors	Signs and symptoms	Detection
	Nickel exposure Leukoplakia	Bloody nasal discharge Nasal obstruction *Salivary glands* Painless swelling Unilateral facial paralysis *Hypopharynx* Dysphagia; Persistent earache Lymphadenopathy *Nasopharynx* Double vision Hearing loss Loss of smell; Hoarseness Adenopathy *Larynx* Hoarseness; Difficulty breathing	
HIV/AIDS related (Kaposi's sarcoma [KS])	All age groups Homosexual or bisexual men highest risk Intravenous drug users Unprotected sexual contact Multiple sex partners	Multifocal, widespread lesions on skin (face, extremities, and torso) Persistent intermittent fever Weight loss, diarrhea Malaise, fatigue Severe cellular immune deficiency Generalized lymphadenopathy	High risk group Appearance of skin lesions HIV (human immunodeficiency virus) serum testing Oral examination

Continued.

Table 3-1 Cont'd.

Site	Associated Risk Factors	Signs and Symptoms	Screening and Detection
		Respiratory infections: *Pneumocystis carinii* Tuberculosis Difficulty breathing; Oral lesions Enlarged liver, spleen	
Leukemia			
Acute	Men higher risk than women Whites higher than African Americans Exposure to radiation Exposure to toxic organic chemicals (benzene) Drugs (alkyating agents, chloramphenicol)	Low grade fever Anemia, pallor Lymphadenopathy Generalized weakness Frequent infections Easy bruising Bleeding (nose, gums) Petechiae lower extremities Bone and joint pain	Complete blood count Platelet count Physical examination
Chronic	Benzene exposure High dose radiation Philadelphia chromosome	Lymphadenopathy Splenomegaly Weight loss; Night sweats Malaise, weakness Recurrent infections, fever	

	Risk Factors	Signs and Symptoms	Screening/Detection
Liver	Exposure to aflatoxin Environmental exposures Viral hepatitis More frequent in males Alcoholic cirrhosis Parasitic infestation Paraneoplastic syndromes Anabolic steroid use	*Early* Bloating Abdominal pain Fever; Weight loss Decreased appetite; Nausea *Advanced* Jaundice; Ascites Extreme weight loss	Annual physical examination Awareness of risk factors Ultrasound
Lung	Cigarette smoking (active and passive) Increase in age; Asbestos Occupational exposure among miners Air pollution (benzopyrenes and hydrocarbons) Genetic predisposition Vitamin A deficiency	Nagging cough Dull ache in the chest Recurrent or persistent upper respiratory infection Wheezing; Dyspnea Hemoptysis Change in volume, color, odor of sputum	None
Lymphoma *Hodgkin's Disease*	Epstein-Barr virus Higher socioeconomic status Small family	Persistent swelling or painless lymph nodes (neck, axilla) Recurrent fevers; Pruritus Night sweats; Weight loss Cough, shortness of breath Leukocytosis	Physical examination Complete blood count

Continued.

Table 3-1 Cont'd.

Site	Associated Risk Factors	Signs and Symptoms	Screening and Detection
Non-Hodgkin's	Occupational exposure (flour and agricultural industries) Abnormalities of the immune system HIV Exposure to radiation or chemotherapy	Lymphadenopathy Fatigue, fever, chills Night sweats Decreased appetite Weight loss	
Multiple myeloma	Older Americans Higher levels of immunoglobin (B-cells) African Americans at at significant increased risk than whites (14 to 1)	*Early* Anemia; Fatigue Bone pain (back, legs), weakness Unexplained bleeding (nose and gums) Recurrent upper respiratory infection *Advanced* Hypercalcemia; Pathologic fractures	Annual physical examination Radiologic tests
Ovary	Familial disposition Late menopause Nulliparity First pregnancy after age 30	*Early* Vague abdominal discomfort Dyspepsia, flatulence, bloating Digestive disturbance *Advanced* Abdominal distention; Pain Abdominal and pelvic masses Ascites; Lower extremity edema	Pelvic ultrasonography (with vaginal probe) Elevated serum markers CEA CA 125

	Risk factors	Signs and symptoms	Detection
Pancreas	Older men Smoking; Diabetes Chronic pancreatitis Ethanol consumption	*Early* Hypoglycemia; Abdominal pain Weight loss, anorexia Cramping pain associated with diarrhea; Pruritus *Advanced* Jaundice; Ascites Lower extremity edema	Blood glucose test Physical examination
Prostate	Occupational exposure Cadmium, heavy metals, chemicals Age (median age of incidence = 70 yrs) Increased fat intake	*Early* Difficult starting urinary stream Unexplained cystitis Urinary bleeding; Dribbling Bladder retention *Advanced* Bladder outlet obstruction Urinary retention Ureteral obstruction with anuria Azotemia; Hematuria; Uremia Anorexia; Bone pain	Digital rectal examination Biochemical markers Prostatic specific antigen Transrectal ultrasound
Skin (Nonmelanoma)	Fair-skinned, freckles Blond hair, blue eyes Sun exposure	Changes in a wart or mole Sore that does not heal The *ABCD*'s of skin cancer:	Extensive examination of the skin Mole mappin

Continued.

Table 3-1 Cont'd.

Site	Associated Risk Factors	Signs and Symptoms	Screening and Detection
	Severe sunburn in childhood Familial conditions Previous skin cancers History of dysplastic nevus	A—Asymmetry (change in size/shape) B—Border irregularity C—Color (change in color) D—Diameter (> than 6 mm)	Annual physical examination Awareness of cancer's early warning signs
Soft tissue sarcoma (bone or muscle)	Familial/genetic syndromes: (Von Recklinghausen disease) High dose radiation Toxic chemical exposure (Agent Orange)	Swelling of extremity Painless mass; Fever Malaise; Weight loss Occasionally hypoglycemia Functional difficulty or pain in joints; Pathologic fractures	
Stomach	Dietary carcinogens (smoked, salt cured, and charcoal foods) Familial/genetic disposition Persons with Type A blood (15-20% increase incidence) Benign gastric ulcers	Feeling of fullness Weight loss; Malaise Loss of appetite Anemia (iron deficiency) GI bleeding; Abdominal pain Persistent epigastric distress	Occult blood testing Complete blood count

Testis	Cryptorchid testes Young white males have rate four times that of African Americans	*Early* Painless mass; Gynecomastia Heavy sensation in the scrotum *Advanced* Ureteral obstruction Abdominal mass Pulmonary symptoms Elevated HCG	Testicular self-examination (monthly) beginning in adolescence Testicular ultrasound
Vulva	Postmenopausal History of genital warts Human papilloma virus Other sexually transmitted diseases Lower socioeconomic status Multiple sex partners Precancerous or cancerous lesions of the cervix	Lump or ulcer Itching Pain Burning bleeding Discharge	Visual and manual inspection of external genitalia Colposcopic exam in women with HPV

Risk Factors

Tobacco

The ACS estimates that cigarette smoking is responsible for 85% of lung cancer deaths among men and 75% among women. Lung cancer now exceeds breast cancer as the leading cause of cancer death in women. Passive exposure to cigarette smoke (side stream and exhaled smoke) appears to increase the risk of lung cancer in nonsmokers who live with smokers. Smoking is associated with cancers of the mouth, pharynx, larynx, esophagus, pancreas, uterine cervix, kidney, and bladder.[3,14,15]

Diet

The recommendations related to cancer, diet, and nutrition are to reduce the intake of fat, both saturated and unsaturated, and to increase the amount of daily intake of natural fiber (components that are not broken down during the digestive process) in the diet. See Box 3-1.

Estimates are that 30% to 60% of all cancers, in men and women respectively, are related to diet. Foods high in fat have been associated with an increased incidence of colon, prostate, and breast cancer. Dietary fat acts as a cancer promoter.[17]

Box 3-1

Dietary Recommendations for Cancer Prevention

1. Reduce the amount of saturated and unsaturated fats in the diet from 40% to 30% of total daily caloric intake.
2. Increase the amount of fiber in the diet by eating fresh fruits, vegetables (especially cruciferous vegetables), and whole grain breads/cereals.
3. Drink alcoholic beverages in moderation (one or two drinks daily) or not at all.
4. Eat limited amounts of broiled, charcoaled, smoked, and salt- or nitrite-cured foods.
5. Maintain ideal body weight.

Adapted from American Cancer Society, *Cancer facts and figures*, 1994, Atlanta.

Alcohol

Excessive consumption of ethyl alcohol can lead to cancers in the head and neck, larynx, and possibly the liver and pancreas.[6]

Genetic Predisposition

The greatest known cancer risk exists when there is a primary relative of a patient with an autosomal dominant inherited cancer.[1,13,19]

Socioeconomic Factors

Issues related to barriers to primary prevention and health care access have been reported as major factors in the differences in cancer incidence, delayed diagnosis, poor survival statistics, and increased mortality from cancer in minority populations.

Five critical issues related to cancer and the poor have been determined.[4,11,12,21]

1. Poor people endure greater pain and suffering from cancer than other Americans.
2. Poor people and their families must make extraordinary personal sacrifices to obtain and pay for health care.
3. Poor people face substantial obstacles in obtaining and using health insurance and often do not seek care if they cannot pay for it.
4. Current cancer education programs are culturally insensitive and irrelevant to many poor Americans.
5. Fatalism about cancer is prevalent among the poor and prevents them from seeking health care.

Sunlight

The sun is the primary source of natural ultraviolet (UV) light exposure that is known to cause the three types of skin cancers: basal cell, squamous cell, and melanoma. Of the three types of skin cancer, melanoma is the most potentially lethal and is increasing in incidence at a rate of 4% per year.

At highest risk for developing skin cancer are persons who work outdoors, who are fair-skinned, with occupational exposure to coal tar, arsenic compounds, and radium. Ultraviolet rays of the sun are strongest between 10 AM and 3 PM. Sun exposure should be limited during those hours and/or protective clothing (hats, scarves, long sleeves) should be worn to offer some protection from the UV rays. Children should be especially protected because of the possible link between severe sunburn in childhood and greatly increased risk of melanoma in later life. Sunscreens should be worn when deliberate sun exposure is expected. A sunscreen with a sun protection factor (SPF) of 15 or higher should be worn on all sun exposed skin surfaces. Sun tanning parlors, which are increasing in popularity among Americans, should be avoided.[7]

Sexual Life-Styles

Sexually transmitted diseases (STDs), genital cancers, and acquired immune deficiency syndrome (AIDS) have a documented direct relationship to sexual life-styles and practices, e.g., cancer of the cervix, vulva, vagina, and AIDS. Several viruses have been implicated in the etiology of cervical neoplasia including herpes simplex virus (HSV) and human papillomavirus (HPV). Penile HPV (genital wart or condyloma) infection in a male partner places the woman at risk of cervical cancer.

Sexual behaviors considered to be high-risk factors associated with AIDS include: unprotected vaginal or anal intercourse, internal watersports (urinating into a body cavity such as the vagina or anus), fisting (inserting a finger, fingers, or fist into the anus), and oral-anal sex, also known as rimming. Sharing of dirty needles by intravenous drug users is also a high-risk factor.[15]

Early Detection and Screening Recommendations

The ACS in 1994 updated screening and early detection guidelines, as listed in Table 3-2.

Nursing Management

Nursing Diagnosis

- Knowledge deficit related to prevention and early detection of site specific cancers.

Assessments

- Patient education and literacy level
- Cultural/ethnic perspectives of patient/significant other
- Beliefs and attitudes towards cancer
- Patient/family history and relative risk of cancer development

Interventions

- Discuss site specific cancer risk factors
- Identify signs and symptoms of site specific cancer
- Health teaching related to diet, nutrition, and lifestyle choices
- Provide appropriate and culturally sensitive printed information to client
- Provide a list of cancer information/support agencies
- Instruct patient in self examination of breast, mouth, skin, cervix, vulva, penis, and testicles
- Review ACS screening guidelines
- Assist patient with access to health care issues for cancer screening and early detection
- Identify sign/ssymptoms that warrant access to the health care system
- Identify community resources available to help patient: Stop smoking, reduce stress, control weight and diet
- Identify occupational and environmental risk factors and reporting agencies: OSHA (Occupational, Safety and Health Administration), EPA (Environmental Protection Agency), NRA (Nuclear Regulatory Agency), FDA (Federal Drug Administration)
- Provide mechanism for necessary referral and follow-up

Outcome Goals

- Patient/significant other will be able to:
- State the 7 warning signals of cancer
- Demonstrate site related self-examination related to breast, oral, skin, vulva, penile, and testicular cancers
- Recognize cancer related signs and symptoms that require follow up in the health care system
- Identify cancer information sources (ACS, Leukemia Society, NCI)
- Identify his/her relative risk for cancer development

Table 3-2 Summary of 1994 American Cancer Society Recommendations for the Early Detection of Cancer in Asymptomatic People (Jan./Feb.)

| Test or Procedure | Population | | Frequency |
	Sex	Age	
Sigmoidoscopy, preferably flexible	M & F	50 and over	Every 3–5 years
Fecal occult blood test	M & F	50 and over	Every year
Digital rectal examination	M & F	40 and over	Every year
Prostate examination	M	50 and over*	Every year
Pap test	F	All women who are or who have been sexually active, or have reached age 18, should have an annual Pap test and pelvic examination. After a woman has had three or more consecutive satisfactory normal annual examinations, the Pap test may be performed less frequently at the discretion of her physician.	

Examination	Sex	Age	Frequency
Pelvic examination	F	18-40	Every 1-3 years with Pap test
		Over 40	Every year
Endometrial tissue sample	F	At menopause, women at high risk§	At menopause
Breast self-examination	F	20 and over	Every month
Clinical breast examination	F	20-40	Every 3 years
		Over 40	Every year
Mammography†	F	40-49	Every 1-2 years
		50 and over	Every year
Health counseling and cancer checkup‡	M & F	Over 20	Every 3 years
		Over 40	Every year

From American Cancer Society: CA 44(1):7, 1994

*Annual digital rectal examination and prostate-specific antigen should be performed on men age 50 and older. If either is abnormal, further evaluation should be considered.

§History of infertility, obesity, failure to ovulate, abnormal uterine bleeding, or estrogen therapy.

† Screening mammography should begin by age 40.

‡To include examination for cancers of the thyroid, testicles, prostate, ovaries, lymph nodes, oral region, and skin.

Bibliography

1.   Albright LA and others: Genetic predisposition to cancer. In DeVita VT, Jr, Hellman S, and Rosenberg SA editors: *Important advances in oncology*, Philadelphia, 1991, JB Lippincott.

2.   American Cancer Society: *Guideline for the cancer related checkup—Update January 1994*, CA 44(1):7, 1994.

3.   American Cancer Society: *Cancer facts and figures—1994*. Atlanta, Ga, 1994, American Cancer Society.

4.   Baquet CR and others: *Socioeconomic factors and cancer incidence among blacks and whites*, J Nat Cancer Inst 83:551, 1991.

5.   Boring CC, Squires TS and Tong T, Montgomery BA: *Cancer statistics*, 1994, CA 44(1):7,1994.

6.   Bridbord K:*Pathogenesis and prevention of hepatocellular carcinoma*, Cancer Detect Prev 14:191,1989.

7.   Croghan IT and Omoto MK: Cancer prevention and risk reduction. In Baird SB, editor: *A cancer source book for nurses*, Atlanta, Ga, 1991, American Cancer Society.

8.   Dodd GD: *American cancer society guidelines on screening for breast cancer: An overview*, CA 42:177, 1992.

9.   *Fighting Cancer in America: achieving the "year 2000 goal,"* Cancer Nurs 12:359, 1989.

10. Fink DJ: Cancer detection: The cancer related checkup guidelines. In Holleb AI, Fink DJ, and Murphy GP, editors: *ACS textbook of clinical oncology*, Atlanta, Ga, 1991, American Cancer Society.

11. Fitzsimmons ML and others: *Hereditary cancer syndromes: nursing's role in identification and education*, Oncol Nurs Forum 16:87, 1989.

12. Freeman HP: *Cancer in the socioeconomically disadvantaged*, CA 39:266, 1989.

13. Graves PL, Thomas CB, and Mead LA: *Familial and psychological predictors of cancer*, Cancer Detect Prev 15:59, 1991.

14. Heath CW: Cancer prevention. In Holleb AI, Fink DJ, and Murphy GP, editors: *ACS textbook of clinical oncology,* Atlanta, Ga, 1991, American Cancer Society.

15. Holleb AI, Fink DJ, and Murphy G: *American cancer society textbook of clinical oncology*, Atlanta, 1991, American Cancer Society.
16. Knopp JM and Croghan IT: Screening, detection and diagnosis. In Baird SB, editor: *A cancer source book for nurses*, Atlanta, Georgia, 1991, American Cancer Society.
17. Kritchewsky D: Diet and cancer. In Holleb AI, Fink DJ, and Murphy GP, editors: *ACS textbook of clinical oncology*, Atlanta, GA, 1991, American Cancer Society.
18. Littrup PJ, Lee F, and Mettlin C: *Prostate cancer screening: current trends and future implications,* CA 42:198, 1992.
19. Lynch HT and Lynch JF: *Familial factors and genetic predisposition to cancer: population studies,* Cancer Detec Prev 15:49, 1991.
20. Phillips J: *Cancer control by the year 2000: implication for action,* J Nation Black Nurses Assoc 5:42, 1991.
21. Stromborg MF and Olsen SJ: *Cancer prevention in minority populations: cultural implication for health care professionals,* St Louis, 1993, Mosby.
22. Watkins MC: *Computerized cancer information sources,* J Med Assoc Georgia 81:143, 1992.

Diagnosis and Staging

4

The diagnosis of cancer involves many aspects of care. Physical examinations are a systematic assessment of major body sites: head, ears, nose, throat, cardiovascular, chest, abdomen, genitourinary system, extremities, lymph nodes, and nervous system. Positive and negative findings are documented and evaluated in terms of the patient's medical history. The diagnostic work-up, planned from the patient's symptoms, history, and physical examination yields a presumptive malignant diagnosis. That diagnosis must be confirmed through histologic and cytologic examination. Staging completes the necessary information for planning treatment. Examples of nursing diagnoses and interventions are listed at the end of the chapter.[2,11]

Diagnostic Work-up

A diagnostic work-up is initiated to determine the cause of a patient's symptoms. A wide range of diagnostic procedures may be used in the individualized work-up for each patient.

- *Radiologic Studies:*—chest x-ray, mammogram, flat plate of the abdomen, x-rays of the extremities, barium studies, intravenous pyelogram, myelogram, computed tomography
- *Magnetic Resonance Imaging*—Provides sensitive images of soft tissues, without interference from bone; including the central nervous system, mediastinal and hilar areas, abnormal vascular states, edema, and other tumors.
- *Ultrasonography*—Visualize internal structures. Abdominal, pelvic, peritoneal, breast, thyroid, and prostate.
- *Nuclear Medicine Scans*—Radioactive isotopes may be injected and tracked to those tissues for which the isotope has an affinity, e.g., greater activity of cells, due to disease, infection, or malignancy. Other scans, including

Table 4-1 Selected Laboratory Studies

Examination	Detects or Assesses
Bone marrow aspiration/ biopsy	Hematologic abnormalities Presence of metastatic disease in the marrow
Chemistry profile: bilirubin, calcium, uric acid, blood urea nitrogen, creatinine, electrolytes, lactic dehydrogenase, serum glutamic oxaloacetic transaminase, alkaline phosphatase, serum glutamic pyruvic transaminase, magnesium	Liver, kidney, bone abnormalities secondary to cancer, therapy, certain chronic illnesses May be used to monitor response to treatment
Complete blood count	Bone marrow abnormalities Toxicity of therapy
Creatinine clearance	Kidney function; especially important when giving nephrotoxic drugs
Hemoccult test	Presence of blood in stool; not specific for cancer
Pap smear	Cervical cancer or premalignant changes
Serum electrophoresis	Serum protein and immunoglobulin levels (multiple myeloma)
Urine catecholamines	Neuroblastoma, pheochromocytoma

Table 4-2 Commonly Used Tumor Markers

Marker	Elevations May Indicate	Useful For
CEA (carcinoembryonic antigen)	Breast cancer, colorectal cancer, lung cancer	Monitoring or management of patients with known disease
PSA (prostate specific antigen)	Prostate cancer, benign prostate enlargement	Monitoring response of patients to treatment; arouse suspicion of prostate cancer
hCG (human chorionic gonadotropin)	Germ cell tumors (testicular, certain types ovarian, others), pregnancy	Differentiation of germ cell tumors
AFP (alpha fetal protein)	Germ cell tumors, liver cancer, benign liver disease, pregnancy	Differentiation of germ cell tumors
CA-125 (antigen)	Ovarian cancer, also elevated in some nonmalignant conditions and in some nongynecologic cancers	Monitoring response
CA-15-3 (2 antigens)	Metastatic or recurrent breast cancer	Monitoring recurrent disease
CA-19-9 (antigens)	Pancreatic cancer, colorectal cancer, gastric cancer, inflammatory bowel, biliary disease	Monitoring response to treatment

thyroid, brain, and liver, are done to evaluate possible primary or metastatic disease in those organs. Radio-labelled
monoclonal antibodies specific to tumor antigens may
also be used to produce gamma camera images of tumors
through a process called immunoscintography[9]

- *Visualization*—Colonoscopy, flexible sigmoidoscopy,
  bronchoscopy, gastroscopy, laparoscopy.

- *Laboratory Studies*—Complete blood count, blood chemistries, liver function tests, renal function tests, urinalysis, serum electrophoresis, calcium and magnesium levels, and levels of tumor-markers. Table 4-1 lists some common laboratory studies used in a diagnostic work-up.

- *Tumor Markers*—Tumor markers are substances that are
  present and measurable in the blood or tissues of patients
  with malignancies that are not present or are present in
  lesser amounts in normal individuals. Table 4-2 lists more
  commonly used tumor markers.[4,6]

Grade

Grade is a classification of tumor cells based on cellular differentiation or resemblance to normal cells in structure, function,
and maturity. Cells may be obtained by cytologic examination
techniques, biopsy, or surgical excision of a suspected mass.

- *Cytology*—Cytology is the examination of cells obtained
  from tissue scrapings, body fluids, secretions, or wash-
  ing. Pap smears are scrapings from the cervix to identify
  abnormal cervical cells. Fluids aspirated by thoracentesis,
  paracentesis, or lumbar puncture may yield cells for examination. Fine needle aspiration may also be used to
  obtain cells for evaluation.[8]

- *Biopsy*—A portion of tissue, generally obtained by surgical procedure, is examined in a biopsy specimen as part
  of an endoscopic procedure or under the guidance of CT
  to ensure that suspicious areas are sampled. Bone marrow biopsy, which uses a special needle to aspirate bone
  marrow tissue, is included in the work-up for hematologic disorders, including lymphomas, and when there is
  suspicion of bone marrow metastasis.[7]

■ *Excision and Analysis*—The pathologist uses a number of techniques to determine the tissue type and the degree of differentiation (grade) of the tumor. Frozen section is a procedure by which a small amount of tissue is quickly frozen, sliced thinly, and stained for immediate examination. A permanent section is prepared using tissue preserved in formalin, sliced thinly, stained, and prepared for microscopic examination. Careful attention is paid to the margins of the excised specimen to determine if margins are free of malignancy.[5,8,10]

Behaviour of a malignancy can be predicted on the basis of grade. The more unlike normal tissue, and less differentiated or mature the cells, the higher the grade. Table 4-3 lists grade classifications.

Table 4-3 Grades

Grade	Definition	Description
X	Cannot be assessed	
I	Well differentiated	Mature cells resembling normal tissue
II	Moderately differentiated	Cells with some immaturity
III	Poorly differentiated	Immature cells with little resemblance to normal
IV	Undifferentiated	No resemblance to normal tissue

Stage

Stage is a classification system based on the apparent anatomic extent of the malignancy. A universal system of staging allows comparison of cancers of similar cellular origin. Classification assist in determination of a treatment plan and prognosis for the individual patient, evaluation of research, comparison of treatment results between institutions, and comparison of worldwide statistics.

The comprehensive staging systems are approved by: The American Joint Committee on Cancer, The College of American Pathologists, The American College of Physicians, The American College of Radiology, The American College of Surgeons, International Union Against Cancer, and The International Federation of Gynecology and Obstetrics.

The TNM system involves assessment of three basic components: the size of the primary tumor (T); the absence or presence of regional lymph nodes (N); and the absence or presence of distant metastatic disease (M). General definitions used throughout the system are included in Table 4-4.[1] Prior to 1992, gynecologic cancers were commonly classified using a separate system developed by the International Federation of Gynecology and Obstetrics (FIGO). Information from the FIGO system has now been incorporated into the TNM system.

Information from the TNM classification is combined to define the stage. Stage classifications have been determined for most cancer sites and are included in Table 4-5. The stage is determined prior to beginning treatment, and is the basis for treatment decisions. The stage is often changed following surgery however, when pathologic measurements more accurately define tumor size and nodal involvement. Stage determined prior to treatment is termed the clinical stage (cTNM or TNM). When stage is changed after surgery, the term pathologic state (pTNM) is used.

Hematologic malignancies cannot be classified using the TNM system. Leukemias are classified according to cell type and differentiation but are not staged further. See Chapter 14.

Table 4-4 General TNM Definitions

T	Primary Tumor	Size, extent, depth of primary tumor
	TX	Primary tumor cannot be assessed
	T0	No evidence of primary tumor
	Tis	In situ
	T1-T4	Increasing size or extent of primary tumor
N	Nodal metastasis	Extent and location of involved regional lymph nodes
	NX	Regional lymph nodes cannot be assessed
	N0	No regional lymph node metastasis
	N1-N3	Increasing numbers and size of involved regional lymph nodes
M	Metastasis	Absence or presence of distant spread of disease
	MX	Distant disease cannot be assessed
	M0	No distant spread of disease
	M1	Distant spread of disease

Table 4-5 Selected TNM Staging Guidelines

Stage	Lung	Breast	Bone
Occult	**TX-N0-M0** TX: primary proven only by cells (sputum)		
0	**Tis-N0-M0** Tis: carcinoma in situ	**Tis-N0-M0** Tis: carcinoma in situ	
I	**T1 or T2-N0-M0** T1: tumor ≤ 3 cm T2: >3 cm and/or involving bronchus or pleura	**T1-N0-M0** T1: tumor ≤ 2 cm	**G1 or 2- T1 or 2** well or moderately differentiated T1, within cortex T2, outside cortex **N0-M0**
II	**T1 or T2-N1-M0** N1: peribronchial or hilar lymph node metastasis; same side as tumor	**T0 or T1-N1-M0** **T2-N0 or N1-M0** **T3-N0-M0** T2: tumor 2-5 cm T3: tumor > 5 cm N1: met. to movable axillary lymph node(s); same side	**G3 or 4- T1 or 2** **N0-M0** G3: poorly differentiated G4: undifferentiated

IIIA	**T1 or T2-N2-M0** **T3-any N-M0** N2: mediastinal or subclavian nodes; same side T3: tumor invades chest wall, diaphragm, mediastinal pleura, pericardium	**T0, T1, T2-N2-M0** **T3-N1 or N2-M0** N2: fixed axillary lymph nodes; same side	**Not defined**
IIIB	**Any T-N3-M0** **T4-any N-M0** N3: metastasis in lymph nodes opposite side T4: invades other organs (heart, mediastinum, etc) or pleural effusion	**T4-any N-M0** **Any T-N3-M0** T4: tumor invades chest wall or skin N3: internal mammary node metastasis; same side	
IV	**Any T, any N, M1** M1: distant metastasis	**Any T-any N-M1** M1: distant metastasis	**Any G & T-N1-M0** **Any G & T-Any N-M1**

From American Joint Committee on Cancer, *Manual for staging cancer*, ed 4, Chicago, 1992, The Committee

Table 4-5 Con't.

Stage	Larynx	Colorectal	Duke's
0	**Tis-N0-M0** Tis: carcinoma in situ	**Tis-N0-M0** Tis: carcinoma in situ	
I	**T1-N0-M0** T1: Tumor limited to vocal cord with normal mobility	**T1 or T2-N0-M0** T1: tumor invading submucosa T2: invading muscle layer	Duke's A
II	**T2-N0-M0** T2: extends to supraglottis and/or subglottis with impaired cord mobility	**T3 or T4-N0-M0** T3: invades through muscle layer, into subserosa T4: directly invades other organs or perforates visceral peritoneum	Duke's B
III	**T3-N0-M0** **T1, T2, or T3-N1-M0** T3: tumor limited to larynx with vocal cord fixation	**Any T-N1, N2, or N3-M0** N1: 1-3 pericolic or perirectal lymph node metastases	Duke's C

N1: single, same-side node
      < 3 cm

N2: ≥ 4 pericolic or perirectal lymph
      node metastases

N3: any nodal metastasis along vascular
      trunk or apical node.

IV   **T4-N0 or N1-M0**   **Any T- any N-M1**   Duke's D
      Any T-N2 or N3-M0   M1: distant metastasis
      Any T, any N, M1
      T4: tumor invades thyroid
            cartilage and/or tissues
            beyond larynx
      N2: single node, same-side, 3-6 cm
      N3: any node > 6 cm
      M1: distant metastasis

Continued.

Table 4-5 Con't.

Stage	Gastric	Prostate
0	**Tis-N0-M0** Tis: carcinoma in situ	**T1a-N0-M0 (G1)** T1a: incidental finding < 5% of tissue G1: well differentiated
IA	**T1-N0-M0** T1: tumor invades lamina propria or submucosa	**T1a, T1b, or T1c-N0-M0** T1b: incidental finding > 5% of tissue T1c: identified by needle biopsy
IB	**T1-N1-M0** **T2-N0-M0** T2: invades muscle layer or subserosa N1: perigastric node within 3 cm of primary site	
II	**T1-N2-M0** N2: perigastric node > 3 cm from primary or any other nodes	**T2-N0-M0** T2: tumor confined within prostate

IIIA	**T2-N2-M0**	**T3-N0-M0**
	T3-N1-M0	T3: extends through prostatic capsule
	T4-N0-M0	
	T3: penetrates visceral peritoneum without invasion of other structures	
	T4: invades other adjacent structures	
IIIB	**T3-N2-M0; T4-N1-M0**	**T4-N0-M0**
		Any T-N1, N2, or N3-M0
IV	**T4-N2-M0**	**Any T-any N-M1**
	Any T, any N, M1	T4: tumor is fixed & invades adjacent structures
	M1: distant metastasis	N1: single node ≤ 2 cm
		N2: single node 2–5 cm
		N3: 1 or more nodes > 5 cm
		M1: distant metastasis

Continued.

Table 4-5 Con't.

Stage	Soft-Tissue Sarcoma	Pancreas	Liver
0			
I	**T1 or 2-N0-M0** T1: tumor < 5 cm T2: tumor > 5 cm	**T1 or 2-N0-M0** T1: limited to pancreas T2: direct extension into duodenum, bile duct, or peripancreatic tissues	**T1-N0-M0** T1: single tumor 2 cm or less
II	**T1 or 2-N0-M0 (G2)** G2: moderately differentiated	**T3-N0-M0** T3: extends directly into stomach, spleen, colon, or large vessels	**T2-N0-M0** T2: single > 2 cm or multiple < 2 cm without vascular or single > 2 cm with vascular invasion

III	**T1 or 2-N0-M0 (G3 or 4)** G3: poorly differentiated G4: undifferentiated	**Any T-N1-M0** N1: regional lymph nodes	**T1 or 2-N1-M0** **T3-N0 or N1-M0** T3: Single > 2 cm with vascular, multiple in one lobe N1: regional lymph nodes involved
IV	**Any T-N1-M0** **Any T- any N- M1** N1: lymph nodes involved M1: distant metastasis	**Any T- any N- M1** M1: distant metastasis	**T4-any N-M0** **Any T- any N-M1** T4: multiple, more than one lobe or major blood vessels M1: distant metastasis

Continued.

Table 4-5 Con't.

Stage	Small Bowel	Esophagus
0	**Tis-N0-M0** Tis: in situ	**Tis-N0-M0** Tis: in situ
I	**T1 or 2-N0-M0** T1: tumor invades lamina propria T2: tumor invades muscularis	**T1-N0-M0** T1: tumor invades lamina propria or sub-mucosa
II	**T3 or 4-N0-M0** T3: invades through muscularis T4: perforates peritoneum or invades other organs	**T2 or 3-N0-M0** T2: invades muscularis T3: invades adventitia into pancreas
III	**Any T-N1-M0** N1: regional lymph nodes involved	**T1 or 2-N1-M0** N1: regional lymph nodes
IV	**Any T- any N- M1** M1: distant metastasis	**T3 or 4-N1-M0** T4: invades adjacent structures **Any T- any N- M1** M1: distant metastasis

Myeloma Staging System

A. Multiple myeloma

Major criteria

I.   Plasmacytoma on tissue biopsy

II.   Bone marrow plasmacytosis with > 30% plasma cells

III.   Monoclonal globulin spike on serum electrophoresis exceeding 3.5 g/dl for G peaks or 2.0 g/dl for A peaks, $\geq$ 1.0g/24 h of κ- or λ-light chain excretion on urine electrophoresis in the presence of amyloidosis

Minor criteria

a.   Bone marrow plasmacytosis 10% to 30% plasma cells

b.   Monoclonal globulin spike present, but less than the level defined above

c.   Lytic bone lesions

d.   Residual normal IgM < 50 mg/dl, IgA < 100 mg/dl, or IgG < 600 mg/dl. Diagnosis will be confirmed when any of the following features are documented in symptomatic patients with clearly progressive disease. The diagnosis of myeloma requires a minimum of one major + one minor criterion or three minor criteria that must include a + b, i.e.:

1. I + b, I + c, I + d (I + a is not sufficient)

2. II + b, II + c, II + d

3. III + a, III + c, III + d

4. a + b + c, a + b + d

Continued.

Table 4-5 Con't.

B. Indolent myeloma (same as myeloma except)
   I. No bone lesions or only limited bone lesions ($\leq$3 lytic lesions); no compression fractures
   II. M-component levels: (a) IgG < 7 g/dl; (b) IgA < 5 g/dl
   III. No symptoms or associated disease features, i.e.:
      a. Performance status > 70%
      b. Hemoglobin > 10 g/dl
      c. Serum calcium normal
      d. Serum creatinine < 2.0 g/dl
      e. No infections

C. Smoldering myeloma (same as indolent myeloma except)
   I. No bone lesions
   II. Bone marrow plasma cell $\leq$ 30%

D. MGUS
   I. Monoclonal gammopathy
   II. M-component level
      IgG $\leq$ 3.5 g/dl
      IgA $\leq$ 2.0 g/dl
      BJ protein $\leq$ 1.0 g/24 h
   III. Bone marrow plasma cells < 10%
   IV. No bone lesions
   V. No symptoms

IgA, immunoglobulin A; IgG, immunoglobulin G; IgM, immunoglobulin M; BJ, Bence Jones light chain. From Salmon SE & Cassady JR: Plasma cell neoplasmas. In DeVita VT Jr, Hellman S, Rosenberg SA, editors, *Cancer: Principles & practice of oncology*, ed 3, Philadelphia, 1989, JB Lippincott, p. 1864.

Table 4-5 con't.

AIDS-Kaposi's Sarcoma Staging

TUMOR (T)

T-0   Confined to skin and/or lymph nodes
           Minimal oral KS
T-1   Tumor associated edema or ulceration
           Extensive oral KS, Gatrointestinal KS
           Other visceral KS

IMMUNE SYSTEM (I)

I-0 T_4 helper cells ≥ 200
I-1 T_4 helper cells ≤ 200

SYSTEMIC ILLNESS (S)

S-0   No history of opportunistic infection or thrush
           No constitutional symptoms
           Karnofsky performance score equal to ≥ 70
S-1   History of opportunistic infection and/or thrush
           Constitutional symptoms
           Karnofsky performance < 70
           Other related HIV illness

Stage	Ann Arbor Staging System for Lymphomas
I	Single lymph node region or localized involvement of single organ
II	Two or more lymph node regions on same side of diaphragm or localized involvement of a single organ plus regional lymph nodes
III	Lymph nodes on both sides of diaphragm involved, may include localized involvement of single organ and/or spleen
IV	Disseminated involvement of extralymphatic organs, or isolated organ plus distant lymph nodes
A	**No systemic symptoms**
B	**Presence of systemic symptoms**

Continued.

Table 4-5 Con't.

Brain Tumor Staging

Supratentorial tumor

T1   Tumor ≤ 5 cm in greatest dimension; limited to one
     side

T2   Tumor > 5 cm in greatest dimension; limited to
     one side

T3   Tumor invades or encroaches on the ventricular system

T4   Tumor crossed the midline, invades the opposite
     hemisphere, or invades infratentorially

Infratentorial tumor

T1   Tumor ≤ 3 cm in greatest dimension; limited to one
     side
T2   Tumor > 3 cm in greatest dimension; limited to
     one side
T3   Tumor invades or enroaches on the ventricular system

T4   Tumor crosses the midline, invades the opposite
     hemisphere, or invades supratentorially

Stage grouping

Stage IA	G1	T1	M0
Stage IB	G1	T2	M0
	G1	T3	M0
Stage IIA	G2	T1	M0
Stage IIB	G2	T2	M0
	G2	T3	M0
Stage IIIA	G3	T1	M0
Stage IIIB	G3	T2	M0
	G3	T3	M0
Stage IV	G1,G2,G3	T4	M0
	G4	Any T	M0
	Any G	Any T	M1

Table 4-5 Con't.

Stage	Basal and Squamous Skin Cancer
I	Tumor is superficial and is 2 cm < at largest dimension
II	Tumor is > 2 cm but ≥ 5 cm in largest dimension, *or* primary tumor is > 5 cm in largest dimension
III	Tumor invades deep extradermal structures such as cartilage, skeletal muscle, or bone, *or* any tumor size with evidence of regional lymph node metastasis
IV	Presence of distant metastasis regardless of tumor size or nodal involvement

Melanoma Staging / TNM	Clark's
Stage I pT1-N0-M0	
pT1: Tumor < 0.75 mm thickness and invading papillary dermis	Clark's level II
pT2: Tumor 0.75-1.5 mm and/ or invades papillary-reticular dermal boundary	Clark's level III
Stage II p-T3-N0-M0	
pT3: Tumor 1.5-4 mm thickness and/or invades reticular dermis	Clark's level IV
Stage III p-T4-N0-M0 any pT-N1-M0	
pt4: Tumor > 4 mm thickness and/or invades subcutaneous tissue and/or satellite lesions	Clark's level V
Stage IV any pT-any N-M1	

Continued.

Table 4-5 Con't.

Stage	TNM	FIGO	Cervical Cancer Staging
0	T0		No evidence of primary tumor
	Tis	0	Carcinoma in situ
I	T1	I	Cervical carcinoma confined to uterus (extension to corpus should be disregarded)
IA	T1a	Ia	Preclinical invasive carcinoma, diagnosed by microscopy only
	T1a1	Iaa1	Minimal microscopic stromal invasion
	T1a2	Ia2	Tumor with invasive component $\leq$ 5 mm in depth taken from the base of the epithelium and $\leq$ 7 mm in horizontal spread
IB	T1b	Ib	Tumor larger than T1a2
	T2	II	Cervical carcinoma invades beyond uterus but not to pelvic wall or to the lower third of vagina
IIA	T2a	IIa	Without parametrial invasion
IIB	T2b	IIb	With parametrial invasion
	T3	III	Cervical carcinoma extends to the pelvic wall and/or involves lower third of vagina and/or causes hydronephrosis or nonfunctioning kidney
IIIA	T3a	IIIa	Tumor involves lower third of the vagina, no extension to pelvic wall
IIIB	T3b	IIIb	Tumor extends to pelvic wall and/or causes hydronephrosis or nonfunctioning kidney
IVA	T4	IVa	Tumor invades mucosa of bladder or rectum and/or extends beyond true pelvis
IVB	M1	IVb	Distant metastasis

Table 4-5 Con't.

Stage	TNM	FIGO	Ovarian Cancer Staging
0	T0		No evidence of primary tumor
I	T1	I	Tumor limited to ovaries
	T1a	Ia	Tumor limited to one ovary; capsule intact, no tumor on ovarian surface
	T1b	Ib	Tumor limited to both ovaries; capsule intact, no tumor on ovarian surface
	T1c	Ic	Tumor limited to one or both ovaries with any of the following: capsule ruptured, tumor on ovarian surface, malignant cells in ascites, or peritoneal washing
II	T2	II	Tumor involves one or both ovaries with pelvic extension
	T2a	IIa	Extension and/or implants on uterus and/or tube(s)
	T2b	IIB	Extension to other pelvic tissues
	T2c	IIc	Pelvic extension (2a or 2b) with malignant cells in ascites or peritoneal washing
III (A + B)			
	T3 and/or N1	III	Tumor involves one or both ovaries with and/microscopically confirmed peritoneal metastsis outside the pelvis and/or regional lymph node metastasis
	T3a	IIIa	Microscopic peritoneal metastasis beyond pelvis
	T3b	IIIb	Macroscopic peritoneal metastasis beyond pelvis ≤ 2 cm in greatest dimension
IIIC	T3c and/or N1	IIIc	Peritoneal metastasis beyond pelvis > 2 cm in greatest dimension and/or regional lymph node metastasis
IVA			T4-any N-M0 T4: invades bladder or rectal mucosa
IVB			Any T-any N-M1 MI: distant metastasis

Continued.

Table 4-5 Con't.

Stage		Uterine Corpus (endometrium)
IA	G123	Tumor limited to endometrium
IB	G123	Invasion to < ½ myometrium
IC	G123	Invasion to > ½ myometrium
IIA	G123	Endocervical glandular involvement only
IIB	G123	Cervical stromal invasion
IIIA	G123	Tumor invades serosa and/or adnexa and/or positive peritoneal cytology
IIIB	G123	Metastases to pelvic and/or para-aortic lymph nodes
IVA	G123	Tumor invasion of bladder and/or bowel mucosa
IVB		Distant metastases including intra-abdominal and/or inguinal lymph nodes
Grade		Histopathology: Degree of Differentiation
	G1	5% or less of a nonsquamous or nonmorular solid growth pattern
	G2	6%-50% of a nonsquamous or nonmorular solid growth pattern
	G3	More than 50% of a nonsquamous or nonmorular solid growth pattern

Stage	TNM	FIGO	Vaginal Cancer Staging
0	T0		No evidence of primary tumor
I	Tis	0	Carcinoma in situ
	T1	I	Tumor confined to vagina
II	T2	II	Tumor invades paravaginal tissue but not to pelvic wall
III	T3	III	Tumor extends to pelvic wall
IV	T4	IVa	Tumor invades mucosa of bladder or rectum and/or extends beyond the true pelvis
	M1	IVb	Distant metastasis

Table 4-5 Con't.

Stage		Vulva Cancer Staging
0	T0	No evidence of primary tumor
I	Tis	Preinvasive carcinoma (carcinoma in situ)
	T1	Tumor confined to the vulva, ≤ 2 cm in greatest dimension
II	T2	Tumor confined to the vulva, > 2 cm in greatest dimension
III	T3	Tumor invades any of the following: urethra, vagina, perineum, or anus
IV	T4	Tumor invades any of the following: bladder mucosa, upper part of the urethral mucosa, rectal mucosa, or tumor fixed to the bone

Nursing Management

Nursing Diagnoses

■ *Fear related to possible cancer diagnosis*
Interventions: Establish rapport; acknowledge validity of feelings; correct misconceptions, provide information; encourage use of support systems[11]

■ *Anxiety related to uncertainty/diagnosis of cancer*
Interventions: Limit time waiting for information; provide information about disease and treatment; encourage exploration and verbalization of feelings; explore previous effective response; teach behavioral interventions, including relaxation and distraction.[2]

■ *Knowledge deficit related to procedure*
Interventions: Explain procedure and rationale; explain what information may be gained; provide written information appropriate to the patient's cognitive and reading level; repeat and simplify information for those persons under stress.[11]

■ *Health-seeking behaviors*
Interventions: Encourage behaviours that are effective in the prevention of cancer or maintenance of a healthy lifestyle (stopping smoking, low-fat diet, increased exercise); answer questions openly and provide information[2]

■ *Ineffective family coping*
Intervention: Identify and encourage effective coping strategies; encourage effective family communication; encourage use of support systems; consult social worker, chaplain, other support services as appropriate.[3]

Bibliography

1. Beahrs O and others: *Manual for staging of cancer*, ed 4, American Joint Committee on Cancer, 1992, JB Lippincott.

2. Clark J, McGee R, and Preston R: Nursing management of responses to the cancer experience. In Clark J and McGee R, editors: *Core curriculum for oncology nursing*, ed 2, Philadelphia, 1992, WB Saunders.

3. Dufault K and others: Ineffective family coping. In McNally J, Somerville E, Miaskowski C and Rostad M, editors: *Guidelines for oncology nursing practice*, ed 2, Philadelphia, 1991, WB Saunders.

4. Flam T and others: *Diagnosis and markers in prostate cancer, Cancer* 70:357, 1992.

5. Greco F and Hainsworth J: *Tumors of unknown origin*, CA 42:96, 1992.

6. Herberman RB: *Tumor markers*. American Association for Clinical Chemistry NCI, Triton Diagnostics, Inc., Alameda, CA, 1991.

7. DeVita V Jr, Hellman S, and Jaffe E: Hodgkin's disease. In DeVita V, Hellman S, and Rosenberg S, editors: *Cancer: principles and practice of oncology*, ed 4, Philadelphia, 1993, JB Lippincott.

8. Markel D: *Introduction to classics in oncology "Spectrophotometer: new instrument of ultrarapid cell analysis* by Kamentsky, Metamed, & Derman,*"* CA 42:57, 1992.

9. Perkins A, Pimm M: *Immunoscintography: practical aspects and clinical application*, 1987, New York, Wiley-Liss.

10. Salmon SE and Cassady JR: Plasma cell neoplasms. In DeVita V, Hellman S, and Rosenberg S, editors: *Cancer: principles and practice of oncology*, ed 4, Philadelphia, 1993, JB Lippincott.

11. Strohl R: Implications of diagnosis and staging on treatment goals and strategies. In Clark J and McGee R, editors: *Core curriculum for oncology nursing*, ed 2, Philadelphia, 1992, WB Saunders.

Section II

Clinical Management
of Major Cancer
Diseases

Bone Cancers and Soft Tissue Sarcomas

5

Bone Cancers

Epidemiology

It is estimated that 2,000 new cases of bone cancer will be diagnosed in 1994. Men will account for approximately 1,100 of these cases and women slightly less with an incidence of 900. The estimated number of deaths is 1,075. This disease exhibits a bimodal pattern with peak occurrences between the ages of 15 to 19 years and after the age of 65.[1,23]

Etiology

Very few risk factors have been associated with primary bone tumors. Paget's disease, fibrous dysplasia, enchondromatosis, bone infarction, or prior exposure to radiation are all conditions known to be associated with bone tumors.

Classification

Primary bone malignancies are classified histologically by the cell or tissue type from which they originate. These include osseous, cartilaginous, fibrous, reticuloendothelial, and vascular as listed in Table 5-1.[9]

Staging

Approximately 30% of patients with malignant lesions present as Stage I lesions, 60% as Stage II, and 10% as Stage III. Stage I lesions are more often intracompartmental (66%), while 90% of Stage II lesions are usually extracompartmental. See Chapter 4 for AJCC Staging information. Diagnostic tests used include imaging techniques (CT scan, MRI), radiography, bone scans, arteriography studies and biopsies.

Table 5-1 Common Malignant Bone Tumors

Tissue Type	Bone Malignancy
Osseous	Classic osteosarcoma (IIB) Parosteal osteosarcoma (IA) Periosteal osteosarcoma (IIA)
Cartilaginous	Primary chondrosarcoma (IIB) Secondary chondrosarcoma (IA)
Fibrous	Fibrosarcoma (IIB) Malignant fibrous histiocytoma (IIB)
Reticuloendothelial	Ewing's sarcoma (IIB) Multiple Myeloma (III)

Adapted from Enneking WF: *Common bone tumors*. Clinical Symposia 41:2, 1989.

Osteosarcoma

Epidemiology

Osteosarcoma (osteogenic sarcoma) constitutes about 20% of all primary malignant bone tumors. The disease most commonly affects adolescents in the second decade of life during the period of maximal growth.

The most commonly affected sites are the distal femur, proximal tibia, and proximal humerus. Less common sites are the pelvis, vertebral column, mandible, clavicle, scapula, or bones in the hands and feet. More than 50% of cases occur in the knee region.[4,8]

Metastasis

In about 50% of adolescent patients, the tumor penetrates the growth plate into the epiphysis. Skip metastases develop in approximately 20% of patients; pulmonary metastases are clinically detectable in about 10% of patients upon initial presentation. Metastatic disease develops by the hematogenous route, and usually appears first in the lungs.[12]

Clinical Features

- Pain and/or swelling in the affected extremity (usually worse at night and increases as disease progresses)
- Unrelated history of trauma or sports-related injury
- Elevated serum alkaline phosphatase level
- May occur in conjunction with Paget's disease of bone[16]

Treatment and Prognosis

The 5-year survival rate for individual's treated with surgery alone or a combination of surgery and radiation is approximately 10% to 20%. Presently, 60% to 80% of patients presenting with osteosarcoma without metastases will be cured following appropriate surgery and chemotherapy.[2]

Chondrosarcoma

Epidemiology

Chondrosarcoma constitutes about 13% of all primary malignant bone tumors. It occurs most often in adults between 40 to 60 years of age and affects males twice as often as females.

The most commonly affected sites are the pelvis, proximal femur, and shoulder girdle. Transformation of a preexisting enchondroma or osteocartilaginous exostosis to a chondrosarcoma occurs in approximately 25% of these cases.[8,23]

Metastasis

Chondrosarcoma is often a slow growing tumor, but can metastasize to distant organs. Tumor growth rates range from slow growing to highly malignant metastasizing tumors.

Clinical Features

- Persistent, dull, aching pain like that of arthritis
- Swollen, firm area over the tumor site

Treatment and Prognosis

The treatment of chondrosarcoma is primarily surgical. Both chemotherapy and radiation therapy have proven to be relatively ineffective in the treatment of this tumor.

Stage I tumors rarely metastasize or recur locally. The estimated 10-year survival rate for this stage is 87%. At 10 years, stage II tumors have an estimated survival rate of 41%, while the stage III rate is 27%.

Fibrosarcoma

Epidemiology/Clinical Feature

Fibrosarcoma accounts for less than 4% of all primary malignant bone tumors and is most often seen in adolescents or young adults. Fibrosarcoma is a malignant fibroblastic lesion usually arising within the medullary cavity. The most commonly affected sites are the femur and the tibia and pain/swelling is the most common symptom.[8]

Treatment and Prognosis

Surgical resection is the optimal treatment for this neoplasm. Excision with a wide margin is indicated for stage IA tumors, whereas stage IIB fibrosarcomas require radical margins or wide margins with adjuvant chemotherapy or radiation therapy. The prognosis is guarded. The reported 5-year survival rate is 21.8%.[18]

Ewing's Sarcoma

Epidemiology

Ewing's sarcoma comprises approximately 6% of all primary malignant bone tumors. Children are affected more commonly than adults. Ewing's sarcoma is seen most frequently in children between the ages of 10 and 15 years. This tumor is more common in males than in females and is rare in the black population.

The bones of the pelvis and lower extremity constitute the majority of sites involved, although any bone and/or portion of that bone may be affected. The femoral diaphysis is the most common site, followed by the ilium, tibia, humerus, fibula, and ribs.[11,14]

Metastasis

Metastases usually occur early and involve the lungs. Other sites of metastases include the bones and regional lymph nodes. While solitary metastases do occasionally occur, it is more common to have multiple metastatic lesions. The presence of metastatic disease has been reported in 14% to 35% of patients at time of diagnosis.[9]

Clinical Features

- Pain and swelling of the affected area
- Symptoms tend to be progressive, with some patients experiencing them for months before they seek medical aid
- Low grade fever
- Flu-like symptoms of malaise, weakness
- Anemia, leukocytosis, and an elevated erythrocyte sedimentation rate

Treatment and Prognosis

Current studies indicate that prognosis is most affected by the presence of disseminated disease and the location or size of the primary lesion. Tumors in the pelvis are often detected late and are therefore larger with a poorer prognosis. The estimated 5-year survival rates now range from 54% to 74%.

Adjuvant systematic chemotherapy, radiation therapy and surgery are all utilized. Initial treatment begins with chemotherapy followed by wide surgical excisions versus radiation therapy for local control if (1) the involved bone is expendable (fibula, rib, clavicle) or can be reconstructed without disabling the patient; (2) radiation therapy would cause significant growth deformity; (3) successful rehabilitation is not feasible; and (4) previous local irradiation was unsuccessful.[15,18]

Soft-Tissue Sarcomas

Epidemiology

The American Cancer Society predicts 6,000 new cases of soft-tissue sarcomas will occur in 1994. Men will account for approximately 3,300 of these cases and women slightly less with 2,700.

The estimated number of deaths is 3,300. Currently, twice as many individuals die of soft-tissue sarcomas each year as die of Hodgkin's disease, even though the incidence of the two neoplasms is similar.[14,23]

Etiology

Approximately 5% of sarcomas occur within ports of prior radiation therapy, which was delivered more than 20 years prior to development of the sarcoma. Chemicals such as asbestos are associated with mesothelioma and polyvinyl chloride, arsenic, and hemochromatosis with angiosarcoma of the liver. Dioxin (in Agent Orange) exposure has been associated with the development of soft-tissue sarcomas.

Individuals with neurofibromatosis have a 7% to 10% risk of developing malignant neurofibrosarcoma. Approximately 50% of all neurofibrosarcomas develop in patients with neurofibromatosis.

Classification

Soft-tissue sarcoma are classified according to cell type or tissue of origin: for example, fat, smooth, and striated muscle as listed in Table 5-2. The majority of soft-tissue sarcomas are found in the lower extremity (40%), trunk (15%), retroperitoneum (15%), and the upper extremity including the head and neck region. Visceral sarcomas arise in the gastrointestinal and gynecologic tracts. Kaposi's and mesotheliomas are classified as miscellaneous sarcomas.

Metastasis

Metastases are usually spread by hematogenous routes or local invasion into surrounding normal tissues by the tumor. This presentation generally indicates a poor prognosis. Presenting symptoms vary due to the anatomic location of the tumor. These may include peripheral neuralgias due to nerve impingement, vascular ischemia, paralysis, bowel obstruction, and various other symptomatology.[7,25]

Table 5-2

Histologic Types of Soft-Tissue Sarcomas	
Tumors of fibrous tissue	Fibrosarcoma
Tumors of adipose tissue	Liposarcoma—well differentiated, myxoid, pleomorphic
Tumors of smooth muscle	Leiomyosarcoma
Tumors of striated muscle	Rhabdomyosarcoma—alveolar, pleomorphic, embryonal
Tumors of vascular origin	Angiosarcoma Lymphangiosarcoma Malignant hemangiopericytoma
Tumors of synovial tissue	Synovial sarcoma
Tumors of mesothelium	Malignant mesothelioma
Tumors of neurogenic origin	Neurogenic sarcoma (malignant schwannoma)
Tumors of "histiocytic" origin	Malignant fibrous histiocytoma Giant cell tumor of soft tissue
Tumors of cartilaginous origin	Extraskeletal chondrosarcoma (choroid sarcoma)
Tumors of uncertain origin	Dermatofibrosarcoma protuberans Epithelioid sarcoma Clear cell sarcoma Kaposi's sarcoma Alveolar soft part sarcoma Ewing's sarcoma in soft tissue

Liposarcoma

- Occur most frequently in adults and tend to involve the proximal lower extremities (thigh, buttocks, groin)
- Primary treatment is surgical resection
- Liposarcomas rarely develop from previous lipomas

Leiomyosarcoma

- Arises from smooth muscle and occurs in visceral regions of the body
- Common sites include the uterus, retroperitoneum, and gastrointestinal tract
- Long-term survival is usually poor due to their early metastatic spread[9]

Rhabdomyosarcoma

Malignant tumors of muscle origin are divided into three types

- Embryonal rhabdomyosarcoma occurs most often in young children
- Alveolar rhabdomyosarcoma occurs in both children and young adults
- Pleomorphic rhabdomyosarcoma occurs in late middle age

Angiosarcoma

- Tumor is of vascular origin and occurs most frequently in the liver, skin, and breast
- Neoplasms are poorly defined and tend to have deep vascular extensions
- Common presenting sign is bruising over the affected area[9]

Synovial Sarcoma

- Arises from mesenchymal cells and occurs most frequently in tendons, bursae, or joints
- Rare tumor that occurs most frequently in young adults and tends to involve the extremities

Malignant Mesothelioma

- Tumor occurs most frequently in the lung pleura and peritoneum and has a poor prognosis due to its unresponsiveness to standard forms of treatment
- Occurs in older male population
- Asbestos exposure has been implicated in this malignancy

Neurogenic Sarcoma

- Also known as neurofibrosarcoma, malignant schwannoma, or malignant neurilemmoma
- Usually arises in the sheath tissue of a peripheral nerve
- Tumors can occur at any age but are common in the first two decades of life
- Tend to recur locally and spread hematogenously to the lungs and bones
- Brachial plexus, sciatic, medial, and spinal nerves are most commonly affected

Diagnosis and Staging

Imaging Techniques

- History and physical examination (individual's age, site and size of the lesion, occupation, and the presence of risk factors that are associated with these malignancies such as Paget's disease of the bone (osteosarcoma) or neurofibromatosis (neurofibrosarcoma) are identified.
- Radiography
- Bone scan
- Computed tomography
- Magnetic resonance imaging
- Arteriography

Biopsy

The purpose of a biopsy is to obtain adequate tissue for an accurate histologic diagnosis and grading. Biopsies can be performed in a number of ways.

1. Open incisional biopsy.
2. Closed percutaneous biopsy, either with a fine needle aspiration cytology or tissue cores from a special cutting needle.
3. Needle biopsy.

Treatment

Surgical Management

Surgical management in conjunction with other treatment therapies is indicated for a majority of primary bone and soft tissue sarcomas. The following surgical techniques are used:[6,7,10,13,21,24]

Surgical Techniques

- *Wide excision*—The goal is to obtain tumor-free histologic margins but spare major neurovascular structures.
- *Amputation*—Indications for primary amputation are late-presenting lesions with neurovascular involvement, pathologic fractures (especially in the proximal femur), infected or inappropriately placed biopsy incisions, or extensive muscle involvement.
- *En bloc resection*—This technique involves wide excision of surrounding normal tissue, removal of entire muscle bundles at points of origin and insertion, and resection of involved bone as well as vascular structures. A whole block or "compartment" is surgically removed. A margin of at least 5 to 7 centimeters above and below the limit of tumor activity is necessary to ensure complete tumor removal.
- *Tikhoff-Linberg Procedure*—This surgical technique is utilized with lesions of the proximal humerus and encompasses en bloc resection of the scapula, part of the humerus, and clavicle. Following this procedure, the functions of the hand and elbow are preserved. This method of resection is performed as an alternative to forequarter amputation.

Reconstructive Options

Patient criteria for limb salvage surgery: age, biopsy incision, and postoperative function of the spared limb ≥ the function of a prosthetic device. Reconstruction can be accomplished by the use of a variety of metal as well as synthetic materials.

Types of Procedures

- *Allograft*—a graft from another individual (usually a cadaver)
- *Autograft*—a graft taken from the patient
- *Vascularized graft*—graft implanted with vessels supplying it intact
- *Arthroplasty*—surgical formation or reformation of a joint
- *Arthodesis*—surgical fusion of a joint
- *Endoprosthesis*—artificial replacement of a joint or bone by a metallic implant

Prosthesis

- *Metallic Endoprosthesis*—Artificial replacement of a joint or bone by a metallic implant
- *Intermedullary Rod*—Similar to an endoprosthesis and is utilized for stability to form a union between two sections of bone following en bloc resection

Joint Reconstruction

- *Arthrodesis*—Fusion of the joint using part of the femur, tibia, or vascularized fibular grafts. This procedure is most useful in the knee, shoulder, hip, and wrist
- *Arthroplasty*—Surgical formation of a joint using a custom metallic implant, bone allograft implant, or a combination of both to maintain joint function

Soft-Tissue Reconstruction

Occasionally, after resection of a soft-tissue or bone sarcoma, a cavity can occur. It may be necessary for a plastic surgeon to perform a muscle flap to close this cavity

Postoperative Rehabilitation

The immediate postoperative treatment for both above-knee (AK) and below-knee (BK) amputation is similar. A rigid dressing is applied at the time of surgery to reduce pain and swelling. Three to four days postamputation, the rigid dressing is removed. A cast is then taken of the amputated limb for the temporary prosthesis.[13,19]

For the AK amputee, the original rigid dressing is reapplied. Extra prosthetic socks may be added to facilitate compression of the stump. In order to prevent hipflexion contractures, range of motion (ROM) and exercises in the prone position are instituted in the immediate postoperative period. The patient receives the temporary prosthesis six to seven days after surgery. Gait training with partial weight bearing is then started. Upon discharge, seven to nine days after surgery, the patient is able to ambulate with assistance of crutches.[13,19]

Once the rigid dressing is removed, the BK amputee receives an immediate postoperative prosthesis (IPOP). Gait training with partial weight bearing is then started. Approximately 3 weeks after surgery, the IPOP is replaced with the temporary prosthesis and full weight-bearing training is begun.[13,19]

Both the AK and the BK amputees remain in temporary prostheses for the period that they are receiving chemotherapy treatments. During this time these individuals may experience weight fluctuations. Also during this period the residual limb matures and shrinks. One month after completion of chemotherapy, the permanent prosthesis is made.[13,19]

Chemotherapy

Chemotherapy may be administered systematically as adjutant (postoperative) therapy, or it may be given as neoadjuvant (preoperative) therapy, either intravenously or intraarterially. Neoadjuvant chemotherapy has become the standard approach to treatment and is designed to produce necrosis and shrinkage of the tumor. The effectiveness of the chemotherapy regimen is evaluated at the time of surgical resection by the amount of necrosis the tumor displays. This necrosis is graded in the following manner: grade I, <50%; grade II, 50% to 90%; grade III >90%; grade IV, 100%. The chemotherapy agents chosen depend on the type of sarcoma and/or the response of the tumor to previous agents. Refer to Box 5-1.[3,15,22,26]

Radiation Therapy

Current trials for soft-tissue sarcomas are now underway utilizing preoperative doxorubicin/cisplatin chemotherapy followed by 2,800 cGy of radiation with subsequent surgical resection. Connective tissue tumors are relatively radioresistant.[12] Other soft tissue sites, such as retroperitoneal and head and neck sarcomas, have not fared well with this mulitmodality approach. Radiation therapy has limited effect on osteosarcoma, chondrosarcoma, and fibrosarcoma and is reserved for palliation of tumors that are inoperable. Ewing's sarcoma tends to be relatively radio-sensitive. [2,17,20]

Box 5-1 Chemotherapeutic Agents for Certain Sarcomas

Soft-tissue sarcoma

- doxorubicin
- dacarbazine
- ifosfamide
- cisplatin

Osteogenic sarcoma/malignant fibrous histocytoma

- doxorubicin
- cisplatin
- methotrexate
- cyclophosphamide
- ifosfamide
- dactinomycin
- bleomycin

Ewing's Sarcoma

- vincristine
- actinomycin D
- doxorubicin
- cyclophosphamide
- ifosfamide
- etoposide

Rhabdomyosarcoma

- vincristine
- actinomycin D
- cyclophosphamide

Nursing Management

Nursing Diagnosis

- *Impaired physical mobility related to limb salvage or amputation*

Interventions

- Assess emotional status
- Determine and evaluate:
    growth and development (age related)
    range of motion (ROM) of joints, muscle strength
    gait, balance, and coordination
    vascular status (circulation and sensation) posture
- Postoperative assessment includes:
    general physical status, vital signs
    proper body positioning
    signs and symptoms of postoperative complications
        related to surgery (hemorrhage, infection,
        compartmental syndrome, pulmonary embolus, skin
        breakdown)
    signs and symptoms of complications related to
        impaired mobility (constipation, skin breakdown,
        pneumonia, urinary retention, anorexia)
        pain management (phantom pain for amputees)
        ability to perform ROM exercises and/or use of
        assistive devices (overhead traction bar, crutches,
        prosthesis, and others)
    ability to care for stump and prosthesis
- Coordinate rehabilitative measures with other
    multidisciplinary members (physical therapist,
    occupational therapist, prosthetist, and others).
- Arrange for contact with rehabilitated patient if
    appropriate
- Patient education:
    Discuss importance of physical therapy (ROM
        exercises, mobility)
    Reinforce importance of proper nutrition and hydration
    Discuss with patient/family possible complications
        associated with amputation/limb salvage (irritation
        of skin, altered fit of cast, increased swelling or pain,
        fever, mechanical problems with prosthesis)
    Emphasize importance of open communication
    Provide information for support groups for patient/
        family

Nursing Diagnosis

- *Knowledge deficit related to surgery*

Interventions

- Describe the surgical procedure:
    incisional biopsy
    local excision
    excision with wide margin
    use of implants and special grafts
    en bloc resection
    amputation
    resection of metastases
    cytoreductive surgery
- Explain common terms and procedure related to pathology specimen
- Discuss potential surgical outcomes:
    change in bodily appearance
    changes in bodily functions
    limitations in mobility
    loss of extremity
- Describe preoperative preparation:
    surgical and bowel prep regimen
    removal of prosthetics and valuables
    dietary restrictions
    preoperative medications
    scheduled time of surgery
- Provide teaching materials/educational videos
- Explain postoperative routine
    pulmonary toilet, mobility, pain management
    potential devices such as drains, surgical wound
        dressings, chest tubes, nasogastric tubes, foley
        catheter, etc.

Bibliography

1. American Cancer Society: *Cancer statistics—1994*, CA 44(1):18, 1994.
2. Antman KH, Eilber FR, and Shiu MH. Soft tissue sarcomas: current trends in diagnosis and management. In Haskell CM, editor: *Current problems in cancer*, Chicago, 1989, Year Book.
3. Bramwell VH: *Chemotherapy for metastatic soft tissue sarcomas—another full circle?* Br J Cancer 64:7, 1991.
4. Carter SR and others: *A review of 13-years experience of osteosarcoma*, Clin Orthop Research 270:45, 1991.
5. Dalinka MK and others: *The use of magnetic resonance imaging in the evaluation of bone and soft-tissue tumors*, Radiol Clin North Am 28:461, 1990.
6. Eckardt JJ and others: *Endoprosthetic replacement for stage IIb osteosarcoma*, Clin Orhtrop 270:202, 1991.
7. Eilber FR and others: *Progress in the recognition and treatment of soft-tissue sarcomas*, Cancer 67:1169, 1990.
8. Enneking WF and Conrad EU: *Common bone tumors*, Clin Symp 41:2, 1989.
9. Enterline H: *Histopathology of sarcomas*, Semin Oncol 8:133, 1981.
10. Finn HA and Simon MA: *Limb-salvage surgery in the treatment of osteosarcoma in skeletally immature individuals*, Clin Orthop 262:108, 1991.
11. Karakousis CP, Emrich LJ, and Vesper DS: *Soft-tissue sarcomas of the proximal lower extremity,* Arch Surg 124:1297, 1989.
12. Klein MJ, Kenan S, and Lewis MM: *Osteosarcoma clinical and pathological considerations*, Orthop Clin North Am 20:327, 1989.
13. Lane MJ and others: *New advances and concepts in amputee management after treatment for bone and soft-tissue sarcomas*, Clin Orthop 256:22, 1990.
14. Lawrence W and others: *Adult soft tissue sarcomas*, Ann Surg 205:349, 1987.
15. Link MP and others: *Adjuvent chemotherapy of high-grade osteosarcoma of the extremity*, Clin Orthop 2770:8, 1991.

16. Meyer WH and Malawer MM: *Osteosarcoma: Clinical features and evolving surgical and chemotherapeutic strategies*, Pediatr Clin North Am 38:317, 1991.

17. Murphy WA: *Imaging bone tumors in the 1990s,* Cancer 67:1169, 1991.

18. O'Connor MI and Pritchard DJ: *Ewing's sarcoma, prognostic factors, disease control, and the re-emerging role of surgical treatment,* Clin Orthop 262:78, 1991.

19. Piasecki PA: *The nursing role in limb salvage surgery,* Orthop Nursing 26:33, 1991.

20. Raney B and others: *Treatment of children with neurogenic sarcoma,* Cancer 59:1, 1987.

21. Rydholm A and Rooser B: *Surgical margins for soft-tissue sarcoma,* J Bone Joint Surg 69-A:1074, 1987.

22. Saleh RA and others: *Response of osteogenic sarcoma to the combination of etoposide and cyclophosphamide as neoadjuvent chemotherapy,* Cancer 65:861, 1990.

23. Santoro A and Bonadonna G: *Soft tissue and bone sarcomas,* Cancer Chemother Biolog Response Modifiers, 10:344, 1988.

24. Simon M: *Limb salvage for osteosarcoma in the 1980s,* Clin Orthop 270:264, 1991.

25. Stotter AT and others: *The influence of local recurrence of extremity soft tissue sarcoma on metastasis and survival,* Cancer 65:1119, 1990.

26. Yasko AW and Lane JM: *Chemotherapy for bone and soft-tissue sarcomas of the extremities,* J Bone Joint Surg 73-A:1263, 1991.

Cancer of the Central Nervous System

6

Cancer of the Central Nervous System

Epidemiology

Cancer of the CNS accounts for 1.5% of all malignancies with 17,500 diagnosed cases in 1994. Peak incidence occurs from birth to 6 years, and after the age of 45. CNS tumors account for the fourth leading cause of cancer death in persons aged 15 to 34.[8]

Etiology and Risk Factors

Genetic factors have been linked with neurofibromatosis, tuberous sclerosis, familial polyposis, Von Hippel-Lindau disease,[16] Turcot syndrome, and familial cancer syndromes of breast, soft-tissue sarcoma, and leukemia.

Chemical exposures that have been implicated include vinyl chloride, radiation, petrochemicals, inks, acrylonitrile, lubricating oils, and solvents. Viruses have also been implicated including the Epstein-Barr virus genome. Traumatic causes and environmental carcinogens have not been indicated at this time.[16,21]

Prevention and Screening Detection

Symptoms appear gradually and do not lend themselves to diagnostic prescreening methods.

Classification

Tumors of the CNS include brain and spinal cord tumors, and are classified as either primary or metastatic in nature. Primary tumors may exist as intracerebral or extracerebral. Major intracerebral tumors include those within the brain: neuroglia, neurons, and cells of the blood vessels of the connective tissue. Extracerebral tumors originate outside of the brain and include meningeomas, acoustic nerve, pituitary, and pineal gland tumors. Metastatic tumors may exist either inside or outside of the brain. (Table 6-1)[6,8,29]

Clinical Features

The clinical features manifested by CNS tumors vary. The most common symptom is headache and seizure activity. Many clinical features vary according to the location of the tumor, see Figure 6-1. Other clinical features are:[28]

- Headaches are commonly bifrontal and biooccipital and occur upon awakening; pain
- Seizure activity; cerebral edema
- Increased intracranial pressure; brain tissue hemorrhages
- Brain herniation
- Structural changes, memory defects, speech, motor, visual changes vary depending on tumor location and size
- Spinal cord tumors related to the site and size of the lesion
- Weakness; loss of bowel and bladder function

Diagnostic and Pathologic Staging

- Computed tomography
- Magnetic resonance imaging
- Positron emission tomography
- Cerebral angiograms and Radionuclide angiograms, x-rays used to evaluate cerebral blood vessel flow near the tumor.
- Tumor markers have only demonstrated usefulness in embryonal tumors in the pineal area.
- Stereotactic needle biopsy
- craniotomy[16,20,21]

Metastasis

The spread of primary CNS tumors beyond the brain and spinal cord is rare. Seeding is the most common method of spread within the CNS and spinal cord. Medulloblastoma tumors have the greatest potential to develop metastatic lesions within the CNS.[16]

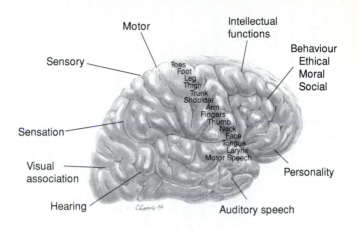

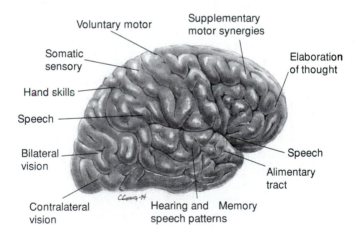

Figure 6-1. A, Principal functional subdivisions of the cerebral hemisphere. **B,** Functional areas of specific cortical areas. (From McCance KL and Huether SE: *Pathophysiology, The biologic basis for disease in adults and children,* St Louis, 1990, Mosby.)

Table 6-1 Brain and Spinal Cord Tumors

Neoplasm	% of Tumors	Location	Characteristics	Cell of Origin
Gliomas				Glial cells (supportive CNS cells)
Astrocytoma	20	Anywhere in brain or spinal cord	Grade I and II Slow growing, invasive	Astrocytes
Glioblastoma Multiforme	30	Common in cerebral hemispheres	Grade III, IV Highly invasive and malignant	Thought to arise from mature astrocytes
Ogliodendro-cytoma	4	Common in frontal lobes deep in white matter; may also arise in brain stem, cerebellum, and spinal cord	Avascular, tends to be encapsulated; more malignant form called *oligodendroblastoma*	Oligodenrocytes
Ependymoma	5	Intramedullary; wall of the ventricles; may arise in caudal tail of the spinal cord	Common in children, variable growth rates; more malignant, invasive form called *ependymoblastoma*; may extend into the ventricle or invade brain tissue	Ependymal cells

Neurilemmoma	4	Cranial nerves (most commonly vestibular division of cranial nerve VIII)	Slow growing	Schwann cells
Neurofibroma	1	Extramedullary—spinal cord	Slow growing	Neurilemma, Schwann cells
Pituitary Tumors	8	Pituitary gland; may extend to or invade floor of the third ventricle	Age-linked, several types slow growing, macro- and microadenomas may be secreting or nonsecreting	Pituitary cells, pituitary chromophobes, basophils, eosinophils
Pineal Region	1	Pineal region; pineal parenchyma (posterior) or third ventricle	Several types (germinoma, pineocytoma, teratoma)	Several types with different cell origins

Continued.

Table 6-1 Cont'd

Neoplasm	% of Tumors	Location	Characteristics	Cell of Origin
Blood Vessel Tumors Angiomas)	3	Predominantly in posterior cerebral hemispheres	Slow growing	Arising from congenitally malformed arteriovenous connections
Neuronal Cell Medulloblastoma	1	Posterior cerebellar vermis, roof of fourth ventricle	Well demarcated, rapid-growing, fills fourth ventricle	Embryonic cells
Mesodermal Tissue Meningioma	20	Intradural, extramedullary; sylvian fissure region, superior parasagittal surface of frontal and parietal lobes, olfactory groove, wing of sphenoid bone, superior surface of cerebellum, cerebellopontine angle, spinal cord	Slow growing, circum-scribed, encapsulated, sharply demarcated from normal tissues, compressive in nature	

Choroid Plexus Papillomas	1	Choroid plexus of the ventricular system, lateral ventricle in children, fourth ventricle in adults	Usually benign, slow in expansion inducing hemorrhage and hydrocephalus; malignant tumor is rare	Epithelial cells
Cranial Nerves and Spinal Nerve Roots				
Hemangio-blastomas	2	Arises from blood vessels Predominant in cerebellum	Benign Slow growing	Embryonic vascular tissue
Lymphoma	1	Cerebral hemispheres	Metastasis common	B cells
Metastatic Tumors	35% of all cancer patients	Cerebral cortex diencephalon	Malignant spread	From lung, breast, colon, kidney, thyroid, prostate

Treatment Modalities

Surgery

Surgery serves as a diagnostic and treatment modality. Surgical intervention provides tissue sampling for histology, decreases the tumor burden for further treatment, and can provide a cure for low-grade tumors. A craniotomy is the most common surgical procedure performed to remove tumor mass or debulk the largest portion of the tumor. Additional surgical procedures may include stereotactic biopsy for the removal of smaller tumors, and placement of radioactive substances to treat nonresectable tumors.[16,17]

Radiation Therapy

Tumors that are inoperable, or have only partial tumor resection, may respond to radiation therapy if the tumor histology is radiosensitive. Tumors that are radiosensitive include medullablastomas, high grade astrocytoma, and metastatic brain tumors of the breast, lung, myeloma, and sarcoma.[6,13,14,17,25]
Other methods of radiation administration include:

- Radioactive sensitizers
- Hyperfractionation
- Heavy particle radiation therapy
- Photodynamic therapy
- Neuron capture therapy

Chemotherapy

Chemotherapy may be utilized in combination with surgery and radiation for the treatment of gliomas and medulloblastomas. Response rate remains as low as 20% to 40% due to the blood-brain barrier mechanism. Common routes of administration include oral and intravenous. Additional methods include intraarterial into the carotid or vertebral artery, via timed-release biodegradable wafers impregnated with chemotherapeutic agent, into the spinal column or the Ommaya reservoir, a surgically implanted pump placed in the ventricles.[7,19,26]

Spinal Cord Tumors

The treatment of spinal cord tumors is similar to brain tumors. Surgical resection is used for diagnosis and tumor removal. Decompression laminectomy is used when tumor compression is present. Postoperative radiation may include the entire spinal column or cord segments. Chemotherapy may be given in the intrathecal route or systemically.[26]

Disease-Related Complications

Major disease related complications include increased intracranial pressure from cerebral edema and displaced brain structures resulting in brain herniation. A major complication of spinal cord tumors is spinal cord compression. Increased intracranial pressure is caused by an increase in intracellular volume from the expanding tumor mass and edema, see Figure 6-2.

Surgery

Postoperative surgical complications are:
- Intracranial bleeding
- Cerebral edema
- Infection
- Neuromotor deficits
- Thrombosis
- Hydrocephalus

Size and location of tumor as well as the overall preoperative state of the patient enhances the potential for complications.[27,28]

Steroidal Therapy

Use of steroids pre- and postoperatively, can also produce a variety of treatment side effects that can produce local as well as systemic effects (hyperglycemia, hypokalemia, hypernatremia, fluid retention, osteoporosis, depressed immune response, and cutaneous striae).[11] Steroids are administered to produce an antiinflammatory response and reduce cerebral swelling. Steroidal therapy may begin after an initial dose of mannitol, which may be used before, during, or after surgery to reduce immediate cerebral edema. Postoperative management with titration will be done with steroids such as dexamethasone.[7,11,22]

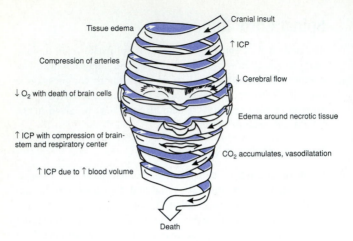

Figure 6-2. Progression of increased ICP. (From Lewis SM and Collier IC: *Medical-surgical nursing*, ed 3, St Louis, 1992, Mosby.)

Prognosis

The ultimate prognosis of CNS tumors is determined by the following factors: histologic type, tumor grade, size and extent of tumor, patient's age, performance status, and residual tumor.[16] Survival rates range from complete cure to rapid deterioration and death. Glioblastoma multiforme (grade IV) has the poorest prognosis and a life expectancy of 6 to 12 months. Younger individuals who are neurologically intact survive longer than the geriatric (elderly) patient.

Nursing Management

Nursing Diagnoses

- *Fear and anxiety related to diagnosis and postoperative outcomes*
- *Knowledge deficit related to limited experience with diagnostic pre- and postoperative routines*

Interventions

- Assessment of past coping mechanisms, and support systems within the family structure
- Education related to treatment modality

Surgery

- Explanation of surgical diagnostic procedures
- Basic review of anatomy and physiology of CNS system
- Tumor location
- Expected signs/symptoms
- Postoperative monitoring
- Equipment
- Postoperative nursing care routines
- Postoperative complications
- Body image concerns

Nursing Diagnoses

- *Self care deficit related to postoperative procedure*
- *Body image changes related to altered physical status*
- *Potential sensory/perceptual alterations related to neurologic deficits*

Interventions[10,22,24,27,28]

- Perform frequent neurologic examinations, measurement of vital signs, supportive nursing care of positioning, administration of medications including pain, steroids, and anticonvulsant therapy
- Observe for increased intracranial pressure and brain herniation
- Neurologic examinations should include measurement of the:
  — level of consciousness
  — orientation
  — emotional response to surgery
  — motor and sensory perception
- Pupils are observed for inequality.
- Vital signs should be observed for decreased respirations, and pulse and widened pulse pressure

- Place patient in a quiet, nonstimulating environment and position according to physician protocol (head of the bed at a 30 degree angle to reduce cerebral edema)
- Monitor dressings and drains for type and amount of drainage
- Coughing, deep breathing techniques, and suctioning are done in a nonaggressive manner so as to reduce increased intracranial pressure

Geriatric Considerations

- Diagnostic difficulties
- Increased assessment (preoperatively and postoperatively)
- Treatment modality complications
- Rehabilitation
- Home care referral

Bibliography

1. Abner B and Collins J: *Cancer chemotherapy and practice*, Philadelphia, 1990, JB Lippincott.
2. Amato CA: *Malignant glioma: coping with devastating illness*, J Neuroscience Nursing 23:20, 1991.
3. American Cancer Society: *Cancer facts and figures—1994*, Atlanta, 1994, American Cancer Society.
4. Association for Brain Tumor Research: *A primer of brain tumors*, The Association, ed 5, 1991.
5. Baird SB and others: *A cancer source book for nurses, Atlanta*, 1991, American Cancer Society.
6. Bernstein M and others: *Interstitial brachytherapy for malignant brain tumors: preliminary results*. Neurosurgery 26:371, 1990.
7. Blaney SM, Balis FM, and Poplack DC: *Pharmacologic approaches to the treatment of meningeal malignancy*, Oncology 5:107, 1991.
8. Boring CC, Squires TS, Tong T, and Montgomery S: *Cancer Statistics*, CA 44(1):7, 1994.

9. Boss BJ, Heath J, and Sunderland PM: Alteration of neurologic function. In McConce KL and Heuther SE, editors: *Pathophysiology the biologic basis for disease in adults and children*, St Louis, 1990, Mosby.

10. Cammermeyer M and Appledome C, editors: *Core curriculum for oncology nursing*, ed 3, Park Ridge, III, 1990, American Association of Neuroscience Nurses.

11. Dropcho EJ and Seng-jaw S: *Steroid-induced weakness in patients with primary brain tumors*, Neurology 41:1235, 1991.

12. Drummond BC: *Preventing increased intracranial pressure: nursing can make a difference.* Focus Crit Care 17:116, 1990.

13. Edwards DK, Stupperick TK, and Welsh DM: *Hyperthermia treatment for malignant tumors: nursing management during therapy.* J Neurosci Nursing 23:34, 1991.

14. Edwards MS and others: *Hyperfractioned radiation therapy for brain-stem glioma: a phase I-II trial*, J Neurosurg 70:691, 1989.

15. Hart S: Neurological care. In Shaw M and others, editors: *Illustrated manual of nursing practice*, Springhouse, PA, 1991, Springhouse Corp.

16. Levin VA, Gutin PH, and Leibel S: Neoplasms of the central nervous system. In DeVita, VT, Hellman S, and Rosenberg SP, editors: *Cancer: principles and practice of oncology*, ed 4, Philadelphia, 1993, JB Lippincott.

17. Loeffler JA and others: *Radiosurgery for brain metastases*, PPU Updates 5:1, 1991.

18. Owens B: Neurological cancer. In Clark J and McGee R, editors: *Core curriculum for oncolgy nursing*, ed 2, Philadelphia, 1992, WB Saunders.

19. Ransohoff R, Koslow M, and Cooper P: Cancer of the central nervous system and pituitary. In Holled AI, Fink DJ, and Murphy GP, editors: *American Cancer Society textbook of clinical oncology*, Atlanta, 1991, American Cancer Society.

20. Robinson C, Roy C, and Seager M: Central nervous sytem cancers. In Baird S, McCorkle R, and Grant M, editors: *Cancer nursing: a comprehensive textbook*, Philadelphia, 1991, WB Saunders .

21. Rowland LP: *Merritt's textbook of neurology*, ed 8, Philadelphia, 1989, Lea and Febiger.

22. Saba MT and Magolan JM: *Understanding cerebral edema: implications for oncology nurses*, One Nursing Forum 18:499, 1991.

23. Saleman M and Kaplan RS: *Intracranial tumors in adults*. In Haskell CM, editor: *Cancer treatment*, ed 3, Philadelphia, 1990, WB Saunders.

24. Schenk E: Management of persons with neurologic problems. In Phipps WS and others, editors: *Medical surgical nursing*, ed 4, St Louis, 1991, Mosby.

25. Shaw EG and others: *Radiation therapy in the management of low grade supratentorial astrocytomas*, J Neurosurg 70:853, 1989.

26. Sunderson N and Suite ND: *Optimal use of the Ommaya reservoir in clinical oncology*, Oncology 3:15, 1989.

27. Walleck C: Intracranial problems. In Lewis SM and Collier IC, editors: *Medical surgical nursing*, ed 3, St Louis, 1992, Mosby.

28. Wegmann JA and Hakius P: Central nervous system cancers. In Groenwald SL and others, editors: *Cancer nursing: principles and practice*, ed 2, Boston, 1990, Jones & Bartlett.

29. Zulch KJ: *Histological typing of tumors of the central nervous system*. International Histologic Classification of Tumors 21:19, 1979.

Breast Cancer

7

Epidemiology

In 1994 the American Cancer Society estimated the average American woman's risk for developing breast cancer is one in eight.[1,5] This translates into 183,000 newly diagnosed female cases in the United States during 1994. Men rarely develop breast cancer by comparison, accounting for only 1,000 new cases during the same year. It is predicted that 46,300 women and 300 men will die from the disease in 1994.[1,5] These numbers reflect cases of invasive breast cancer. Breast cancer remains the most common site of cancer in American women.

The highest rates of breast cancer in the world are in the United States (by country), and, specifically, by population group: Hawaiians in Hawaii, white women in Hawaii, and white women in Alameda County in Northern California. While black women generally have a lower incidence rate of breast cancer than white women in the United States, incidence rates have been increasing at a greater rate for black women.[1]

Risk Factors[2,14,29]

- Gender
- Age
- Personal history of cancer
- Family history of cancer
- Genetics
- Early menarche and late menopause
- Reproductive history
- Benign breast disease
- Obesity and dietary fat
- Radiation exposure
- Exogenous hormones
- Alcohol consumption

Prevention, Screening, and Detection

Early detection is the most important means of control of breast cancer. Research has shown that survival is directly related to the stage of the disease at diagnosis. The American Cancer Society (ACS) has developed *screening guidelines* for asymptomatic women that incorporate three methods of early detection.[3,7,9,10]

1. *Breast self-examination* (*BSE*) should be performed monthly by all women beginning at age 20.
2. *Clinical breast examinations* (*CBE*) by a health professional should be done every 3 years for women age 20 to 40 and annually after age 40.
3. *Mammography* should begin at age 40. Routine screening mammography should be performed every 1 to 2 years for women ages 40 to 49, and then every year beginning at age 50.

Breast Self Examination

BSE includes inspection and palpation of the breasts in both a standing and a lying position. Attention is focused on evaluating for change. A thorough BSE will usually take 20 to 30 minutes. The components of BSE for proficiency in practice include: *inspection* of the breasts in front of a mirror, *palpation* of the entire area of the breast using the flat *pads of the fingers* at different levels of *pressure*, in a specific *pattern* and *motion* within that pattern, see Figure 7-2.

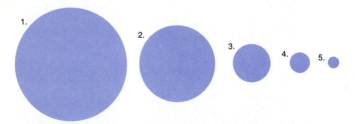

Figure 7-1. 1; Average-size lump found by women untrained in BSE. **2**; Average-size lump found by women practicing occasional BSE. **3**; Average-size lump found by women practicing regular BSE. **4**; Average-size lump found by first mammogram. **5**; Average-size lump found by regular mammograms. (From Spence W: *Breast care: the good news,* Waco, TX, 1986, Health Edco, Inc.)

Mammography

Mammography is the only proven means of detecting breast cancer before it can be detected by physical examination or BSE. Screening mammography is used to detect cancer in *asymptomatic* women, see Figure 7-1. Ultrasound is helpful in conjunction with mammography for diagnostic purposes to help differentiate a fluid-filled cyst from a solid mass.

Classification

- Carcinoma in situ
- Ductal carcinoma in situ (DCIS)
- Lobular carcinoma in situ (LCIS)
- Infiltrating ductal carcinoma
- Infiltrating lobular carcinomas
- Paget's disease
- Inflammatory carcinoma

Clinical Features

Clinical features of breast cancer are:

Most common symptoms at presentation

- Mass (particularly if hard, irregular, nontender) or thickening in the breast or axilla
- Spontaneous, persistent, unilateral nipple discharge that is serosanguineous, bloody, or watery in character
- Nipple retraction or inversion
- Change in size, shape or texture of breast (asymmetry)
- Dimpling or puckering of the skin
- Scaly skin around the nipple

Symptoms of local or regional spread

- Redness, ulceration, edema, or dilated veins
- Peau d'ange skin changes
- Enlargement of lymph nodes in the axilla

Evidence of metastatic disease

- Enlargement of lymph nodes in the supraclavicular (collar bone) cervical area
- Abnormal chest x-ray with or without pleural effusion
- Elevated alkaline phosphatase, elevated calcium, positive bone scan, and/or bone pain related to bone involvement
- Abnormal liver function tests

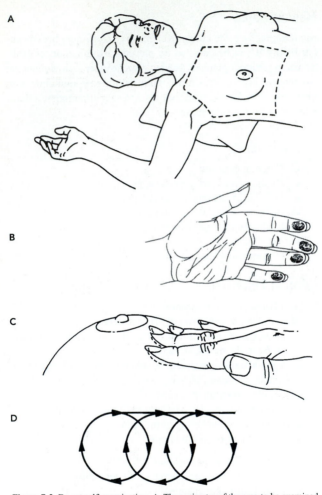

Figure 7-2. Breast self-examination. **A,** The perimeter of the area to be examined should include all breast tissue. This area is bounded by a line that extends vertically from the middle of the axilla (armpit) to the rib just beneath the breast and continues horizontally along the underside of the breast to the mid sternum (middle of the breast bone). It continues up the mid sternum to the clavicle (collarbone), and along the lower border of the clavicle to the shoulder and back to the mid-axilla. **B,** Palpation is performed with the pads of the fingers. **C** and **D,** Move your fingers (e or 4) in small circles about the size of a dime. Varying levels of pressure (light, medium, and firm) should be applied to each spot palpated. Moderate pressure is illustrated. The following patterns can be used for the examination: **E,** Vertical strip. **F,** Wedge. **G,** Circle. (Courtesy American Cancer Society.)

E

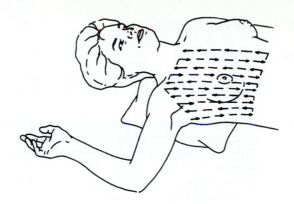

F

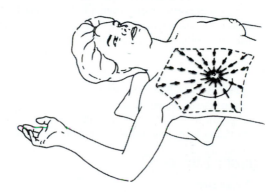

G

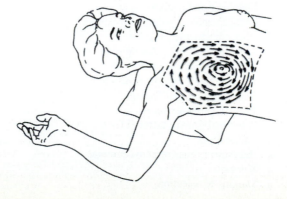

Diagnosis and Staging

Tissue Diagnosis

Breast cancer can be diagnosed following cytologic (cells) or histologic (tissue) evaluation. Examination of tissue will give a definitive diagnosis.[18,30]

- *Fine needle aspiration (FNA) biopsy* for cytology is easily performed when dominant masses are palpable.
- *Core needle biopsy* provides a core of tissue from a dominant mass.
- *Incisional biopsy* is performed when the mass is large, and involves removal of only a portion of the mass.
- *Excisional biopsy* involves removal of the entire mass and a margin of normal tissue around it. Non palpable masses detected mammographically can also be removed by excisional biopsy *(needle localization biopsy)*.

Staging

Breast cancer is most frequently staged according to the TNM classification system, which evaluates the tumor size (T); involvement of regional lymph nodes (N); and distant spread of the disease or metastases (M) (discussed in detail in Chapter 4).

Prognostic Factors[12,29,33]

- Tumor size
- Lymph node status
- Histologic and nuclear grade
- Estrogen and progesterone receptors
- DNA content analysis:
    Ploidy (normal), Aneuploidy (abnormal)
    S phase fraction (SPF)
- Vascular and lymphatic invasion
- Oncogene (e.g., HER-2/*neu*)
- Tumor suppressor genes
- Epidermal growth factor (EGF)
- Cathepsin D
- Heat shock stress response proteins
- Necrosis
- Margins of resection

- Inflammatory response
- Multicentricity
- Extensive intraductal component (EIC)
- Demographic characteristics

Tumors that are ER positive and PR positive have shown more responsiveness than ER and PR negative tumors, see Table 7-1.

Tumor type and size, lymph node status, estrogen and progesterone receptor status, histologic and nuclear grade, and DNA content (ploidy and SPF) are the most commonly considered evaluations in use today for determining prognosis and treatment plans.

Metastasis

The most frequent sites of systemic or distant spread are bone, lung, pleura, liver and adrenals. Other less common sites are the brain, thyroid, leptomeninges, eye, pericardium, and ovary.

Prognosis

The median survival from the appearance of metastasis is approximately 2 to 3.5 years, though some patients (25% to 35%) may live for 5 years, and others (10%) may live for more than 10 years. Patients who were diagnosed with metastases a longer time after their initial breast cancer diagnosis and who have metastases to the bone or soft tissue areas have a better prognosis.[8,12]

Treatment Modalities

Surgery

Primary Therapy

The type of surgery selected is based on clinical stage of the disease (tumor size, fixation, histology, nodes, metastases), mammographic findings (including evidence of cancer cells in other areas of the breast separate from the primary), the tumor location, patient history, available surgical and radiotherapeutic expertise, breast size and shape, and patient preference.[13,17,18,26]

Surgical Procedures

- *Lumpectomy (or excision; tumorectomy)*—The tumor is removed and the major portion of the breast is left.

Table 7-1 Clinical and Biologic Differences between ER Positive and Negative Tumors

Biologic Parameter	ER Positive	ER Negative
Tumor differentiation	Well-differentiated (low-grade)	Poorly differentiated (high-grade)
DNA content	Normal (diploid)	Abnormal (aneuploid)
Nuclear grade	Cell nuclei well-differentiated	Poorly differentiated cell nuclei
S phase fraction	Low percentage of cells in S phase (DNA synthesis)	High percentage of cells in S phase
Age/menopausal status	≥50, postmenopausal	<50, premenopausal
Clinical course of disease	Prolonged disease-free survival and overall survival	Shorter time to recurrence and shorter overall survival
Type of metastases	Bone and soft tissue	Visceral involvement (lung, liver, brain)
Response to endocrine therapy	Responsive	Unresponsive

Adapted from Osborne CK: *Receptors*. In Harris JR and others, editors: *Breast diseases*, ed 2 Phildelphia, 1991, JB Lippincott.

- *Wide excision (limited resection, partial mastectomy)*— Excision of the tumor with grossly clean margins of normal breast tissue.[36]
- *Quadrantectomy*—The entire quadrant of the breast containing the tumor is removed along with the overlying skin and the lining over the pectoralis major muscle.
- *Total mastectomy*—All the breast tissue, including the nipple-areolar complex and the lining over the pectoralis major muscle is removed. There is no axillary node dissection. Chest wall muscles are not removed.
- *Modified radical mastectomy*—The entire breast is removed along with axillary lymph nodes and the lining over the pectoralis major muscle. The pectoralis major muscle is not removed. The pectoralis minor muscle may or may not be removed.

Considerations in Patient Selection for Breast Conserving Treatment[26]

- *Tumor size*
- *Tumor location*
- *Breast size*
- *Patient preference and attitude*
- *Contraindications*
    stage III or IV disease
    multifocal/multicentric disease
    large pendulous breast
    prior irradiation to breast region

Metastatic Disease

Surgery also has a role in the management of metastatic disease. Examples include procedures to excise local recurrences, drain pleural effusions, debulk and decompress spinal cord metastasis, and remove ovaries to eliminate that source of endogenous estrogen.

Breast Reconstruction

The goals of reconstructive surgery are to (1) construct a breast mound, (2) achieve symmetry with the opposite side, and (3) build a nipple-areolar complex. Considerations for type of surgery include the quality and amount of skin, the size and shape of the opposite breast, the initial surgical operation for cancer, the patient's goals, and general health.[17,22,31]

Radiation Therapy

External beam radiotherapy begins 2 to 4 weeks after adequate healing following wide excision and axillary node dissection. Treatment planning is done to ensure homogeneity of dose through consistent reproducible positioning of the patient and the use of supervoltage equipment. Each field should be treated daily, Monday through Friday, to a total whole breast dose of 4,500 to 5,000 cGy at 180 to 200 cGY per fraction. This generally takes 4 to 5 weeks. A radiation boost (electron beam) and iridium-192 implant may also be used.[36]

Systemic Therapy

Systemic treatment of breast cancer involves the use of chemotherapy or endocrine manipulation to treat patients with (1) axillary node involvement, (2) poor prognosis node-negative disease, (3) advanced local-regional disease, or (4) distant metastases. The specific therapy recommended is influenced by the prognostic factors, and the patient's general medical condition. Dosages used and the duration of therapy vary. Common regimens used for breast cancer management:

CMF	Cyclosphosphamide (Cytoxan) Methotrexate 5-Fluorouracil (5-FU)
FAC/CAF	5-FU Doxorubicin (Adriamycin) Cytoxan
CMF ±VP	Cytoxan Methotrexate 5-FU Vincristine Prednisone

Adjuvant Chemotherapy

The regimens most commonly used in adjuvant therapy contain a combination of cyclophosphamide (C), methotrexate (M), and 5-flurouracil (F). Because doxorubicin is one of the most active single agents for the treatment of metastatic breast cancer, it is often used in the adjuvant setting in combination regimens.[15]

Adjuvant Endocrine Therapy

Tamoxifen delays recurrence in postmenopausal breast cancer patients. In studies of node negative patients it also reduces the incidence of cancers in the opposite breast. In premenopausal patients, however, the long-term risks of tamoxifen therapy secondary to endocrine abnormalities are not fully known. The optimal duration of therapy has yet to be established.[19]

Treatment of Advanced Disease

The goal of therapy in metastatic disease is control of the disease and palliation of symptoms. Metastatic breast cancer is incurable with either chemotherapy or hormone manipulation. These modalities are able to achieve temporary regression of the disease in a majority of patients, but these responses rarely last a long time.

Hormonal Manipulation

Receptor-positive patients respond 50% to 60% of the time while only 10% of receptor-negative patients will respond. A variety of endocrine approaches can be classified as *additive* or *ablative therapies.*

- Ablative therapy via bilateral oophorectomy, radiation therapy, or luteinizing hormone-releasing hormone (LHRH) agonists or antagonists
- Antiestrogen therapy (Tamoxifen)
- Additive therapies (estrogens, androgens, and progestins)

Nursing Management[6,7,8,20]

Nursing Diagnosis

■ *Potential for injury (infection, delayed wound healing, immobility) related to surgical wound and impaired lymph drainage secondary to breast cancer surgery, complicated by failure to view and care for wound/drains.*

Interventions

■ Inform patient and family about hospital and operative routines.

■ Describe postoperative activity before surgery so that patient will be prepared to participate appropriately.

■ Position arm on operative side slightly elevated with flat pillow or folded towel behind upper arm, until patient fully awake and ambulatory. Maintain position when reclining.

■ Reinforce importance of early ambulation, coughing and deep breathing.

■ All intravenous access or venipunctures should be managed on the nonoperative side.

■ Monitor wound for inflammation, tenderness, swelling, or purulent drainage. Change dressing when ordered using aseptic technique.

■ Monitor drains: intact, secured to the skin or clothing so as not to dangle, color and amount of fluid output.

■ Provide information on normal sensory sensations patient will experience postoperatively such as paresthesias of the inner aspect of the upper arm, and increase skin sensitivity. "Phantom breast" experiences have also been reported.

■ Assess readiness to look at incision, and offer support when patient decides to view the incision. Description of the wound appearance may be helpful to some patients prior to actual viewing. Discuss possible response of patient's spouse/significant other toward viewing the incision and patient's readiness for this.

■ Instruct patient in arm care and postsurgical arm exercises. This will usually require further follow-up instruction in the outpatient setting, because the exercises should continue for a minimum of 6 weeks after surgery but may need to be continued for up to 6 months for full recovery and flexibility.

■ Instruct patient to avoid strenuous household tasks such as vacuuming, sweeping, moving or rearranging furniture, and lifting objects more than 10 pounds until full surgical wound healing has occurred, and range of motion is improved.

■ Instruct in use of temporary prosthesis and wearing of bra, and possible options for the woman postmastectomy for sense of symmetry and balance pending fitting for a weighted prosthesis or reconstruction.

■ Educate about possible complications related to surgery, radiation therapy and/or chemotherapy.

Lymphedema

Lymphedema after breast cancer surgery is the accumulation of lymph fluid in the tissues of the upper extremity, extending from the upper arm potentially to the hand and fingers. It occurs in less than 6% to 7% of all patients undergoing modified radical mastectomy. Risk of developing lymphedema is increased by complete lymph node dissection (levels I, II, and III), radiation therapy to the axilla, obesity, poor nutritional status, increased age, and

---

Box 7-3

Arm Care Precautions after Axillary Lymph Node Dissection

Avoid sunburns or heavy sun exposure (and wear sunscreen).

Avoid burns while cooking, baking, or smoking.

Wear protective gloves when gardening.

Use the *unaffected* arm for injections, blood samples, intravenous access, or blood pressures.

Use thimble when sewing.

Watches, jewelry, and clothing should fit loosely on the arm and hand.

Use creams and lotions to keep cuticles soft; do not pull cuticles.

Treat cuts promptly and monitor for signs of infection.

No chemotherapy is to be given in the affected arm.

wound infection. It may occur at any time after surgery. Prevention of cosmetic deformity, functional impairment, and discomfort are the goals. Mechanical decompression with a pneumatic pump and arm sleeve may be indicated to reduce swelling. With new onset of lymphedema the medical assessment includes evaluation for infection and other obstructive problems (vein thrombosis or tumor recurrence). Specific arm care precautions to prevent trauma and infection in the arm on the operative side are listed in Box 7-3.[16,27]

Nursing Diagnosis

- *Anxiety related to fear of side effects of additional treatment with chemotherapy and/or radiation therapy.*

Interventions

- Explain the rational for adjuvant systemic therapy.
- Describe the specific treatment regimen schedule, route(s) of administration, anticipated side effects, and prevention or management of side effects.
- For premenopausal women, discuss effects of chemotherapy on menstrual function: irregularities, amenorrhea, and potential for pregnancy, with options for birth control while undergoing treatment.
- Postmenopausal women, or premenopausal women undergoing tamoxifen therapy, need information about potential side effects such as hot flashes and vaginal discharge and dryness. Patients should be informed to report such symptoms and subsequently be given guidance on the management of these problems.
- Encourage discussion of other psychosocial concerns such as role functions in the home, return to work, vocational retraining, and family and social relationships.

Patient Teaching Priorities

Prevention and early detection

- Risk factors
- Breast self-exam
- Clinical breast exam
- Mammography

- Signs and symptoms to report to health care professional (e.g., mass in breast or axilla; dimpling, puckering, and/or scaly skin; spontaneous, persistent nipple discharge)
- Follow ACS guidelines for health care exam

Treatment options
- Biopsy procedures
- Surgery
    Breast conserving treatment
    Breast reconstruction
- Radiation therapy
- Chemotherapy
- Hormonal therapy

Disease and treatment related complications
- Disease recurrence, infection, impaired wound healing, lymphedema, shoulder dysfunction, marrow suppression, alopecia, stomatitis, hemorrhagic cystitis, weight gain, "flare reaction," pain, anorexia
- Prosthesis options
- Support groups
- Recovery and long-term follow-up

Geriatric Considerations[9,14,20]

Prevention and detection
- Health assessments need to incorporate cognitive function, physical limitations/sensory deficits, and support network.
- Education efforts should address knowledge, skill, and confidence in BSE, mammography and CBE, and benefits of early detection.
- Continuity and participation may be enhanced when health care is coordinated by one or few providers (e.g., advocate, case manager).
- Community-based breast cancer screening is beneficial.
- The effectiveness of rescreening after age 70 is controvertial.
- Education of health care providers should emphasize continuing need for scheduled screening of elderly women in light of current data.

Diagnosis and treatment

- The importance of patient involvement in decision making needs to be considered irrespective of age.
- Age in and of itself ought not to determine type or extent of surgery or subsequent therapy.
- Care throughout the operative phase includes careful preoperative assessment and intra- and post-operative physiologic monitoring.
- Early *comprehensive discharge planning* should involve the patient and significant other.
- Side effects with radiation and chemotherapy may be enhanced or prolonged.
- Most trials of systemic therapy have excluded women over 70 years of age.

Rehabilitation

- Return to or maintenance of pre-cancer level of functioning is a reasonable goal.
- Care should be taken to incorporate psychosexual assessment and intervention as appropriate for all ages.
- Physical illness can impair developmental task completion.
- Depression in the elderly may be masked by physical symptoms.

Metastatic disease

- Differential diagnosis of symptoms must differentiate normal or pathologic changes from signs of metastatic disease.
- Chronic pain may be indirectly expressed via other physical changes (e.g., anorexia, irritability, aching, insomnia).
- Recurrent disease may exacerbate other felt losses of the elderly.

Bibliography

1.   American Cancer Society: *Cancer facts and figures 1994,* Atlanta 1994, American Cancer Society, 1994.
2.   American Cancer Society: *Cancer facts and figures for minority Americans 1994*, Atlanta, 1994, American Cancer Society.

3. *American Cancer Society: Special touch breast health trainer's guide*, ed 2, Oakland, CA 1990, American Cancer Society, California Division.

4. Bassett LW: Mammographic features of malignancy. In Mitchell GW and Bassett LW, editors: *The female breast and its disorders,* Baltimore, 1990, Williams & Wilkins.

5. Boring CC, Squires TS, Tong T, and Montgomery S: *Cancer statistics*, CA 44 (1):7, 1994.

6. Brown M, Eyles H, and Bland KI: Nursing care for the patient with breast cancer. In Bland KI and Copeland EM III, editors: *The breast: comprehensive management of benign and malignant diseases*, Philadelphia, 1991, WB Saunders.

7. Coleman CM and Crane R: Knowledge deficit related to prevention and early detection of breast cancer. In McNally JC, Somerville ET, Miaskowski C, and Rostad M, editors: *Guidelines for oncology nursing practice*, ed 2, Philadelphia, 1991, WB Saunders.

8. Cooley ME and Erikson B: Rehabilitation. In Fowble B and others, editors: *Breast cancer treatment: a comprehensive guide to management*, St Louis, 1991, Mosby.

9. Costanza ME: *Breast cancer screening in older women: synopsis of a forum,* Cancer 69:1925, 1992.

10. Dodd GD: *American Cancer Society Guidelines on screening for breast cancer*, Cancer (Supplement) 69:1885, 1992.

11. Dupont WD and Page DL: *Menopausal estrogen replacement therapy and breast cancer,* Arch Intern Med 151:67, 1991.

12. Fisher B: *A biological perspective of breast cancer: contributions of the National Surgical Adjuvant Breast and Bowel Project clinical trials*, CA 41:97, 1991.

13. Ganz PA and others: *Breast conservation versus mastectomy*, Cancer 69:1729, 1992.

14. Garber JE: Familial aspects of breast cancer. In Harris JR and others, editors: *Breast diseases,* ed 2, Phildelphia, 1991, JB Lippincott.

15. Goodman M: *Adjuvant systemic therapy of stage I and II breast cancer*, Sem Oncol Nurs 7:175, 1991.

16. Gottlieb LJ and Patel P-KK: Lymphedema following axillary surgery: elephantiasis chirurgica. In Harris JR and others, editors: *Breast diseases*, ed 2, Philadelphia 1991, JB Lippincott.

17. Handel N: *Current status of breast reconstruction after mastectomy*, Oncology 5:73, 1991.

18. Harris JR: Clinical management of ductual carcinoma in situ. In Harris JR and others, editors: *Breast diseases,* ed 2, Philadelphia 1991, JB Lippincott.

19. Henderson BE and Bernstein L: *The role of endogenous and exogenous hormones in the etiology of breast cancer.* In Harris JR and others, editors: *Breast diseases*, ed 2, Philadelphia, 1991, JB Lippincott.

20. Johnson JB and Kelly AW: *A multifaceted rehabilitation program for women with cancer,* Oncol Nurs Forum 17:691, 1990.

21. Kaplan KM and others: *Breast cancer screening among relatives of women with breast cancer*, AJPH 81:1174, 1991.

22. LaRossa D: Reconstructive surgery. In Fowble B and others, editors: *Breast cancer treatment: a comprehensive guide to management,* St Louis, 1991, Mosby.

23. Love SM: *Dr. Susan Love's breast book*. Reading, Massachusetts, 1990, Addison-Wesley.

24. Marchant D: Surgery for breast cancer. In Mitchell GW Jr and Bassett LW, editors, *The female breast and its disorders*, Baltimore, 1990, Williams & Wilkins.

25. McGuire WL and Clark GM: *Prognostic factors and treatment decisions in axillary-node-negative breast cancer*, N Engl J Med 326:1756, 1992.

26. Morrison BW: Oncogenes and breast cancer. In Harris JR and others, editors: *Breast diseases,* ed 2, Philadelphia, 1991, JB Lippincott.

27. Rosato EF and Curcillo PG II: Surgical considerations in the management of breast cancer. In Fowble B and others: editors, *Breast cancer treatment: a comprehensive guide to management,* St Louis, 1991, Mosby.

28. Schnitt SJ and Connolly JL: Benign breast disorders. In Harris JR and others, editors: *Breast diseases,* ed 2, Philadelphia, 1991, JB Lippincott.

29. Stampfer MJ, Bechtel SD, and Hunter DJ: *Fat, alcohol, selenium, and breast cancer risk,* Contemporary OB/GYN 37:42, 1992.

30. *Treatment of early-stage breast cancer.* National Institutes of Health consensus development conference statement, 1990, June 18-21:8(6).

31. Vinton AL, Traverso LW, and Zehring RD: *Immediate breast reconstruction following mastectomy is as safe as mastectomy alone,* Arch Surg 125:1303, 1990.

32. Vogel CL: *Treatment of metastatic breast cancer,* Sem Oncol Nurs 7:194, 1991.

33. Weiss MC and Kelsten ML: Biologic markers of breast cancer prognosis. In Fowble B and others, editors: *Breast cancer treatment: a comprehensive guide to management,* St Louis, 1991, Mosby.

Colorectal Cancer

8

Epidemiology

Colorectal cancer is the third most common malignant tumor in the United States, second only to lung cancer in its incidence and mortality. An estimated 14,900 new cases develop each year with an annual death rate of 56,000. Colorectal cancer affects both sexes equally, with the incidence increasing significantly in persons over the age of 50. The mean age at the time of diagnosis is 62. The disease occurs most frequently in Western industrialized countries of Northern America, Northern Europe, and New Zealand.[1,4]

Diet

Diets low in animal fats and high in fiber demonstrate a significantly lower incidence of disease. Other dietary factors that serve as promoters of the carcinogenic process include genetoxic carcinogens such as charbroiled meats, fish, and fried foods.[10]

Genetic Factors

Persons with first-degree relatives who have colorectal cancer have a threefold risk of having the disease themselves. Polyposis syndromes such as Gardner's, Turcot's, and Plutz-Jegher's are linked with increased risks for the development of colorectal cancers.[21] Other predisposing factors include ulcerative colitis, Crohn's disease, adenomas polyposis, and villainous adenomas.

Prevention, Screening, and Detection

The American Cancer Society recommends specific protocols for the screening and prevention of colorectal cancers, which include diet and diagnostic examinations, see Table 8-1. Dietary recommendations for cancer prevention are reduction in amount of saturated and unsaturated fats, increased fiber, and foods rich in Vitamins A, C and E.[1]

Classification

The site of presentation is primarily the sigmoidorectal area. The vast majority (40% to 50%) of lesions occur in the rectum, and 20% to 35% occur in the descending and sigmoid colon. Only 8% occur in the transverse colon and 16% in the cecum and ascending colon. A small percentage (4% to 8%) may occur as a second primary site. The majority of bowel cancers are adenocarcinomas and are moderately to well differentiated cancers. Other forms of colorectal cancers consist of epithelioma, squamous cell carcinomas, sarcoma, lymphoma, leiomyosarcoma, and melanomas.[5,12]

Clinical Features

- General: Change in bowel habits, blood in the stool, abdominal pain, anorexia, flatulence, and indigestion (Fig 8-1)
- Late symptoms: Weight loss, fatigue, decline in general health
- Right-sided lesions: Dull, vague abdominal pain radiating to the back, dark/mahogany red blood in stool, weakness, anemia, malaise, indigestion, weight loss, and liquid stool
- Left-sided lesions: Change in bowel habits—cramps, gas pains, decrease in the caliber of the stool, bright red bleeding, constipation, rectal pressure, and incomplete evacuation of stool[17]
- Transverse colon: Palpable masses, obstruction, changes in bowel habits, and bloody stools
- Rectal: Changes in bowel habits, bright red bleeding, tenesmus, severe pain in groin, labia, scrotum, legs, or penis

Diagnosis and Staging

Persons at high risk for disease or who have symptoms and are fecal occult blood positive require additional diagnostic testing:

- Barium enema
- Colonscopy
- Chest X-ray
- CBC, SGOT, LDH, (CEA), alkaline phosphate
- Liver scan
- Bone scan

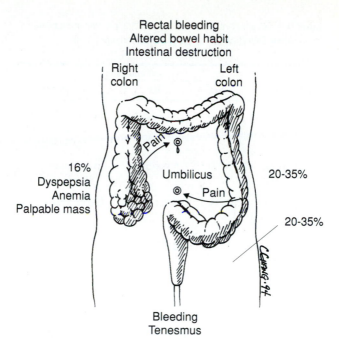

Figure 8-1. Signs and symptoms related to colon cancer. (From Beare P and Myers J: *Principles and practice of adult health nursing*, ed 1, St Louis, 1990, Mosby.)

Staging

See Chapter 4 for AJCC staging guidelines.

Metastasis

Most colorectal cancers spread by direct extension and penetration into layers of the bowel. Local invasion occurs to surrounding organs. Lymph node involvement and invasion into the vascular bed allow for disseminated disease. Lymphatic disease is present in 50% of all diagnosed cases. Nodal chains follow the pathway of the superior and mesenteric arteries. Venous invasion permits distant metastasis, with the liver and lung as the most common site. Additional sites include brain, bone, and adrenal glands.[5,12,17]

Table 8-1 Summary of American Cancer Society Recommendations for the Early Detection of Cancer in Asymptomatic People

Test or Procedure	Population		
	Sex	Age	Frequency
Sigmoidoscopy	M & F	50 and over	Every 3–5 years based on advice of physician
Fiscal occult blood test	M & F	Over 50	Every year
Digital rectal examination	M & F	Over 40	Every year
*Colonscopy or double contrast barium-enema X-ray exam	M & F	35–40	Every 5 years

*First-degree family member or parent with colorectal cancer dies at age ≤55.

Treatment Modalities

Surgery

Colon resection with disease-free margins remains the surgical goal. Tumor and associated blood vessels are resected en bloc with the vascular and lymphatic structures to prevent seeding of malignant cells. A biopsy of the liver and regional lymph nodes is taken at the time of surgery to evaluate the extent of disease.

Tumor size, location, and additional metastasis determine the type and the extent of surgery. Three major surgeries performed for colorectal cancer include resection of the tumor with reanastomosis (colectomy), a colostomy (temporary or permanent), and an abdominal perineal resection see Figure 8-2.[7,12,17,19]

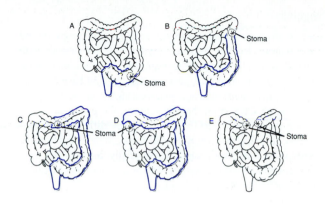

Figure 8-2. A, Sigmoid colostomy. **B**, Descending colostomy. **C**, Transverse colostomy. **D**, Ascending colostomy, **E**, Double-barrel colostomy. (From Beare P and Myers J: *Principles and practice of adult health nursing*, ed 1, St Louis, 1990, Mosby.)

Chemotherapy

Chemotherapy continues to be considered an adjunct to the initial surgical intervention. Various forms of combination drug therapy include:

- 5 Fluorouracil
- Floxuradine
- Mitomycin C
- Vincristine
- Cisplatin
- Methotrexate
- Levamisole
- Leucovorin

Radiation Therapy

Radiation therapy is often used for patients with extensive microscopic tumor penetration, lymph node involvement, and direct tumor extension into the viscera or perineum. Various combination approaches have been attempted including preoperative radiation, postoperative radiation, and a combination of both known as the "sandwich technique."[5]

Prognosis

Spread to distant organs has a direct impact on the prognosis and ultimate survival of the person. Survival time for persons with metastasis is usually less than one year. Age is an additional factor that affects the survival rate; persons under age 30 have a poorer prognosis and patients over age 70 have a higher surgical morbidity rate. High CEA titers before surgery, the presence of obstruction at the time of diagnosis, and poorly differentiated cancers also decrease the survival rate. Rectal tumors continue to be associated with poor prognosis, especially those located near the lower one third of the rectum. The overall survival rate of all stages is 40%.[6]

Nursing Management[2,4,13,14,16]

Nursing Diagnoses

- *Knowledge deficit related to lack of experience in surgical routine and procedure.*
- *Fear related to the diagnosis of cancer and operative procedure outcomes.*
- *Knowledge deficit related to ostomy.*

Interventions

- Provide support.
- Explain the rationale of the bowel-prep routine.
- Observe the patient's tolerance of laxatives and enemas.
- Report the side effects of nausea, vomiting, abdominal discomfort, excessive diarrhea, and the symptoms of electrolyte imbalance.
- Review of the preoperative routine; preoperative medications, IVs, recovery room procedures, placement of a Foley catheter, nasogastric tube, and abdominal dressings.
- Review and practice postoperative exercises such as coughing and deep breathing, wound splinting and leg exercises.
- Review anatomy, necessary for the person to understand the surgical procedure and colostomy placement.

- Review of past coping mechanisms to provide the individual with the opportunity to evaluate strengths and weaknesses.
- Refer to an enterostomal therapist or appropriate resource for colostomy care.
- Review the type of surgery, various pouching methods available, and marking of the stoma site.

Nursing Diagnoses

- *Alteration in bowel elimination related to loss of normal bowel function.*
- *Alteration in skin integrity related to abdominal incision and stoma drainage.*

Interventions

- Observe the patient for initial complications including the assessment of vital signs and lung and bowel sounds.
- Monitor the incision, the nasogastric tube, and Foley catheter for the amount of drainage, color, and patency.
- Record intake and output.
- Observe stoma site each shift for color and size.

Geriatric Considerations

Education needs:
- Awareness of screening recommendations
- Knowledge of signs and symptoms
- Understanding of risk factors

Treatment complications:
- *Surgery*
   Pulmonary
   Circulatory
   Bowel

- *Chemotherapy and radiation*
   Fluid and electrolyte imbalance
   Infection
   Skin impairment

- ■ *Teaching concerns*
  Vision/hearing impairment
  Dexterity for pouch applications

- ■ *Community resources*
  Financial/home care referral

Bibliography

1. American Cancer Society: *Cancer facts and figures—1994,* Atlanta, 1994, American Cancer Society.

2. Boarini J: Gastrointestinal cancer: colon, rectum, and anus. In Groenwald SL, Frogge MH, Goodman M, and Yanbro HC, editors: *Cancer nursing principles and practice,* Boston, 1990, Jones and Bartlett Publishers.

3. Boring CC, Squires TS, Tong T and Montgomery S: *Cancer statistics,* CA 44(1)7, 1994.

4. Clark JC and Gwin RR: *An overview of cancers in bowel and bladder diversions,* Progressions 4:15, 1992.

5. Cohen AM, Minsky BD and Schilsky RL: Colorectal cancer. In DeVita VT, Hellman S, and Rosenburg SA, editors, ed 4, *Cancer: principles and practice of oncology,* Philadelphia 1993, JB Lippincott.

6. Douglass HO: Adjuvant therapy of colorectal cancer. In Moossa AR, Schimpff SC, and Robson MC, editors, ed 2, *Comprehensive textbook of oncology,* Baltimore, 1991, Williams & Wilkins.

7. Fazio VW: *Surgery of colonic carcinoma: techniques and tactics,* Sem in Colon Rectal Surg 2:36, 1991.

8. Haskell CM, Selch MT, and Ramming KP: Colon and rectum. In Haskell CM, editor, ed 3, *Cancer treatment,* Phildelphia, 1990, WB Saunders.

9. Heuther SE, McCance KL, and Tarmina MS: The digestive system. In McCance KL and Heuther SE, editors: *Pathophysiology: the biologic basis for disease in adults and children,* ed 2, St Louis, 1994, Mosby.

10. Kritechvsky D: *Diet and Nutrition,* CA 41:328, 1991.

11. Long BC and Roberts RA: Management of persons with problems of intestinal nature. In Phipps WS and others, editors, ed 4, *Medical surgical nursing,* St Louis, 1991, Mosby.

12. Luk GD: *Colorectal cancer*, Gastroenterol Clin North Am 17:654, 1988.

13. Masson M: Gastrointestinal care. In Shaw M and others, editors, *Illustrated manual of nursing practice*, Springhouse, PA, 1991, Springhouse.

14. Rhedume A and Gooding BA: *Social Support, coping strategies, and long-term adaption to ostomy among self-help members*, J Enterstom Ther 18:11, 1991.

15. Shank B, Cohen AM, and Kelsen D: Cancer of the anal region: In DeVita VT, Hellman S and Rosenberg SA, editors, ed 4, *Cancer: principles and practice of oncology,* Philadelphia, 1993, JB Lippincott.

16. Shell JA: *The psychosexual impact of ostomy surgery*, Progressions 4:3, 1992.

17. Sleisenger MH and Fortran JS: *Gastronintestinal disease, pathology, diagnosis and management*, ed 4, Philadelphia, 1989, WB Saunders.

18. Strohl RA: Colorectal cancers: In Clark JC and McGee RF, editors, *Core curriculum for oncology nursing,* ed 2, Philadelphia, 1992, WB Saunders.

19. Swatske ME, Whittaker K, and Young M: *Care of the intestinal stoma: preoperative, postoperative, long-term*, Semin Colon Rectal Surg 2:148, 1991.

20. Weinhouse S and others: *American Cancer Society guidelines on diet, nutrition, and cancer*, CA 41:324, 1991.

21. Winawer SJ, Schottfeld D, and Flehinger BH: *Colorectal cancer screening*, J Natl Cancer Inst 83:1, 1991.

Gastrointestinal Cancers

9

Cancer of the Esophagus

Epidemiology

In the United States the estimated number of new cases of cancer of the esopahagus in 1994 is 11,000, and 10,400 of these patients will die of their disease. Esophageal cancer is most common in elderly males, and the male-to-female ratio is approximately 3:1. The incidence and mortality rates are over three times higher among blacks than whites.[5,9]

Etiology and Risk Factors

- Smoking
- Alcohol ingestion
- Previous history of squamous cell carcinoma of the head and neck
- History of lye ingestion
- Esophageal achalasia
- Plummer-Vinson syndrome
- Tylosis

Prevention, Screening, and Detection

Prevention of the disease focuses on counseling regarding alcohol and tobacco usage and instructing patients with risk factors to report any problems with dysphagia (difficulty in swallowing) or odynophagia (pain on swallowing).

Classification

The most common types of esophageal carcinomas are squamous cell carcinoma (60%) and adenocarcinoma (35%). Squamous cell carcinomas arise from the surface epithelium and are found most often in the middle and lower esophagus. Adenocarcinoma most often occurs in the lower third of the esophagus and probably arises from the gastric fundus.[1,14,20]

Clinical Features

The most common clinical features are:

- Dysphagia
- Weight loss
- Pain on swallowing

The symptoms of advanced disease are usually due to the invasion or involvement of surrounding organs and structures:

- Dysphonia
- Diaphragmatic paralysis
- Coughing when swallowing
- Superior vena cava syndrome
- Palpable supraclavicular or cervical nodes
- Malignant pleural effusion
- Malignant ascites
- Bone pain

Diagnosis and Staging

- Barium swallow and an upper GI endoscopy
- Biopsies and brushings can be obtained through the endoscope to confirm the diagnosis
- Endoscopic ultrasonography
- Computed tomography

The American Joint Committee on Cancer's Tumor, Node, Metastasis (TNM) staging system is used for staging both cervical and thoracic esophageal carcinomas. See Chapter 4.

Metastasis

Esophageal cancer can spread to almost any part of the body. Primary sites of metastasis include the lung, stomach, peritoneum, kidney, adrenal gland, brain, and bone.[1,14,20]

Treatment Modalities

Surgery

The choice of surgical approach to an esophagectomy and esopagogastrostomy depends on the extent and location of the tumor. Lesions involving the esophagogastric junction or lower thoracic esophagus are approached by a left thoracotomy. For lesions of the upper esophagus, a total esophagectomy using an upper midline incision and right thoracotomy (Ivor Lewis) or a transhiatal approach may be used.[1,14,20]

Radiation Therapy

Both squamous cell carcinoma and adenocarcinoma of the esophagus are sensitive to radiation therapy, which is used most often as palliation for obstruction and for pain control for patients who are not candidates for surgical procedures. Radiation therapy is seldom used as a primary therapy, because a course of treatment usually lasts 6 to 8 weeks and median survival for these patients is only a few months.

Chemotherapy

Single agent and combination chemotherapy have shown some effectiveness in treating squamous cell carcinoma but not in adenocarcinoma of the esophagus and cardia.
Agents commonly used are:

- Cisplatin
- Bleomycin
- Mitomycin
- Doxorubin
- Methotrexate
- 5-fluororouacil

Prognosis

The prognosis for persons with esophageal cancer is very poor. For the period from 1981 to 1987 the 5-year survival rate reported was 9% for whites and 6% for blacks. Therefore, 90% to 95% of patients are in need of palliative care at diagnosis or shortly thereafter.

Cancer of the Stomach

Although cancer of the stomach has shown a significant decline in incidence, about 60% from the 1930s to the 1970s, it remains the eighth most common cause of cancer deaths in the United States. The United States reports an incidence of 10 per 100,000 population, Japan's incidence is 90 per 100,000.[5,9]

Epidemiology

Projections for 1994 are 24,000 new cases and 14,000 deaths will be attributed to this disease. Gastric cancer is more common in men than women; the ratios range from 3:2 to 2:1. It is found more commonly in people between 50 and 70 years of age, and is three times more common in semiskilled and unskilled labor groups than in executive and professional groups.[5,9,17]

Etiology and Risk Factors

High consumption of smoked or salted foods or foods contaminated with aflatoxin has been associated with increased incidence of stomach cancer. Occupational risk factors have also been associated with higher incidence of stomach cancer. Workers in coal mining, farming, nickel refining, rubber processing, timber processing, and asbestos processing have all been shown to have higher than normal incidence.

Prevention, Screening, and Detection

Nutrition counselling to prevent gastric cancer should stress the importance of consuming a balanced diet high in fresh fruits and vegetables and moderate in amount of animal protein and fats. Salted, smoked, and pickled foods should be consumed in low quantities.

Classification

Adenocarcinomas represent almost 90% of the malignant tumors of the stomach. Lymphoma accounts for up to 8%, leiomyosarcoma makes up from 1% to 3%. Other, rarer types of malignant gastric tumors include carcinoids, plasmacytomas, and metastatic cancers.[12,18]

Clinical Features

Symptoms are vague and may have been present for several months.

They include:

- Indigestion
- Epigastric discomfort
- Postprandial fullness
- Back pain
- Vomiting after meals

- Early satiety
- Malaise
- Loss of appetite
- Dysphagia
- Hematemesis

Diagnosis and Staging

Physical examination of the patient suspected of having gastric cancer should include palpation of the abdomen for masses and nodules around the umbilicus. A digital rectal examination should be performed to assess for the presence of a shelf of metastatic deposits and diagnostic tests.

- Upper GI endoscopy
- Double-contrast upper GI series

- CT scans
- Ultrasonography

The American Joint Commission on Cancer's Staging TNM criteria for classification and staging of cancer of the stomach are discussed in Chapter 4.

Metastasis

Cancer of the stomach metastasizes most frequently to the liver, lungs, bone, and brain. Stomach cancer also spreads to local lymph nodes.

Treatment Modalities

Surgery

Surgery is the major treatment modality, usually a subtotal or toal gastrectomy, and is used for both cure and palliation. See Figure 9-1. It is recommended that any patient with biopsy-proven gastric cancer and no evidence of distant metastasis should undergo an exploratory laparotomy or celiotomy to determine whether the patient should undergo a curative procedure or a palliative one. Treatment related complications are infection, hemorrhage, ileus, and anastomotic leak.[25]

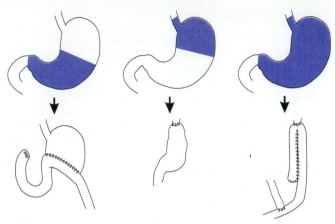

Figure 9-1. Surgical resections and reconstruction for the three locations of gastric cancer. (From Lawrence W Jr: Gastric neoplasms. In Holleb AI, Fink DJ, and Murphy GP, editors: *Textbook of clinical oncology,* Atlanta, 1991, American Cancer Society.)

Chemotherapy

Chemotherapy is now being used as adjunct therapy for fully-resected tumors, for advanced gastric cancer, and in combination with radiation therapy. Examples:

- 5-Fluororouacil
- Doxorubicin
- Mitomycin-C
- Etoposide
- Cisplatin
- Leucovorin

Radiation Therapy

Although radiation therapy has been used alone with some response, it has greatest benefit when combined with chemotherapy. A tolerable dose is 45 to 50 Gy delivered in 1.8 Gy fractions per day. Intraoperative radiation therapy (IORT) has been useful in the control of microscopic disease with a maximum tolerated dose of 15 to 20 Gy.[18,20]

Prognosis

The prognosis for patients with gastric cancer depends on the extent of the disease and on the treatment. The 5-year survival rate reported for the period of 1981 to 1987 is 16%.

Cancer of the Liver

Epidemiology

Hepatocellular carcinoma (HCC) is relatively uncommon in the United States but is one of the most common malignancies in some parts of the world, especially parts of Africa and Asia. The estimated number of new cases in the United States, of liver and biliary tract cancers in 1994 is 16,100, which will result in 13,200 deaths.[3,5,9]

Etiology and Risk Factors

- Hepatitis B and C virus
- Hemochromatosis
- Cirrhosis
- Aflatoxins, alcoholism
- Occupational exposure to pesticides and herbicides

Prevention, Screening, and Detection

High-risk patients with chronic hepatitis B or cirrhosis may be screened for the tumor marker alpha-fetoprotein (AFP) and by abdominal ultrasonography.

Classification

The histopathologic types of primary cancers of the liver include hepatomas or hepatocellular carcinomas, intrahepatic bile duct carcinomas or cholangiocarcinomas, and mixed types. Almost 95% of all primary liver tumors are malignant. The benign liver tumors include adenomas, focal nodular hyperplasia, hamartomas, and hemangiomas.[2,7,8]

Clinical Features

- Abdominal pain
- Weight loss
- Anorexia
- Nausea/vomiting
- Abdominal mass
- Gastrointensstinal bleeding
- Abdominal mass/hepatomegaly
- Diarrhea
- Jaundice
- Ascites
- Fever
- Weakness, fatigue, malaise

Diagnosis and Staging

- Ultrasound
- CT scan
- Laboratory tests AFP and hepatitis surface antigens

- Anteriogram
- Biopsy

See Chapter 4 for staging information.

Metastasis

The usual sites for HCC metastasis are the regional nodes, lung, bone, adrenal gland, and brain. Approximately 40% of the HCC patients have tumor cells in the regional nodes, but other meta-static sites are rare.

Treatment Modalities

Surgery

Surgery is the only potentially curative treatment modality for patients with HCC. Unfortunately, only 25% of the patients meet the criteria for liver resection. Hepatic resection involves either a bilateral subcostal or a thoracoabdominal incision. Following the incision, there are four recognized resection techniques: the right and left lobectomy, the trisegmentectomy, and the lateral segmentectomy. The lateral segmentectomy involves the removal of the outer portion of the left lobe. The trisegmentectomy is the removal of the right lobe and the inner portion of the left lobe.[13,16,19,26]

Chemotherapy

Regional chemotherapy involves infusion of agents that are highly metabolized by the liver via the hepatic artery. This greatly in-creases the dose of drug delivered to the tumor but minimizes the systemic side effects. Intraarterial chemotherapy can be ad-ministered through temporary catheters placed into the axillary or femoral arteries. Complications of this method include thrombosis of the hepatic and other intraabdominal arteries, cath-eter displacement, sepsis, and hemorrhage. Drugs may also be administered via an implantable pump, which offers the advan-tages of allowing the patient to remain ambulatory and reducing catheter-related complications. The agents used most commonly for intraarterial chemotherapy are floxuridine (FUdR) and 5-FU. Other drugs used include cisplatin, doxorubicin, mitomycin-C, and dichloromethotrextate.[2,4]

Embolization and Chemoembolization

Embolization is the selective occlusion of hepatic vessels by injecting nondegradable particles, typically Gelfoam and Ivalon. Embolizations usually need to be repeated because of the formation of collateral circulation. Chemoembolization involve occlusion by particles into which chemotherapeutic agents have been absorbed. Drugs used in this application include doxorubicin, cisplatin, mitomycin-C, aclarubicin, and carmustine (BCNU).[2,4,13]

Radiation Therapy

Even though HCC is considered a radiosensitive tumor, the use of radiation therapy is restricted by the relative intolerance of the normal liver parechyma. The whole liver will tolerate 3000 cGy. At this dose the incidence of radiation hepatitis is 5% to 10%. A cure or long-term remission of HCC requires significantly higher doses.[2,6,7]

Prognosis

Overall prognosis for the patient with primary liver cancer is poor. The relative 5-year survival rate for cancer of the liver is 5%.[9] For those with resectable disease this rate increases to 10%.

Cancer of the Pancreas

Epidemiology

The estimated number of new cases of cancer of the pancreas reported in 1993 is 27,000, which will result in 25,900 deaths. This represents 3% of the cancers diagnosed and 5% of the cancer deaths in women, and 2% of the cancers diagnosed and 4% of deaths in men. Pancreatic cancer is the second most common GI cancer and the fourth leading cause of cancer death in the United States. The incidence is about 35% higher in the black population than in the white population; the American black male is the person at highest risk worldwide.[2]

Etiology and Risk Factors

Cigarette smoke is the most clearly identified carcinogen in pancreatic cancer. High-risk dietary components include excessive consumption of meat, coffee, and alcohol. Occupational exposure to solvents and petroleum compounds is associated with increased risk of pancreatitis and diabetes mellitus.

Prevention, Screening, and Detection

No specific risk factors have been conclusively identified for pancreatic cancer. Avoiding cigarette smoke and eating a healthy balanced diet will reduce potential risk. The occupational exposure is decreased if safety precautions are employed when working with known carcinogens.

Classification

Ninety-five percent of cancers involving the pancreas arise from the exocrine gland. Ductal adenocarcinoma accounts for 80% of all pancreatic cancers. Other less common types include squamous cell carcinomas, giant cell carcinomas, and carcinosarcomas. The majority of the carcinomas occur in the proximal gland, which includes the head, neck, and uncinate process of the pancreas. Twenty percent occur in the body of the pancreas, and 5% to 10% occur in the tail.[8,10]

Clinical Features

The following are clinical features of pancreatic cancer:

- Weight loss
- Pain
- Anorexia
- Nausea
- Vomiting
- Diarrhea
- Jaundice
- Jaundice
- Palpable liver
- Palpable gall bladder
- Abdominal tenderness
- Abdominal mass
- Ascites

Diagnosis and Staging

Ultrasonography is an effective means of demonstrating a mass in the pancreas, but CT may be necessary for the diagnosis of pancreatic cancer. The CT can show a mass in the pancreas, involvement of the liver or bile ducts, ascites, and the presence of metastases. Endoscopic retrograde cholangiopancreatography (ERCP) is used to identify tumors of the ampulla or obstructed stenotic or sclerosed ducts. Angiography is helpful in determining any abnormal vasculature and whether the tumor is resectable. To confirm the diagnosis of pancreatic cancer, a biopsy is needed. See Chapter 4 for staging information.[13,19]

Metastasis

Early invasion of adjacent organs by pancreatic tumors is common. These adjacent organs include the major vessels, duodenum, stomach, bile duct, retroperitoneum, spleen, kidney, and colon. Widespread carcinomatosis and ascites are common because of intraperitoneal seeding.[2] Distant metastasis occurs most commonly to the liver. Other sites are the lung, bone, and brain.

Treatment Modalities

Surgery

The majority of pancreatic cancers occur in the head of the pancreas. Patients who are amenable to curative resection will undergo either a pancreatoduodenectomy (or Whipple operation) or a total pancreatectomy. The pancreatoduodenectomy involves the removal of the distal stomach, the gallbladder, the common bile duct, the head of the pancreas, the duodenum, and the upper jejunum. A total pancreatectomy is an extension of the pancreatoduodenectomy and involves, in addition, removal of the body and tail of the pancreas and the spleen and a more extensive regional lymphadenectomy. Complications include hemorrhage, thrombosis, infection, and gastric retention.

Chemotherapy

Pancreatic cancer cells are relatively chemoresistant. 5-FU and mitomycin-C are the most responsive single agents, but combinations now in use show improved responses. These include streptozotocin (Adriamycin), mitomycin-C, and 5-FU; 5-FU, doxorubicin (Adriamycin), and mitomycin-C; and/or with the addition of streptozotocin.

Radiation Therapy

The use of radiation therapy in treating cancer of the pancreas is limited by the close proximity of the pancreas to dose-limiting structures such as the kidneys, bowel, liver, and spinal cord. It is the primary treatment for patients with unresectable disease. Adjuvent radiation therapy is being studied for resectable tumors. Researchers are using postoperative external beam radiation with or without 5-FU as a radiosensitizer. Intraoperative radiation therapy has the advantage of being able to deliver tumor-specific high-dose radiation therapy while avoiding adjacent normal tissue.

Prognosis

The prognosis for persons with cancer of the pancreas is relatively poor. The reported 5-year survival rate for pancreatic cancer is 3%. Median survivals in patients who have had a pancreatoduodenectomy range from 16 to 30 months.

Cancer of the Small Intestines

Neoplasms of the small intestines are rare. They comprise only 1% of GI malignancies. The estimated number of new cases for 1994 is 3,600, which will result in 950 deaths. Small bowel cancers have been reported in patients from 1 year to 84 years of age, but the average age is 57 years. The types of neoplasms found in the small intestines include adenocarcinoma, lymphoma, leiomyosarcoma, liposarcoma, neurofibrosarcoma, malignant schwannoma, carcinoid, fibrosarcoma, hemangiosarcoma, and lymphangiosarcoma. Risk factors that have been associated with small bowel cancers include inflammatory bowel disease, Crohn's disease, Peutz-Jeghers syndrome, familial polyposis, Gardner's syndrome, celiac disease, and neurofibromatosis.[5,9]

Symptoms may include pain, small bowel obstruction, bleeding, and weight loss. Because the signs and symptoms are not

specific, diagnosis may not be confirmed until surgery is performed. Treatment depends on the histologic type of tumor, but
surgery is indicated in all symptomatic tumors. Radiation therapy
and chemotherapy have little impact on primary small intestinal
cancer, although adjuvent therapy is currently being investi-
gated.[22,24]

Nursing Management

Nursing Diagnosis

- *Altered nutrition (less than body requirements) related to
  gastrectomy*

Interventions

- Weigh daily
- Accurate intake and output every 24 hours
- Monitor laboratory values including electrolytes and leu-
  kocyte count
- Provide patient/caregiver dietary instructions:
    Six small feedings per day
    Limit fluids at meal time, drink fluids between meals
    Progress slowly from liquid to soft diet
    Choose high protein and moderate carbohydrate foods
    Avoid greasy foods
    Eat slowly
- Provide instructions on signs and symptoms to report to
  health care team:
    Diarrhea
    Clay colored stools
    Fatty stools
    Abdominal cramps
    Weakness
    Faintness
    Rapid heartbeat
- Provide instructions for diet if diarrhea occurs:
    Choose low-residue, bulk-forming foods
    Avoid foods such as whole-grain breads or cereals,
    fresh fruits and vegetables, gas-forming foods, citrus
    fruits, and juices

> Eat slowly
> Notify health care team of need for antidiarrheal and/ or antispasmodic agents

- Provide instructions for diet if dumping syndrome occurs:
  > Choose foods high in protein and fat, low in carbohydrates
  > Avoid concentrated sweets
  > Drink liquids between meals
  > Rest after meals for at least 30 minutes
  > Notify health care team if symptoms continue

Nursing Diagnosis

- *Knowledge deficit: management of hepatic artery infusion therapy related to lack of exposure*

Interventions

- Assess the patient's understanding of treatment goals, and the patient's ability to manage care post-operatively, the availability of support from family and friends
- Provide both verbal and written instructions regarding the implanted pump and chemotherapy:
  > Purpose of the pump and where the catheter is placed anatomically in the liver
  > Management of the pocket site: keep incision clean and dry until healed; resume usual activities when healed; avoid activities that may lead to blunt trauma to the pump pocket or those which may cause increased temperature, pressure, or altitude
  > What to report to health care team: temperature greater than 101 degrees fahrenheit for more than 24 hours; air travel; or change in residence requiring a change in altitude
  > Side effects of the chemotherapy drug(s) being infused and other medications
- Provide written list of phone numbers of health care team members and schedule of treatment cycles

Patient Teaching Priorities

Prevention and early detection:
- Risk factors
- Dietary habits
- Avoidance of cigarette smoking
- Moderate or no alcohol consumption
- Signs and symptoms to report to health care professional (e.g., dysphagia, odynophagia, chronic indigestion, jaundice, weight loss not associated with dieting, and change in bowel habits)
- Annual physical examination, and cancer checkup

Diagnostic procedures:
- Purpose of procedure
- Preparation needed by patient
- Procedure description
- Post procedure care by patient

Treatment modalities:
- Surgery—preoperative instructions include operative experience and immediate postoperative period; discharge instructions include self care needs and any further treatment plans
- Chemotherapy—name of agent, possible side effects and measures to control, route of administration, dose, schedule, and any directions needed for self administration
- Radiation therapy—description of the procedure and schedule and duration of treatment, skin care measures, and management of any side effects

Supportive care:
- Community resources (e.g., home health care agencies, inpatient and outpatient hospice care)
- Use of any medical equipment in the home
- Referrals necessary for psychosocial support for patient and caregiver
- Referrals for financial assistance if needed

Geriatric Considerations

Factors related to cancer prevention and early detection:

- Encourage low fat high fiber diet within ethnic, social, and economic limitations
- Encourage smoking cessation and avoidance of exposure to other health hazards (e.g., sun, chemicals, petroleum products)
- Be suspicious of symptoms such as malaise, fatigue, anorexia, weight loss, and altered bowel habits as possible indicators of cancer and not automatically attributed to nonmalignant illnesses associated with aging

Factors related to modalities of therapy:

- Alterations in hepatic and renal function may necessitate adjustment of dosage and schedule of chemotherapy protocols
- Decreased bone marrow cellularity may place the patient at risk of prolonged myelosuppression following chemotherapy with toxic effects on the bone marrow
- Decreased nurtitional intake may be exacerbated due to the nausea and taste changes associated with many of the chemotherapeutic agents commonly used for GI malignancies
- Fatigue may be increasing problem following courses of therapy requiring additional assistance with ADLs
- Co-morbid disease (e.g., obesity, poor nutritional status, lung and cardiovascular disease, altered immune function) places the older adult at greater risk regarding surgical morbidity and mortality
- Teaching should be tailored to take into account the older adult's life experiences and cognitive and physical impairments (e.g., reading comprehension, decreased vision and hearing, altered tactile sense, misconceptions regarding cancer and cancer treatment, past experience with cancer and family members)

From Boyle DM and others: *Oncology nursing society position paper on cancer and aging: the mandate for oncology nursing*, Oncol Nurs Forum 19:913, 1992.

Bibliography

1. Ahlgren JD: Esophageal cancer: chemotherapy and combined modalities. In Ahlgren JD and McDonald JS, editors: *Gastrointestinal oncology,* Philadelphia, 1992, JB Lippincott.

2. Ahlgren JD, Hill MD, and Roberts IM: Pancreatic cancer: patterns, diagnosis, and approaches to treatment. In Ahlgren JD and McDonald JS, editors: *Gastrointestinal oncology,* Philadelphia, 1992, JB Lippincott.

3. Ahlgren JD, Wanebo HF, and Hill MC: Hepatocellular carcinoma. In Ahlgren JD and McDonald JS, editors: *Gastrointestinal oncology,* Philadelphia, 1992, JB Lippincott.

4. Ahmed T and Friedland ML: Chemotherapy of primary and metastatic hepatic neoplasms. In Hodgson WJB, editor: *Liver tumors: multidisciplinary management,* St. Louis, 1988, Warren H. Green.

5. American Cancer Society: *Cancer facts and figures,* Atlanta, 1994, The American Cancer Society.

6. Anderson BB and others: *Primary tumors of the liver,* J Natl Med Assoc 84:129, 1992

7. Beazley RM and Cohn I Jr: Tumors of the liver. In Holleb AI, Fink DJ, and Murphy DP, editors: *Textbook of clinical oncology,* Atlanta, 1992, American Cancer Society.

8. Beazley RM and Cohn I Jr: Tumors of the pancreas, gallbladder, and extrahepatic ducts. In Holleb AI, Fink DJ, and Murphy DP, editors: *Textbook of clinical oncology,* Atlanta, 1991, American Cancer Society.

9. Boring CC, Squires TS, and Tong T: *Montgomery's cancer statistics,* CA Cancer J Clin 44(1):7, 1994

10. Brennan MF, Kinsella T, and Friedman M: Cancer of the pancreas. In DeVita VT Jr, Hellman S, and Rosenberg SA, editors: *Cancer: principles and practice of oncology,* ed 4, Philadelphia, 1993, JB Lippincott.

11. Caudry M: Gastric cancer: radiotherapy and approaches to locally unresectable or recurrent disease. In Ahlgren JD and McDonald JS, editors: *Gastrointestinal oncology,* Philadelphia, 1992, JB Lippincott.

12. Cuschieri A: Tumors of the stomach. In Moossa AR, Schimpff SC, and Robson MC, editors: *Comprehensive textbook of oncology,* ed 2, Baltimore, 1991, Williams & Wilkins.

13. Edmondson HA and Craig JR: Neoplasms of the liver. In Schiff L and Schiff ER, editors: *Diseases of the liver,* ed 6, Philadelphia, 1987, JB Lippincott.

14. Ellis FH, Levitan N, and Lo TCM: Cancer of the esophagus. In Holleb AI, Fink DJ, and Murphy GP, editors: *Textbook of clinical oncology,* Atlanta, 1991, American Cancer Society.

15. Grady R, Farnen J, and Ascheman P: Nutrition, alteration in: less than body requirements related to dysphagia. In McNally JC, Somerville ET, Miaskowski C, and Rostad M, editors: *Guidelines for oncology nursing practice,* ed 2, Philadelphia, 1991, WB Saunders.

16. Jordan GL Jr: *Pancreatic resection for pancreatic cancer,* Surg Clin North Am 69:569, 1989.

17. McDonald JS, Hill MC, and Roberts JM: Gastric cancer: epidemiology, pathology, detection, and staging. In Ahlgren JD and McDonald JS, editors: *Gastrointestinal oncology,* Philadelphia, 1992, JB Lippincott.

18. Alexander HR, Kelsen DP, and Tepper JE: Cancer of the stomach. In DeVita VT Jr, Hellman S, and Rosenberg SA, editors: *Cancer: principles and practice of oncology,* ed 4, Philadelphia, 1993, JB Lippincott.

19. Moossa AR: Tumors of the pancreas. In Moossa AR, Schimpff SC, and Robson MC, editors: *Comprehensive textbook of oncology,* ed 2, Baltimore, 1991, Williams & Wilkins.

20. Roth JA and others: Cancer of the esophagus. In DeVita VT Jr, Hellman S, and Rosenberg SA, editors: *Cancer: principles and practice of oncology,* ed 4, Philadelphia, 1993, JB Lippincott.

21. Sandor C: Nutrition, alteration in: less than body requirements related to disease process and treatment. In McNally JC, Somerville ET, Miaskowski C, and Rostad M, editors: *Guidelines for oncology nursing practice,* ed 2, Philadelphia, 1991, WB Saunders.

22. Coit DG: Cancer of the small intestines. In DeVita VT Jr, Hellman S, and Rosenberg SA, editors: *Cancer: principles and practice of oncology,* ed 4, Philadelphia, 1993, JB Lippincott.

23. Smith JW and Brennan MF: *Surgical treatment of gastric cancer,* Surg Clin North Am 72:381, 1992.

24. Smith LE and Hill MC: Cancer and other tumors of the small bowel. In Ahlgren JD and McDonald JS, editors: *Gastrointestinal oncology,* Philadelphia, 1992, JB Lippincott.

25. Vezeridis MP and Wanebo HJ: Gastric cancer: surgical approach. In Ahlgren JD and McDonald JS, editors: *Gastrointestinal oncology,* Philadelphia, 1992, JB Lippincott.

26. Lotze MT, Flickinger JC, and Carr BI: Cancer of the hepatobiliary system. In DeVita VT Jr, Hellman S, and Rosenberg SA, editors: *Cancer: principles and practice of oncology,* ed 4, Philadelphia, 1993, JB Lippincott.

Genitourinary Cancers

10

Prostate Cancer

Epidemiology

Prostate cancer is the most common tumor among men in the United States. Approximately 200,000 new cases are diagnosed each year.[3] The second leading cause of cancer deaths in men, with an estimated annual mortality of 38,000, it has a devastatingly morbid, as well as mortal impact, on the aging American male population. Of particular concern is the higher rate of prostate cancer in black males, with a correspondingly higher mortality also documented. It is projected that one in nine black North American males will develop prostate cancer, while one in 11 white North American males will develop the disease.[3,4,16]

Etiology and Risk Factors

The influence of endogenous hormones is the only clear factor implicated in the promotion and subsequent development of prostate cancer. Various promoting and initiating factors, including genetic influences, sexual history, exposure to viruses, pathogens, cadmium, industrial chemicals, and urbanization, have been postulated. Dietary habits, specifically the high-fat Western diet, which alters hormone metabolism, are suggested as associative factors. Documented familial patterns may reflect genetic or lifestyle influences. Prostate cancer is associated with the aging process because fewer than 1% of the cases occur under age 50.[16]

Prevention, Screening, and Detection

The major challenge in prostate cancer is the promotion of early detection when the cancer is confined to the prostate gland and is curable. This can be accomplished most easily by a simple, cost-effective, and high-yield examination, the digital rectal exam (DRE). The American Cancer Society (ACS) suggests annual DRE of the prostate gland for men beginning at age 40. Recent guidelines issued by ACS recommend prostate specific antigen (PSA) level quantification annually for men 50 years of age and older.[5]

Classification

Ninety-five percent of prostate cancers are adenocarcinomas. Ductal carcinomas, including transitional and squamous cell carcinomas, endometrioid carcinomas, and sarcomas, account for the remainder. The classically employed Gleason system ascertains a degree of glandular differentiation and tumor growth pattern in relation to prostate stroma. A score is assigned both to the predominant pattern of differentiation, ranging from well-formed to undifferentiated tumor, and to any secondary pattern of differentiation observed microscopically.[5]

Diagnosis and Staging

Clinically, prostate cancer is staged A through D by the Whitmore-Jewett System. The Tumor, Node, Metastasis (TNM) System was adopted by the American Joint Committee for Cancer Staging (AJCC), and End Results Reporting in 1975. Both systems are described in Chapter 4.

Diagnostic evaluation includes:
- Digital rectal exam (DRE)
- Laboratory tests (PSA, acid phosphatase)
- Transrectal ultrasonography
- MRI
- CT Scan
- Prostatic needle biopsy

Clinical Features

Early Symptoms: Painful and frequent urination, hematuria
Late Symptoms: Bone, back, and joint pain; fatigue, weight loss

Biological Markers

Laboratory quantification of acid phosphatase levels provides a marker for monitoring response to therapy. This enzyme is rarely elevated in early disease and may also be within normal limits in up to 40% of patients with metastatic disease. PSA, a glycoprotein produced by normal and neoplastic ductal epithelium, serves to lyse the seminal coagulum. PSA has been found in seminal fluids, in benign hypertrophied prostate tissue, and in cancerous tissue. Monoclonal and polyclonal antibodies that react with PSA have been developed to provide laboratory determination of the level of PSA present. A rising PSA after radical prostatectomy suggests clinical recurrence. In men without prostatic disease, the normal range in the Tandem-R assay is 0 to 40 ng/mL.[2,16]

Treatment Modalities

Surgery

Surgery is the primary therapy for prostate cancer in the form of radical prostatectomy for localized cancer, transurethral resection for a tumor causing bladder outlet obstruction, or bilateral orchiectomy for the management of metastatic disease. Stage A, B_1, B_2, T1 and T2 lesions may be treated surgically by radical prostatectomy.[5,21]

Radiation Therapy

For males who are not candidates for radical prostatectomy based on performance status, concomitant medical conditions, or preference, external beam radiotherapy with or without interstitial radiation implantation may result in long-term complete remissions, with disease-free survival rates paralleling those achieved with radical prostatectomy for clinical stage A, B_1, B_2, T1 and T2 disease.[20]

Hormonal Therapy

Established therapeutic interventions, including orchiectomy and oral estrogens, have effectively managed the disease process for long periods of time without compromising the quality of life for the majority of patients. Removal of the testes as a source of

95% of testosterone, the major circulating androgen, through bilateral orchiectomy is a cost-effective, well-tolerated intervention that interrupts the gonadal portion of the axis.[20]

Administration of exogenous estrogens such as diethylstilbestrol (DES) profoundly inhibit pituitary LH secretion, thereby reducing circulating testosterone to castrate level while increasing sex steroid-binding globulin and promoting prolactin secretion. This mechanism has led to widespread application of DES in varying daily doses in the treatment of metastatic prostate cancer.

The long-term administration of LHRH analogues results in a enduring inhibition with corresponding gonadal down-regulation, including inhibition of prostatic growth. LHRH agonists (e.g., Leuprolide, Zoladex) have been established as effective options in the treatment of advanced prostate cancer. Antiandrogens, both steroidal and nonsteroidal agents, such as flutamide (Eulexin), compete with dihydrotestosterone for binding sites on prostatic cells.[8,14]

Chemotherapy

Single agents, including cyclophosphamide, 5-fluorouracil, doxorubicin, methotrexate, and cisplatin, have been associated with subjective responses and disease stabilization in 25% to 50% of patients. Combination chemotherapy does not appear to offer any significant clinical advantages and is associated with significant morbidity.[5]

Metastasis

Prostate cancer spreads by direct extension to the seminal vesicles and contiguous structures, the bladder, membranous urethra, and pelvic sidewalls. Lymphatic spread to pelvic nodes or hematogenous deposition to bone is frequently encountered.

Prognosis

Survival for prostate cancer is related to the stage of the disease:

Stage A - 87%	Stage C - 64%
Stage B - 81%	Stage D - 30%

Testicular Cancer

Epidemiology

Although testicular tumors are rare, accounting for 1% of all cancer in U.S. males, they are the most common cancers in young men between the ages of 15 and 35. Testis tumors occur more commonly in white males than black males in the United States.[3]

Etiology and Risk Factors

Testicular tumors are more likely to occur in an atrophic testis or a cryptorchid (undescended) testis. With 12% of all testis tumors originating in cryptorchid testis, the likelihood of subsequent development of a testis cancer in an undescended testis is 40 times greater than in a normal testis. Orchiopexy, surgical descent of the cryptorchid testis, before a boy is 2 years old may reduce the probability of subsequent development of testis tumor. Testis tumors occur more commonly in white males than in black males in the United States.

Prevention, Screening, and Detection

As recommended by the ACS, young men from puberty through age 40 need to be taught and encouraged to perform monthly testicular self-examination. The examination is facilitated by the heat of a warm bath or shower. Each testicle is examined with both hands. The index and middle fingers are placed one side of the testicle; the thumbs are placed on the other side. A gentle rolling motion allows for complete palpation of each testicle. The epididymis, which collects and carries sperm, is felt as a cordlike structure at the back of each testicle. Any new lump or worrisome area needs to be reported.

Classification

Ninety-seven percent of all testicular tumors are germ cell tumors originating in the primordial germ cells essential for spermatogenesis. The remaining 3% are nongerminal in origin or metastatic foci of other tumors, primarily lymphomas and leukemias. Pure seminomas account for 40% of testis tumors; 15% to 20% are pure embryonal carcinoma. The rest of the tumors are usually mixed types. Approximately 70% of patients with seminoma have the disease confined to the testis.[6]

Clinical Features

Clinical features of testis cancer are:

- Non-tender, enlarged testis
- Trauma
- Mumps orchitis
- Episodic testicular pain or heaviness

Symptoms
- Abdominal aching
- Low back pain
- Gynecomastia
- Breast tenderness

Diagnosis and Staging

Approximately 60% of males have evidence of lymphatic or other sites of metastatic involvement at diagnosis. CT has replaced lymphangiography for assessment of nodal status and definition of areas of abnormality. Whole lung tomography and lung CT scans are sensitive diagnostic methods for evaluation of the lungs. A standard chest x-ray is also necessary. Intravenous pyelography (IVP) may be used to assess the kidneys, ureters, and bladder.

Biologic Markers

The α-fetoprotein (AFP) and β subunit of human chorionic gonadotropin (hCG) as serum markers provide valuable information for the assessment of testicular malignancies. Any elevation in AFP or hCG in a patient with a testicular mass raises the clinical index of suspicion. Serum marker proteins need to be obtained before an orchiectomy so that the efficacy of the removal of the primary testicular malignancy may be assessed. The half-life of AFP is approximately 5 days; the half-life of hCG is approximately 16 hours. Elevation in serum marker proteins after appropriate attention is given to the half-life curve, indicates the persistence of metastatic disease. Elevated hCG is possible with pure seminoma. An elevated AFP is never observed in pure seminoma. If the AFP is elevated, the tumor is not pure seminoma but rather a mixed cell type. High levels of hCG are suspicious in the patient considered to have pure seminoma.[8]

Treatment Modalities

Seminoma Therapy

Seminomas exhibit dramatic radiosensitivity. Stage A seminoma confined to the testis is treated with regional radiation designed to eliminate a micrometastatic tumor. After orchiectomy, radiotherapy is delivered to the periaortic area and ipsilateral pelvic lymph nodes. An approximate dose of 165 cGy daily is given for a total dose of 2,500 cGy over 3 weeks. Generally, stage B seminoma is cured with radiotherapy. However, Stage B_3 patients with a palpable tumor demonstrate a less successful response to radiotherapy. Chemotherapy is the treatment of choice for stage C disease, advanced supradiaphragmatic adenopathy, or metastases to brain, bone, lung, or liver.[8]

Nonseminoma Therapy

Radical retroperitoneal lymph node dissection (RPLND) has been the classic therapy for pathologic staging of nonseminomatous disease, and removal of all nodes involved in lymphatic drainage of the testis. Surveillance programs for follow-up are usually monthly for 12 months, including a physical examination, tumor markers (AFP, hCG, and LDH) and chest x-ray. For patients who have experienced a relapse, salvage combination chemotherapy can be successfully employed. Critical to surveillance programs is patient compliance.

Chemotherapy

A number of single agents demonstrated activity in disseminated testicular cancer, most notably actinomycin D, methotrexate, chlorambucil, vinblastine, mithramycin, and bleomycin. However, lasting complete remissions occurred in less than 20% of the patients. With the introduction of cisplatin-based chemotherapy, this percentage dramatically increased to 80%-90%. The coupling of cisplatin with vinblastine and bleomycin has made a substantial number of patients disease free. Etoposide and ifosfamide have demonstrated exciting activity in germ cell tumors.

Fertility after Treatment

Many of the patients successfully treated for testis tumors are interested in parenthood, and the effects of therapy including surgery, radiation, and chemotherapy on fertility. Reviews indicate that combination chemotherapy does affect spermatic function, rendering most patients azoospermic. A high degree of recovery of spermatogenesis is experienced 2 to 3 years after initiation of chemotherapy. Subsequent to successful pregnancies, no increased incidences of fetal abnormalities or tumors in offspring have been reported.[9]

Metastasis and Prognosis

Testicular cancer metastasizes primarily by the lymphatic route,. Metastasis may occur in the lungs, retroperitoneum, and bones.The overall survival rate for all stages of testicular cancer is above 80% and approaches 100% for patients with low stage disease.

Testicular Cancer Disease and Treatment-Related Complications

Potential organ system, body image, and reproductive capacity complications associated with testis cancer and treatment are serious and significant. Compliance is paramount to achievement of optimal success in the management of testis tumors. With cure a likely expectation, the individual with a testis tumor, his support network, and his clinicians are encouraged to maintain an outcome-focused approach, while mandating compliance with proven therapeutic regimens with their acceptable and generally reversible profile of complications.

Renal Cell Cancer

Epidemiology

Approximately 28,000 tumors of the kidney are diagnosed in the United States each year, representing 2% of all malignancy in adults[3] and 20% of childhood malignancy.

Wilms' tumors, usually diagnosed in children under age 5, account for approximately 4% of all kidney cancers. In adults, kidney cancer occurs more commonly in men than women (2:1 ratio). Cancer of the kidney is most commonly encountered in adults over age 40, with a median age at diagnosis of 64.3 years for whites and 58.2 years for blacks.[7]

Etiology and Risk Factors

Etiologic factors include cigarette, cigar, or pipe smoking, chewing tobacco, urbanization, obesity, and exposure to petrochemical products. Studies report an increased risk of 1.5% to 2.2% for tobacco users. A high-fat diet may be responsible for the obesity and renal cell cancer relationship.

Classification

Renal cell or clear cell adenocarcinoma (hypernephroma) is the most common kidney cancer. Transitional cell cancers, the most commonly occurring cancer of the renal pelvis, also occur in the kidney. Squamous cell carcinoma and nephroblastoma are also identified. The growth of the kidney carcinoma may be well defined, surrounded by perinephric fat rather than infiltrating.

Clinical Features

Clinical features of renal cell cancer are:

- Pain
- Hematuria
- Anemia
- Fever
- Fatigue

Diagnosis

A renal mass may be detected by:

- IVP
- CT
- Angiography
- Ultrasonography

Treatment Modalities

Surgery

For tumors suspected to be confined to the kidney, nephrectomy is the therapy of choice. The potential for surgical cure depends on a number of factors including stage, size, grade, and histologic type of tumor, and the procedure performed. Involvement of regional lymph nodes indicates a significantly decreased survival rate.[1,12]

Systemic Therapy

A number of chemotherapeutic agents have been employed in the management of metastatic renal cell carcinoma. Vinblastine continues to be the most active single agent with objective responses, defined as shrinkage of measurable tumor dimensions by at least 50%, observed in about 15% of patients.[7] Combinations of chemotherapeutic agents do not appear to offer any advantage.

Interleukin-2, a glycoprotein primarily produced by activated T-helper cells, has been approved for the treatment of metastatic renal cell cancer. The durability of responses to IL-2, most notable in the complete responders, has led to continuing research investigation with this cytokine alone or in combination with autologous tumor vaccine or alpha interferon.[1,12,18]

Metastasis

Metastasis may spread by the lymphatics or by the venous route. The most common sites are lung, bone, liver, and brain.

Prognosis

The median survival of patients with metastases is eight months, with a five-year survival rate of less than 10%.

Bladder Cancer

Epidemiology

With approximately 51,200 new cases anticipated each year, primary bladder cancer is responsible for approximately 4% of cancer deaths reported in the United States annually.[3] Of historic interest, there has been a 50% increase in bladder cancer in the past four decades. Previously bladder cancer was predominantly a disease of aging men; it is now being seen increasingly in women and in younger patients, both males and females.[3]

Etiology and Risk Factors

Tobacco habits are clearly implicated in the initiation and promotion of 30% to 40% of bladder cancers. As many as one-third of all bladder cancers are felt to be related to industrial chemical exposure. Benzidine, 2-naphthlamine,4-aminodiphenyl, and 4-nitrobiphenyl are implicated.[13]

Classification

Approximately 90% of all cancers of the bladder are transitional cell carcinomas. The remainder are squamous cell.

Clinical Features

Clinical features of bladder cancer are: bladder spasms, hematuria, infection, and a history of tobacco use.

Diagnosis and Staging

The primary goals in the management of superficial papillary tumors are to prevent tumor invasion into the bladder wall muscle, and to reduce or prevent recurrences. In a patient with unexplained hematuria or suspected tumor of the bladder, IVP is performed. This is done before cystoscopy so that the upper urinary tracts, the kidneys, and the ureters, can be visualized. IVP can indicate a persistent bladder filling defect, or the presence of abnormality of the upper urinary tract. CT is reserved as an additional staging examination in patients with invasive tumors.

Cystoscopy remains the main diagnostic method in patients suspected of having a bladder tumor. All areas of the bladder may be visualized during cystoscopy, with biopsies taken of suspicious areas. In addition to tissue biopsies, cells may be captured from bladder mucosa by bladder wash or voided urine for cytologic evaluation.[13]

Metastasis

The bladder is a common site for contiguous spread from anaplastic lesions of the neighbouring viscera, most notably the uterine cervix and prostate. These tumors may invade the bladder by direct extension. Also the bladder may be invaded by carcinoma of the sigmoid colon, rectum, or the uterine body.

Treatment Modalities

Noninvasive Bladder Cancer

Transurethral surgical resection of superficial tumors is used in the management of low-grade, early-stage malignancies. It offers the advantage of preserving bladder and sexual functioning, while being associated with low morbidity and mortality. Intravesical chemotherapy or direct intracavity administration of drugs into the bladder may be used for the treatment of existing low-grade superficial tumors, or prophylaxis against tumor recurrence of superficial transitional cell carcinoma, or CIS. The most commonly employed drugs are thiotepa, doxorubicin, mitomycin, and *Bacille* bilié de Calmette-Guérinbacillus (BCG), an attenuated strain of *Mycobacterium bovis*. Interferons may also have a role in the management of superficial bladder cancer.[10,17,19]

Invasive Bladder Cancer

Therapeutic management of bladder cancer penetrating into the muscularis of the bladder wall involves a radical surgical procedure to remove the bladder. In the male patient undergoing radical cystectomy, a radical cystoprostatectomy is performed.

In a female patient, a total abdominal hysterectomy may be performed as well. The standard of care for urinary diversion after radical cystectomy has been creation of an ileal conduit from a piece of small bowel. The ureters are anchored into the ileal conduit, which protrudes through the skin as a bud stoma in the right lower quadrant, for application of an external ileostomy drainage device. Treatment related complications for bladder cancer are loss of bladder function, body image and sexuality assaults.[13]

Prognosis

Recent advances in combination therapy have resulted in responses ranging from a disease stabilization, to partial, to complete remission in the management of metastatic bladder cancer.

Nursing Management

Nursing Diagnosis

Urinary elimination, alteration in patterns
- *Decreased bladder capacity*
- *Urinary diversion*
- *Obstruction*
- *Retention*
- *Incontinence*

Interventions

- Promote acceptance of change in body, secondary to disease or treatment process
- Provide information and assure continuing care for the individual with a urinary diversion
- Provide resource and referral information for persons on a bladder catheterization program and those experiencing any degree of incontinence

Nursing Diagnosis[5,6,15]

Sexuality pattern alteration
- *Pathophysiologic changes associated with cancer or treatment:*
    - *Diagnostic procedures*
    - *Surgery*
    - *Radiation therapy*
    - *Hormonal manipulation*
    - *Chemotherapy*
    - *BRM therapy*
- *Self-image and self-esteem assaults*
- *Physiologic function*
    - *Males   - Potential for fertility impairment*
    - *- Dry orgasms after removal of prostate*
    - *Females - Inadequate vaginal lubrication and infertility*

Interventions

- Assess patterns of sexuality expression prior to diagnosis as a guide to predicting or planning for similar pattern maintenance, or attainment during and after treatment
- Consider technique of permission granting general discussion regarding disease and treatment, followed by individual specific questions
- Review anticipated physiologic impact of disease and treatment on libido and potency
- Consider general themes associated with age, sex, disease, and treatment modalities while focusing on the person's perception of cancer and potential impact on lifestyle
- Maintain an awareness of personal biases and values and allow for possibility of nontraditional partner or expressions of sexuality
- Encourage enhancement of satisfaction and pleasure from everyday encounters
- Review options for management of impotence including injectable drugs, oral drugs, vascular reconstructive surgery, vacuum devices, and surgically implanted rigid or inflatable penile prosthetics

Patient Teaching Priorities

Health seeking behaviors

- Prevention
  - Avoid or limit exposure to exogenous carcinogens
  - Discourage development of tobacco habits
  - Maintain low-fat diet
- Early detection
  - Encourage early investigation of GU findings
  - Mass
  - Pain
  - Hematuria
  - Alteration of urinary patterns
- Follow ACS screening guidelines
  - Monthly testicular self examination
  - Annual DRE (males 40 years and older)
  - Annual PSA (males 50 years and older)
- Risk modification
  - Encourage cessation or moderation of tobacco habits
  - Avoid obesity
  - Limit exposure to petrochemicals

Geriatric Considerations

As approximately 87% of prostate cancer patients are 65 years of age or older, awareness of the concerns of this population is appropriate. With the transition to older adulthood and accommodation to the gradual shift in family responsibilities, retirement, and declining economic opportunities as described by Havighurst, the aging adult is challenged to achieve ego integrity as defined by Erikson.

Along with the acceptance of age-related limitations, the senior adult is adjusting to physiologic aging, retirement, reduced income, deaths of relatives, friends and conceivably spouse, while maintaining a safe and solvent environment often in a relocation setting. The older person is customarily concerned about finances, loss of independence, and placing a burden on family or society. Frequently the senior adult approaches the health care system and care providers from a docile perspective and may not aggressively pursue or report symptoms, thus resulting in delay of diagnosis or lack of symptom resolution. The older adult with Medicare has acute-care coverage but may not have comprehensive coverage for preventive or supportive care, including oral and subcutaneous medications. Intellectual function is usually maintained in older adulthood although short-term memory may gradually decline, underscoring the need for application of recall and repetitive techniques. Special attention to establishing a framework for open communication, and identifying components of the individual's dilemma, such as reimbursement, are suggested for facilitating compliance and rehabilitation for the older adult.[6]

Bibliography

1. Belldegrun A and others: *Renal cell carcinoma: basic biology and current approaches to therapy*, Semin Oncol 18(5):96, Suppl 7, 1991.
2. Brawer MK and Lange PH: *Prostate-specific antigen and premalignant change: implicatiors for early detection*, Ca 39:361-375, 1989.
3. *Cancer statistics*, 1994, Ca 44:7,1994.
4. Catalina WJ: *Epidemiology and etiology in prostate cancer,* Orlando, Fla, 1984, Grune & Stratton.
5. Crawford ED and Dawkin CA: *Diagnosis and management of prostate cancer,* Hosp Prac 21(3):159, 1986.
6. Dansak DA: Psychiatric oncology: In Crawford ED and Borden TA, editors: *Genitourinary cancer surgery*, Philadelphia, 1982, Lea & Febiger.
7. Dayal HH and Wilkinson GS: *Epidemiology of renal cell cancer*, Semin Urol VII(3):139-143, 1989.
8. Donohue JP: *Selecting initial therapy*, Cancer 90(3) (suppl):23, 1987.
9. Drasga RE and others: *Fertility after chemotherapy for testicular cancer*, J. Clin Oncol 1(3):37, 1983.
10. Maldazys JD and deKernion JB: Management of superficial bladder tumors and carcinoma in situ. In deKernion JB and Paulson DP, editors: *Genitourinary cancer management*, Philadelphia, 1987, Lea & Febiger.

11. Papsidero LD and others: *A prostate antigen in sera of prostatic cancer patients,* Cancer Res 40:2428, 1980.

12. Pritchett TR, Lieskovsky G, and Skinner DG: Clinical manifestations and treatment of renal parenchymal tumors. In Skinner DG and Lieskovsky G, editors: *Genitourinary cancer,* Philadelphia, 1988, WB Saunders.

13. Fair WR, Fuks ZY and Scher HI: Carcinoma of the bladder. In Devita VT Jr, Hellman S, and Rosenberg SA, editors: *Cancer principles and practices of oncology,* ed 4, Philadelphia, 1993, JB Lippincott.

14. Rosenberg SA and others: *A progress report on the treatment of 157 patients with advanced cancer using lymphokine activated killer cells and interleukin-2 or high dose interleukin-2 alone,* N Engl J Med 316:889, 1987.

15. Schmale AH: *Psychological reactions to recurrences, metastases, or disseminated cancer,* Int J Radiat Oncol Biol Phys 1:1515, 1976.

16. Schmidt JD and Benson RC: *Prostatic carcinoma epidemiology.* In *Prostatic carcinoma: current concept and management,* Monograph of University of California, San Diego.

17. Smith JA: *Laser treatment of bladder cancer,* Semin Urol 3:2, 1985.

18. Sufrin G and others: *Paraneoplastic and serologic syndromes of renal adenocarcinoma,* Semin Urol 7(3):159, 1989.

19. Torti FM and others: *Aplha-interferon in superficial bladder cancer.* A Northern California Oncology Group Study, J Clin Oncol 6:476, 1988.

20. Waisman J: Pathology of neoplasms of the prostate gland. In Skinner DG and Lieskovsky G, editors: *Genitourinary cancer,* Philadelphia, 1988, WB Saunders.

21. Walsh PC: Radical prostatectomy, preservation of sexual function, cancer control: the controversy. In Donahue JP, editor: *Controversies in urologic oncology,* Urol Clin North Am 14:663, 1987.

Gynecologic Cancers

11

Cervical Cancer

Epidemiology

The ACS estimates that 15,000 women were diagnosed with cervical cancer in 1994. Patterns of occurrence have been described based on age and socioeconomic status. Invasive cervical cancer occurs most commonly among women between the ages of 35 and 50 years old. Invasive cervical cancer is usually preceded by a 10 to 20 year history of preinvasive cellular changes ranging from mild dysplasia to carcinoma in situ (Figure 11-1). If untreated, a small proportion of women with mild dysplasia will eventually develop invasive cancer. Even with the widespread use of the Papanicolaou (Pap) smear for early detection of preinvasive and invasive cervical disease, an estimated 4,600 women will die of cervical cancer in 1994.[1,6]

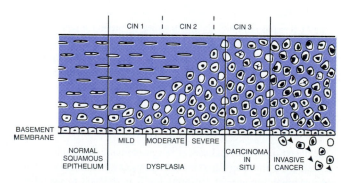

Figure 11-1. Progression of cervical intraepithelial neoplasia. (From Jones HW, Wentz AC, and Burnett LS: *Novak's textbook of gynecology*, ed 11, Baltimore, 1988, Williams & Wilkins Co.)

Etiology and Risk Factors

Sexual practices associated with an increased risk for cervical cancer include onset of sexual intercourse prior to 18 years of age and multiple sexual partners. The number of sexual partners of the male partner(s), may also play a significant role in the development of cervical cancer. A history of infection with sexually-transmitted viruses, such as herpes simplex virus, type 2 (HSV-2), and the human papilloma virus (specifically types HPV-16 and HPV-18), initial pregnancy prior to 18 years of age, and multiple pregnancies place an individual woman at increased risk for cervical cancer.[1]

Prevention, Screening, and Detection

Prevention

For women of all ages, the limitation of the number of sexual partners, and the use of barrier-type contraceptives, such as condoms and diaphragms, are recommended to reduce the risk of cervical cancer. Dietary modifications that may reduce the risk of cervical cancer include increased ingestion of foods high in vitamins A and C and folic acid. In addition, strategies to prevent initiation or to encourage discontinuation of tobacco and/or alcohol use could be included.[1,5,7]

Screening

The ACS recommendations for screening of asymptomatic women for cervical cancer include an annual Pap smear and pelvic examination for all women who are or have been sexually active or who are 18 years of age. After three or more normal, consecutive, annual Pap smears, the Pap smear and pelvic examination can be performed less frequently at the discretion of the physician.[1]

Detection

The detection of cervical cancer in symptomatic women is determined by a thorough history and physical examination. The rectovaginal, bimannual examination is performed to visualize the cervix, obtain a Pap smear, conduct a colposcopic examination, and palpate the cervix and adjacent tissues.

A colposcopic examination may be performed in women with significant symptoms or grossly suspicious lesions on the cervix. The clinician obtains a colposcopically-directed biopsy from the most abnormal areas for evaluation. Refer to Figure 11-2.

Classification

More than 90% of cervical carcinomas are of the squamous cell type. Squamous cell carcinomas have been divided further into keratinizing, non-keratinizing, and small cell types based on histological descriptors. Adenocarcinomas and adenosquamous carcinomas account for an increasingly greater proportion of cervical cancers (11% to 16%), particularly in women under 35 years of age. [2,6,11]

Clinical Features

Clinical features of cervical cancer are:
- Abnormal vaginal bleeding—increase in amount, frequency, and/or length
- Contact bleeding related to intercourse
- Urinary urgency, dysuria, and hematuria

Diagnosis and Staging

Staging for cervical cancer is done clinically. Data obtained from the clinical examination (inspection, palpation, and colposcopy), radiographic examinations (chest, skeleton, kidneys, sigmoid colon, and rectum), and pathologic evaluation of biopsy and curettage materials, are used to determine the extent of disease and ultimately plan treatment. See chapter 4. [6,9]

Metastasis

Cervical carcinomas are slow-growing tumors that invade by direct extension to adjacent tissues of the uterus, vagina, rectum, bladder, and parametrial tissues. Lymphatic invasion also occurs in regional and distant lymphatic channels. Cervical cancer rarely spreads hematologically; however, metastatic disease can occur in the lungs or liver.

Normal colposcopic findings

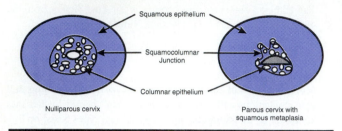

Abnormal colposcopic findings: **White epithelium**
Abnormal vascular patterns:
Mosaic and punctate vessels

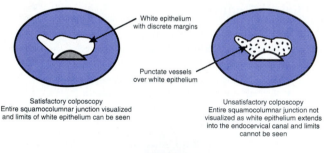

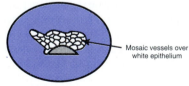

Figure 11-2. Graphic representation of cervical findings using the colposcope.

Treatment Modalities

The treatment of pre-invasive cervical disease is based on the extent of disease (Figure 11-3). Women with preinvasive disease may be treated conservatively with cryosurgery, electrocautery, laser vaporization, loop electrosurgical excision procedure (LEEP), or ionization of the cervix. Localized cervical carcinoma (stages I to IIA) may be treated with surgery alone, radiation therapy alone, or a combination of surgery and radiation therapy. Surgical treatment of women with invasive cervical cancer most commonly includes a radical hysterectomy with bilateral pelvic lymphadenectomy. Advanced cervical carcinoma (stages IIB to IV) is treated primarily with radiation therapy alone. Chemotherapy, radiosensitizing agents, hyperbaric oxygen, and hyperthermia is administered in conjunction with radiation.[2,6,10]

Treatment During Pregnancy

Pregnant women with abnormal Pap smears are evaluated with colposcopy and biopsies. If the squamocolumnar junction can be visualized entirely on colposcopy and directed biopsies are sufficient to rule out the presence of invasive cancer, the clinician can follow the woman to term with interval Pap smears and colposcopy examinations.

Women with stage IA disease can usually be followed with Pap smears, colposcopy, and biopsies to term. In the presence of invasive cancer, immediate treatment is recommended. For women at less than 24 weeks of gestation, the pregnancy is terminated. Radical hysterectomy or radiation therapy can be used as primary treatment.[2,6,9,10]

Prognosis

Prognosis in cervical cancer is determined primarily by the stage of the disease. The 5-year survival rate for patients diagnosed with carcinoma in situ approaches 100%; with local disease, 88%; regional disease, 52%; and distant metastasis, 14%.

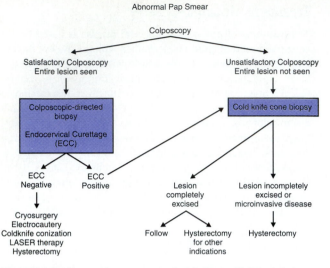

Figure 11-3. Decision tree for management of cervical intraepithelial neoplasia. (From Flannery M: Reproductive cancers. In Clark JC and McGee RF, editors: *Core curriculum for oncology nursing.* Philadelphia, 1992, WB Saunders.)

Endometrial Cancer

Epidemiology

Endometrial cancer is the most common gynecologic malignancy among women over 50 years of age. Of the estimated 31,000 women diagnosed with endometrial cancer in 1994, approximately 70% were over 50 years of age.[1]

Etiology and Risk Factors

Risk factors for cancer of the endometrium include advancing age, early onset of menstruation, late menopause, and concurrent conditions. Women who have a history of postmenopausal bleeding and have never been pregnant are at higher risk for cancer of the endometrium. Concurrent conditions, such as obesity, diabetes, hypertension, Stein-Leventhal syndrome, endometrial hyperplasia, or previous history of breast, colon, or ovarian cancer, also increase the risk of endometrial cancer.[1]

Prevention, Screening, and Detection

Prevention/Screening

Maintenance of ideal body weight is recommended to avoid obesity and to decrease the risk of hypertension and diabetes. Treatment of premalignant changes of the endometrium such as endometrial hyperplasia with progesterone is suggested as a prevention strategy. To control the symptoms of menopause in women with an intact uterus, the addition of cyclic progesterone to the estrogen replacement regimen is recommended to reduce the risk of development of endometrial cancer.[1,5,7] The ACS recommends that asymptomatic, high-risk women have an endometrial tissue sampling done at menopause.[1]

Detection

The detection of endometrial cancer in symptomatic women is guided by a complete history, physical examination, and diagnostic evaluation. The uterine size, shape, and consistency is determined by palpation on the rectovaginal, bimanual examination. The depth of the uterine cavity is determined by inserting a uterine sound. An endometrial biopsy is obtained for histologic confirmation of the disease.[2,7]

Classification

Five primary types of endometrial cancers are seen: adenocarcinoma, mixed mullerian tumors, sarcomas, clear cell carcinoma, and epidermoid carcinoma. More than 90% of endometrial cancers are adenocarcinomas. Variants of adenocarcinoma include adenocanthoma (benign squamous elements) and adenosquamous carcinoma (malignant squamous elements). Mixed müllerian tumors, sarcomas, clear cell carcinomas, and epidermoid carcinomas are rare and are associated with higher incidences of local and distant metastases and lower survival rates than adenocarcinomas.[2,6]

Clinical Features

Clinical features of endometrial cancer include:

- Prolonged, excessive premenopausal or postmenopausal bleeding
- Yellow, watery vaginal discharge
- Pyometria
- Hematometria
- Pain in hypogastric or lumbosacral areas or pelvis
- Advanced disease symptoms may be intestinal obstruction, ascites, jaundice, respiratory distress, or hemorrhage

Diagnosis and Staging

Cervical biopsies, endocervical curettage, endometrial biopsy, and/or a fractional dilatation and curettage (D & C) are done to rule out the presence of a cervical malignancy and to obtain a tissue sample for diagnosis. Laboratory studies routinely include a complete blood count (CBC), blood chemistry profile (SMA), and liver and renal chemistries. Additional radiographic studies to determine the presence of metastatic disease may include a chest x-ray, magnetic resonance imaging (MRI), and computed tomography (CT Scan). If involvement of the bladder or rectum is suspected, intravenous pyelogram (IVP), barium enema (BE), proctosigmoidoscopy, and cystoscopy may be done. Endometrial cancer is staged surgically. Staging is based on the depth of myometrial invasion, degree of cellular differentiation, and the extent of metastatic disease. See chapter 4.

Metastasis

The majority of endometrial cancers originate in the fundus of the uterus and spread by direct extension to the entire endometrium. The disease may also spread outside the uterus to the structures of the parametria and the abdominal cavity, such as the ovaries, fallopian tubes, vagina, bladder, rectum, omentum, or bowel. Lymphatic metastases occur primarily to the pelvic and para-aortic lymph nodes. The endometrium is highly vascular; therefore, hematogenous spread, particularly with sarcomas, is common. Lung, liver, bone, and brain metastases may occur.[2,6]

Treatment Modalities

Surgery

Surgery, usually a total abdominal hysterectomy and bilateral salpingo-oophorectomy, is the most common primary treatment for women with early stage disease. If more extensive disease is present, bilateral pelvic lymphadenectomy is also done.

Radiation Therapy

Radiation therapy is used as primary treatment for women with other health problems that increase the risks of surgical complications. In women with bulky disease, poorly differentiated tumors, or greater depth of myometrial invasion, the addition of preoperative or postoperative radiation therapy may be recommended. Radiation may consist of brachytherapy, teletherapy, or a combination of the two.

Hormone Therapy

Depo-provera, provera, dilalutin, and megace are the most common progestational agents currently used for women who are estrogen and progesterone receptor positive. Response rates with hormonal manipulation range from 30% to 70% with the highest response rate occurring in women with well-differentiated tumors.[2,6]

Chemotherapy

Antineoplastic agents are reserved for women who have estrogen/progesterone negative tumors, who have failed hormone therapy, or who have disseminated disease. Agents commonly used include doxorubicin, 5-fluorouracil, vincristine, cistplatin, and cyclophosphamide.

Prognosis

The 5-year survival rate for patients with all stages of endometrial cancer is 83%; with localized disease, 93%; with regional disease, 70%; and with distant metastasis, 27%.

Ovarian Cancer

Epidemiology

The 24,000 new cases of ovarian cancer account for only 25% of all gynecologic cancers diagnosed in the United States in 1994. Yet the disease is the leading cause of death (13,600 deaths in 1994) in women diagnosed with gynecologic cancers. The highest incidence of ovarian cancer is reported in highly industrialized countries. The ACS estimates that 1 out of every 70 women will develop ovarian cancer during her lifetime. This statistic is particularly alarming, since early disease is not symptomatic and no cost-effective, reliable, and valid screening tests are available.[1]

Etiology and Risk Factors

Age, genetics, history of other cancers, and menstrual history have been associated with an increased incidence of the disease. The majority of ovarian cancers are diagnosed in the 50-to-59-year age group. A familial or personal history of other cancers, including breast, colon, and uterine, increases the risk of ovarian cancer. The incidence of ovarian cancer is greater among women who are single, nulliparous, and infertile; the incidence is lower among women who use oral contraceptives.[9,11]

Prevention, Screening, and Detection

Prevention and Screening

Women in higher risk categories, as described previously, are encouraged to seek routine gynecologic care including an annual pelvic examination. Palpatation of a normal-sized ovary in postmenopausal women is cause for further diagnostic evaluation.

Detection

Most women with early stage ovarian cancer are asymptomatic. A careful personal and family history is important to identify women at higher risk for the disease. Attention to generalized, vague complaints among women during their middle years will often alert the clinician to the possibility of ovarian cancer.

Finally, a pelvic examination and palpation of an adnexal mass or a postmenopausal ovary raise suspicions for ovarian cancer.

Classification

Ovarian carcinomas are classified as epithelial, sex cord-stromal, or lipid cell tumors. Epithelial tumors, most frequently found in women 40 to 65 years of age, account for 85% of all ovarian malignancies diagnosed in the United States. Sex cord-stromal tumors occur much less frequently than epithelial tumors. Lipid cell tumors account for less than 5% of all ovarian malignancies. These tumors, particularly dysgerminoma, endodermal sinus tumors, and embryonal carcinoma, occur most frequently in younger women.[6,9,16]

Clinical Features

Clinical features of ovarian cancer include:

- Dyspepsia
- Indigestion
- Anorexia
- Early satiety
- Urinary frequency
- Constipation
- Pelvic pressure and discomfort
- Increased abdominal girth
- Pain
- Shortness of breath
- Intestinal or ureteral obstruction
- Muscle wasting

Diagnosis and Staging

Diagnosis and staging of women with ovarian cancer is achieved by tissue sampling and inspection of the abdominal cavity at the time of exploratory laparotomy. A CBC biochemical profile, and CA-125 are obtained. In addition, a chest x-ray, cystoscopy, proctoscopy, intravenous pyelogram, barium enema, CT, MRI, or ultrasound may be ordered.[16] See Chapter 4.

Metastasis

Ovarian carcinoma spreads by direct extension to adjacent pelvic organs such as the opposite ovary, uterus, fallopian tubes, bladder, rectum, and peritoneum, and by seeding the peritoneal cavity, and through lymphatic and vascular channels. Common sites of metastatic disease include the omentum and surfaces of the bowel, uterus, bladder, and peritoneum.

Lymphatic invasion can occur in the pelvic, paraaortic, and aortic nodes even in the early stage of the disease. Partial or complete obstruction of lymphatic channels in the diaphragm results in the accumulation of malignant ascitic fluid. The most common sites of hematogenous spread include the liver, lung, and pleura.[2,6,9,16]

Treatment Modalities

Surgery

In addition to the exploratory laparotomy required for staging, surgery is used as primary treatment for women with borderline and malignant tumors of the ovary. For younger women with tumors of borderline malignant potential, conservative treatment with unilateral oophorectomy may be considered as the definitive treatment. With a total abdominal hysterectomy and bilateral salpingo-oophorectomy, the surgical resection of the bulk of the remaining tumor is attempted. Resection of the bladder, colon, or omentum may be indicated. The extent of the debulking procedure is based on evaluation of potential risks of more extensive resection and potential benefits in terms of survival and quality of life.[16]

Radiation Therapy

Teletherapy to the pelvis and abdomen and the instillation of radioactive isotopes in the peritoneal cavity have been used in the treatment of women with early stages (I and II) of ovarian cancer. Radioactive isotopes (P^{32}) have been used to treat residual disease in the peritoneal cavity. Women who have limited residual disease, less than 2 cm, are the most likely candidates for P^{32} therapy.[16]

Chemotherapy

Systematic melphalan, 5-FU, thiotepa, and cyclophosphamide have shown activity. Altretamine, cisplatin, carboplatin, doxorubicin, ifosfamide, and etoposide have also been used with response rates ranging from 27% to 78%. In general, systematic combination therapy with taxol, cisplatin, and cyclophosphamide has resulted in improved response rates, increased disease-free survival, and/or increased survival.[16]

Other Therapies

Studies with hormonal therapy, megace, tamoxifen, and leuprolide acetate are in progress. Biologic response therapy with interferon, interleukin-2, monoclonal antibodies, and lymphokine-activated killer cells have been used in the treatment of ovarian cancer with varying results.[16]

Prognosis

Although the relative 5-year survival rates improved significantly, the rates remain dismally low (39%). Prognosis improves (87%) when the disease is diagnosed at an early stage and rated aggressively. Since early ovarian cancer is commonly asymptomatic, only 23% of patients are diagnosed with localized disease. Patients with distant metastasis at the time of diagnosis have a 19% 5-year survival rate.[9,16]

Vulvar Cancer

Epidemiology

Vulvar carcinoma accounts for approximately 5% of all gynecologic malignancies. Vulvar intraepithelial neoplasia (VIN) occurs most commonly in women in their 40s, carcinoma in situ in women in their 50s, and invasive disease in women in their 60s. The most frequent sites for vulvar carcinoma include the labia majora, labia minora, and the clitoris.[1]

Etiology and Risk Factors

Several factors associated with an increased incidence include con-current diseases such as hypertension, diabetes, cardiovascular disease, obesity, cervical cancer, early menopause, and chronic vulvar irritation.[1,16]

Prevention, Screening and Detection

Emphasis is placed on teaching women vulvar self-examination as a strategy for screening in asymptomatic women. A thorough history and physical examination are required to identify women with existing risk factors and to inspect and palpate vulvar tissue, groin, and pelvis for abnormalities.[4,5]

Classification

Invasive cancers of the vulva are classified as squamous cell, basal cell, adenocarcinoma, and malignant melanoma. Ninety percent of all malignancies of the vulva are squamous cell carcinomas.[6,9,11]

Clinical Features

Clinical features of vulvar cancer include:
- Vulvar lump or mass
- Pain
- Pruritus
- Reddened, white, warty, or abnormally pigmented vulva tissues
- Vulvar bleeding
- Discharge
- Dysuria

Diagnosis and Staging

Diagnosis of vulvar cancer is made by biopsy of abnormal areas noted on inspection, palpation, or colposcopic examination. A metastatic workup includes cystoscopy, proctoscopy, barium enema, intravenous pyelogram, lymphangiogram, CT, and MRI. Staging for vulvar carcinoma is done clinically. See chapter 4.

Metastasis

Carcinomas of the vulva follow a predictable, slow pattern of spread by extension to local tissues and by lymphatic spread to inguinal and pelvic lymph nodes. Approximately one-third of women with disease confined to the vulva will have nodal metastasis.

Treatment Modalities

Treatment of women with vulvar cancer is based on the size and extent of the lesion as well as depth of invasion. For women with preinvasive disease, VIN, or carcinoma in situ in a limited area, a conservative approach with topical 5-FU, cryotherapy, laser therapy, wide local excision, skinning vulvectomy, or simple vulvectomy can be used for primary treatment. In women with invasive disease less than 2 cm in diameter, less than 5 mm of invasion, and negative inguinal lymph nodes on frozen section, wide local excision alone may be done. If the inguinal lymph nodes are positive, a radical vulvectomy with complete, bilateral groin dissection is done. For women who are not candidates for surgical intervention, radiation therapy for early stage disease has been used successfully.[6,9] The treatment plan for women with locally advanced disease can consist of a combination of surgery, radical surgery (vulvectomy, anterior exenteration, posterior exenteration), and preoperative or postoperative radiation therapy. For women with distant metastasis, a combination of radiation therapy to control central disease and chemotherapy for systemic disease is commonly used as palliative treatment. Chemotherapy (mitomycin C, 5-FU, cisplatin) has been used to treat limited numbers of women with vulvar cancer.[6,9]

Prognosis

Survival of patients with vulvar cancer is associated with the stage of disease at diagnosis and more specifically the status of pelvic lymph nodes. Survivial for patients with Stages I and II range from 90% to 98%. If nodes were negative, regardless of stage, survival rates range from 69% to 100%. A marked decrease in survival (21% to 53%) is noted for patients with positive nodes.

Vaginal Cancer

Epidemiology, Etiology and Risk Factors

Carcinoma of the vagina account for approximately 2% of all gynecologic cancers. The disease, preinvasive and invasive, occurs primarily in the fifth and sixth decades of life, respectively. Prior radiation to a field including the vagina, DES exposure in utero, and increasing age, place a woman at higher risk for the disease.[1]

Prevention, Screening, and Detection

Prevention and Screening

A thorough physical examination including inspection and palpation of the vaginal tissues, cervical cytology, and bimanual examination should be done routinely as part of a gynecologic examination for women who are sexually active or 18 years of age or older.[5]

Detection

Detection of preinvasive and invasive lesions is accomplished by a thorough inspection of the vaginal tissues, colposcopic examination, and palpation of the tissues along the length of the vaginal wall. Preinvasive lesions of the vagina may only be visualized by colposcopic examination that reveals areas of whitened tissues or atypical vascular patterns. Lesions occur most commonly on the posterior wall and the upper third of the vagina.[6,9]

Classification

The majority of carcinomas of the vagina are squamous cell cancers (93% to 97%). Other cell types include clear cell carcinomas associated with exposure to DES in utero, malignant melanomas, and sarcomas.[6,9]

Clinical Features

Clinical features of vaginal cancer include:

- Abnormal perimenopausal, postmenopausal or postcoital vaginal bleeding
- Dyspareunia
- Foul-smelling vaginal discharge
- Advanced disease may present changes in pattern of urination and pelvic pain

Diagnosis and Staging

Diagnosis of preinvasive and invasive carcinoma of the vagina is made by biopsy. Staging is done clinically based on inspection of the vagina, and palpation of pelvic structures on rectovaginal, bimanual examination. Laboratory and radiographic studies including biochemical profile, chest x-ray, intravenous pyelogram, barium enema, cystoscopy, and proctoscopy, MRI, CT, and lymphangiography may be used to rule out metastatic disease. See Chapter 4.[6,9]

Metastasis

Squamous cell carcinoma of the vagina spreads primarily by direct extension to adjacent tissues including the urethra, bladder, rectum, parametria, and the pelvic side wall. In addition, spread can occur through extensive lymphatic channels surrounding the vagina and can extend to the rectal, pelvic, paraaortic, femoral lymph nodes, the supraclavicular nodes, and lungs.

Treatment Modalities

Treatment of vaginal neoplasia is based on the stage of disease and general health status of the woman. For women with premalignant lesions of the vagina, a local excision, CO_2 laser, or topical chemotherapy (5-FU), may be used for primary treatment. Partial or total vaginectomy may be done for treatment of women with multifocal disease involving more than a single portion or the full length of the vagina. Radiation therapy for treatment of preinvasive vaginal neoplasia is reserved for women who are poor surgical candidates.[6,9,11]

Surgery

Surgery is recommended as treatment for women with early stage disease (stage I). Based on the location, size, and extent of the lesion, a total hysterectomy, radical hysterectomy, partial vaginectomy and pelvic lymphadenectomy, or in very selected cases anterior or posterior exenteration, may be recommended.

Radiation Therapy

Radiation therapy alone or in combination with surgery is recommended as treatment for women with stage II and higher carcinoma of the vagina. Teletherapy with or without brachytherapy may be used.

Chemotherapy

Cisplatin, 5-FU, vincristine, cyclophosphamide, and doxorubicin have been used as single agents and in combined protocols with minimal response rates.

Prognosis

Survival at 5 years after diagnosis for all stages ranges from 42% to 56%. The most promising results occur in women who have been diagnosed with stage I (65% to 100%) and stage II (42% to 75%) disease.

Fallopian Tube Cancer

Epidemiology, Etiology and Risk Factors

Cancer of the fallopian tubes accounts for only 0.1% of all cancers of the female reproductive system. The disease occurs in women 19 to 80 years of age, with the majority of women being diagnosed between 40 and 65 years of age. Fallopian tube carcinoma occurs in both tubes in 5% to 31% of women diagnosed with the disease.[8,10,11] Chronic inflammation of the tubes and tubal tuberculosis may contribute to the development of the disease.

Prevention, Screening and Detection

The presence of persistent positive cervical cytology in a woman without evidence of cervical, endometrial, or vaginal cancers, should alert the clinician to the possibility of cancer of the fallopian tubes. Clinical examination is done to detect the presence of ascites and a pelvic mass. A pelvic mass is palpable in over 50% of women with fallopian tube cancer.

Classification

Adenocarcinoma is the most common histologic type of cancer of the fallopian tube. Sarcomas, mixed mesodermal tumors, lymphomas, hydatidiform moles, and choriocarcinoma have also been reported.[15]

Clinical Features

Clinical features of fallopian tube cancer include:

- Vaginal bleeding
- Intermittent, colicky, dull, aching pain
- Profuse, watery, vaginal discharge
- Sense of heaviness on bladder or rectum
- Ascites
- Abdominal fullness and pressure

Diagnosis and Staging

Diagnosis of fallopian tube carcinoma is made at the time of surgery for definitive treatment of a pelvic mass. Although many clinicians use the FIGO system for ovarian cancer, no official staging system for cancer of the fallopian tube exists.

Metastasis

Carcinoma of the fallopian tube metastasizes primarily by direct extension to adjacent tissues and organs, seeding of the abdominal cavity, and lymphatic spread to local and regional nodes. For women with lesions in the proximal portion of the tube, metastasis is more likely to occur in the myometrium and endometrium. For women with lesions in the lateral position of the tube, metastasis is more likely to occur to the ovaries and aortic nodes.

Treatment Modalities

Surgery, total abdominal hysterectomy, bilateral salpingo-oophorectomy, and omentectomy, is the treatment of choice for fallopian tube carcinoma. Debulking of the tumor burden is the primary goal. For women with residual disease, treatment with interperitoneal radioactive isoptopes (P^{32} or Au^{198}), pelvic and/or abdominal teletherapy, or systemic single agent or combination chemotherapy with cyclophosphamide, doxorubicin, progestins, cisplatin, or chlorambucil, is recommended.[6,8,9]

Prognosis

The prognosis for patients with cancer of the fallopian tube is similar to that of patients with ovarian cancer, and is related to the stage of disease in general and to the depth of penetration of the tubal wall, specifically. The survival rate for all stages has been reported as 38%, with the rate as high as 88% in patients with stage I disease.

Gestational Trophoblastic Disease

Epidemiology

Gestational trophoblastic disease (GTD) can occur with a molar pregnancy or after an abortion, ectopic pregnancy, or normal term delivery. Although the disease accounts for only 1% of all cancers of the female reproductive system in the United States, incidence rates in Asia and South America have been reported as high as 1:120 pregnancies.[8,9,15]

Etiology and Risk Factors

GTD includes a variety of tumors that originate in the trophoblastic layer of the chorionic villae during pregnancy. The tumors may range from benign hydatidiform moles to locally invasive moles to choriocarcinomas. Empirical data indicates that low protein diets, poverty, and increasing age may contribute to development of the disease.

Prevention, Screening, and Detection

No recommendations for prevention or screening of asymptomatic women for GTD are available. The detection of GTD is based on a careful review of findings on history, clinical examination, and laboratory studies. Disparities in gestational dates, uterine size, and hCG levels are keys to the early detection of GTD.

Classification

GTD is classified morphologically as either hydatidiform moles, invasive moles, or choriocarcinoma. Invasive moles and choriocarcinoma have a higher incidence of metastasis to surrounding tissues and thus carry a poor prognosis.

Clinical Features

Clinical features of GTD include:
- Vaginal bleeding, particularly during the first trimester
- Hyperemesis
- Enlargement of the uterus in excess of the estimated length of gestation

- Fetal heart sounds are absent
- Fetal parts cannot be palpated
- Elevations of the human chorionic gonadotropic (hCG) titers that exceed those found during the course of a normal pregnancy and postpartum period

Diagnosis and Staging

Diagnosis of GTD is confirmed by tissue examination from expulsion of grape-like villae, vaginal bleeding, or evacuation of tissues from the uterus. Clinical examination of the uterus, pelvis, and vagina prior to and during surgery for evidence of metastasis is recommended. The lungs, brain, and liver are evaluated by laboratory and radiographic studies to rule out the presence of metastatic disease. Staging classification for GTD.[6,9]

- Stage O — Molar pregnancy
  A. Low risk
  B. High risk
- Stage I — Confined to uterine corpus
- Stage II — Metastases to pelvis and vagina
- Stage III — Metastasis to lung
- Stage IV — Distant metastasis

Metastasis

Metastasis from GTD occurs primarily by local extension to surrounding tissues of the pelvis or through hematogenous spread. The most common sites of distant metastasis include the lungs, brain, and liver.

Treatment Modalities

Surgery

Surgery, including evacuation of the uterus and dilatation and curettage, is the primary treatment for women with hydatidiform moles. Surgery, including hysterectomy, also plays a role in the treatment of women with other types of GTD.[6]

Chemotherapy

Treatment with antineoplastic agents is used for women with hydatidiform moles who have a plateau or elevation of weekly β-hCG titers postevacuation or the development of metastatic disease, and for women with invasive moles or choriocarcinoma who present with metastatic disease. The most effective agents include methotrexate, with or without leucovorin rescue, actinomycin D, and chlorambucil. Salvage treatment with combination drug regimens including methotrexate, cisplatin, vincristine, or vinblastine, bleomycin, and etoposide has been recommended.

Radiation Therapy

Women with metastasis to the brain or elevated levels of hCG in the spinal fluid receive whole brain radiation. Metastatic lesions to the liver may be treated with radiation therapy.

Response to Therapy

For women with metastatic disease, β-hCG levels are evaluated prior to each course of treatment. Once the β-hCG levels have returned to normal and have remained within normal levels for 3 weeks, monitoring at monthly intervals is begun and is continued for 1 year. Current recommendations include measures to prevent pregnancy during the 1-year follow-up period.

Prognosis

For patients with nonmetastatic disease, remission (hCG levels within normal range for 3 consecutive weeks) rates with single agent chemotherapy range from 90% to 100%. Patients with metastatic disease to the lungs or vagina have higher remission rates (74%) than those with metastatic disease at other sites.

Nursing Management

Nursing Diagnosis

- *Altered sexuality patterns related to the impact of structural, functional, and psychological changes associated with treatment for gynecologic cancers.*[8]

Interventions

- Review normal anatomy and physiology of the reproductive system with woman and significant other.
- Describe strategies recommended for minimizing effects of treatment that can influence sexuality patterns.
- Discuss the potential structural, functional, or psychological effects of treatment—surgery, radiation therapy, and/or chemotherapy.

Surgery

- Only a small portion of the vagina is resected as a component of either a simple or radical hysterectomy. The edges of the vagina are sutured to form a closed tube. The vagina has the ability to stretch during penile/vaginal intercourse.
- Removal of the ovaries results in lack of estrogen.

Radiation Therapy

- Radiation also can affect the vaginal tissues making them thinner, dryer, and less elastic over time. If the woman is not sexually active, vaginal stenosis may occur after radiation therapy.
- Teach use of vaginal dilators to prevent vaginal stenosis.

Chemotherapy

Common side effects of chemotherapy including hair loss, stomatitis, nausea, vomiting, and fatigue can influence both perceptions of body-image and self-concept as well as the desire for sexual intimacy. Review signs and symptoms of altered sexuality patterns to be reported to the health care team: feelings of decreased self-worth, negative feelings about body-image or self-concept, any changes in expression of sexuality that are not satisfying or pleasurable to self or to partner. Refer for sexual counseling if problems persist.

Nursing Diagnosis

- *Fluid volume excess: ascites related to intra-abdominal metastasis.*[8]

Interventions

- Position patient with head elevated 30 to 90 degrees to allow for maximum respiratory expansion with minimal effort.
- Monitor intake and output ratio each day.
- Encourage wearing of loose clothing around the trunk and abdomen: larger size bra, bikini-cut panties, pantyhose made for pregnant women.
- Encourage compliance with low-salt diet.
- Monitor for signs and symptoms of respiratory or gastrointestinal distress that requires medical intervention: marked shortness of breath, protracted nausea or vomiting, acute changes in pattern of pain.
- Provide supportive care as physician performs palliative paracentesis.
- Observe site post procedure for continued drainage, discharge, redness, pain, or warmth.

Nursing Diagnosis

- *Altered urinary elimination related to disease or treatment for gynecologic cancers.*[12,13,14]

Interventions

After hysterectomy or radical hysterectomy innervation to the bladder may be damaged. Decreased sensation of need to void and incontinence are common effects. A suprapugic catheter is usually placed after surgery. Bladder retraining occurs with the catheter in place until residual urines of 50mL are achieved after voiding.

- Encourage to drink as much fluid as possible
- Limit fluid intake after 7:00 PM
- Establish a regular schedule for voiding

For women undergoing a total or anterior pelvic exenteration, a urinary diversion will be constructed.

- Teach skills to evaluate the condition of the stoma, application of collection devices, care of the peristomal skin.
- Discuss critical changes in the character of the urine, condition of stoma or peristomal skin, or functioning of the diversion to report to the health care team.

Nursing Diagnosis

- *Impaired skin integrity related to surgey or radiation theraphy for treatment of vulvar cancer.*

Interventions

Surgery

- Key elements of wound care for these patients are keeping the wound clean and dry.
- Irrigate surgical wounds with one-half strength hydrogen peroxide.
- Pack wounds with gauze.
- Dry perineum with a hair dryer on the coolest setting.
- Use bed cradles and positioning to increase circulation of air to the wound.

Radiation Therapy

- Suggest comfort measures such as wearing loose cotton panties or no panties, avoiding pantyhose, using cool compresses to perineum, and taking pain medication as ordered by the physician.
- Recommend measures to keep tissues clean and dry.
- Discourage use of any topical agents other than those recommended by the radiation oncologist.
- Review signs and symptoms of infection and skin breakdown that should be reported to the health care team.

Nursing Diagnosis

- *Alteration in health maintenance related to lack of endogenous estrogen in presence of an estrogen/progesterone dependent malignancy.*

Interventions

- Discuss rationale for avoiding estrogen replacement therapy in presence of an estrogen-progesterone dependent cancer.
- Describe potential risks to health maintenance from lack of estrogen.

Geriatric Considerations

Vulvar and vaginal cancer disease onset occurs in the late fifth decade to the sixth decade of life. Teaching the patient the need for annual ongoing health examinations that include bimanual pelvic exam with a through inspection and palpation of the perineal and vaginal areas. Other chronic diseases (hypertension, diabetes, arthritis) may exacerbate with the onset/progression of the disease and/or the side effects of the multiple therapies. Age-related modifications may require drug/therapy reduction. Elderly women may live alone and have limited financial/social/healthcare resources—assess needs and intervention strategies and consult with multiple referral systems (American Cancer Society, Social Services, Meals on Wheels, Home Health Care Agencies).

Bibliography

1. American Cancer Society: *Cancer facts & figures—1994*, Atlanta, 1994 American Cancer Society.
2. Barber HRK: *Manual of gynecologic oncology*, ed 2, Philadelphia, 1989, JB Lippincott.
3. Clark J: Mucous membrane integrity, impairment of: Related to vaginal changes. In McNally JC, Somerville ET, Miaskowski C, and Rostad M, editors: *Guidelines for oncology nursing practice*, ed 2, Philadelphia, 1991, WB Saunders.
4. Clark JC, McGee RF, and Preston R: Nursing management of responses to the cancer experience. In Clark JC and McGee RF, editors: *Core curriculum for oncology nursing,* Philadelphia, 1992, WB Saunders.
5. Davis M: Secondary prevention in oncology nursing practice. In Clark JC and McGee RF, editors: *Core curriculum for oncology nursing*, Philadelphia, 1992, WB Saunders.
6. DiSaia PJ and Creasman WT: *Clinical gynecologic oncology*, ed 4, St Louis, 1993, Mosby.
7. Fanslow J: Knowledge deficit related to prevention and early detection of cervical and uterine (endometrial) cancer. In McNally JC, Somerville ET, Miaskowski C, and

Rostad M, editors: *Guidelines for oncology nursing practice,* ed 2, Philadelphia, 1991, WB Saunders.

8. Flannery M: Reproductive cancers. In Clark JC and McGee RF, editors: *Core curriculum for oncology nursing,* Philadelphia, 1992, WB Saunders.

9. Hoskins WJ, Perez C, and Young RC: Gynecologic tumors. In DeVita VT Jr., Hellman S, and Rosenberg SA, editors: Cancer: *Principles and practice of oncology* ed 4, Philadelphia, 1993, JB Lippincott.

10. Martin LK and Braly PS: Gynecologic cancers. In Baird SB, McCorkle R, and Grant M, editors: *Cancer nursing: A comprehensive textbook,* Philadelphia, 1991, WB Saunders.

11. Otte DM: Gynecologic cancers. In Groenwald Sl, Frogge MH, Goodman M, and Yarboro CH, editors: *Cancer nursing: Principles and practice,* ed 2, Boston, 1990, Jones and Bartlett.

12. Spencer MM: Bowel elimination, alteration in: Diversional methods. In McNally JC, Somerville ET, Miaskowski C, and Rostad M, editors: *Guidelines for oncology nursing practice,* ed 2, Philadelphia, 1991, WB Saunders.

13. Spencer MM: Urinary elimination, alteration in: Diversional methods. In McNally JC, Somerville ET, Miaskowski C, and Rostad M, editors: *Guidelines for oncology nursing practice,* ed 2, Philadelphia, 1991, WB Saunders.

14. Swihart J: Bowel elimination, alteration in: Bowel obstruction. In McNally JC, Somerville ET, Miaskowski C, and Rostad M, editors: *Guidelines for oncology nursing practice,* ed 2, Philadelphia, 1991, WB Saunders.

15. Tombes MB: Gynecologic malignancies. In Baird SB, Donehower MG, Stalsbroten VL, and Ades TB, editors: *A cancer source book for nurses,* Atlanta, 1991, American Cancer Society.

16. Young RC, Fuks A, and Hoskins WJ: Cancer of the ovary. In DeVita VT Jr., Hellman S, and Rosenberg SA, editors: *Cancer: Principles and practice of oncology,* ed 4, Philadelphia, 1993, JB Lippincott.

Head and Neck Cancers

12

Epidemiology and Etiology

Carcinoma of the upper aerodigestive tract accounts for 5% of all human tumors, with 95% of cases being of squamous cell histology. These tumors typically occur in patients between the ages of 40 and 70 years. The most common sites are the oral cavity and the larynx. At the time of diagnosis, the majority of patients have locally advanced (Stage III and IV) cancer.

Various etiologic factors implicated in the incidence of head and neck cancer are mustard gas, nitrosamines, tobacco use, asbestos, ethyl alcohol and radiation exposure.

Prevention, Screening, and Detection

Major risk factors for the development of cancer in the oral cavity, pharynx, and larynx include the use of tobacco products (smoked and smokeless) and alcohol. Each factor alone accounts for a two- or threefold increase in risk; jointly they can increase the risk more than 15 times that of persons who neither smoke nor drink. Evidence indicates that certain types of human viruses, such as the papilloma virus and herpes simplex virus (HSV), may be involved in the development of cancers in the aerodigestive tract. Because there are no effective screening and detection methods, prevention related to minimizing risks and exposures to above mentioned etiology factors are the key.

Classification

Carcinomas arising in the head and neck region are classified according to anatomic regions rather than cell type. These regions include: (1) nasal cavity, (2) nasopharynx, (3) oral cavity, (4) oropharynx, (5) larynx, and (6) hypopharynx. Each region is subdivided into specific sites (Table 12-1).

Table 12-1 Major Subdivisions of Aerodigestive Tract

Site	Function	Anatomic Relationship	Clinical Features
Oral cavity	Maintain oral competency for swallowing, articulation	Sensory-motor innervation of tongue is bilateral. Central chamber of salivary system. Sensory innervation mediated by lingual nerve (V). Motor innervation to muscles by hypoglossal nerve (XII). Lymphatic drainage to submaxillary and upper cervical lymph nodes and retropharyngeal lymph nodes	Early symptoms: painless "white spot," persistent ulcerations, difficulty with denture fit, difficulty swallowing, blood-tinged sputum
Oropharynx	Mouth and pharynx perform together in alimentary functions of swallowing, emesis, and respiratory functions of crying, speaking, coughing, and yawning	Boundaries include soft palate, tonsils, tonsillar fossa, base of tongue. Glossopharyngeal nerve (IX) mediates motor and sensory innervation to pharynx and posterior one third of tongue. Soft palate and pharynx innervated by vagus nerve (X)	Irregular ulcerations of the mucosal surfaces, painless growth, dysphagia, pain on swallowing, otalgia, persistent sore throat

		Lymphatic drainage to jugulodigastric (tonsillar) node, retropharyngeal lymph nodes	Late symptoms: speech difficulties, palatal resultant incompetence with nasal regurgitation, dysphagia with or without aspiration, trismus
Nasal cavity	Conditions inspired air before entrance— olfaction humidification, temperature control, cleansing, antibacterial and antiviral protection	First cranial nerve (olfactory) innervates mucous membranes to mediate a sense of smell Drain into submandibular nodes	Similar to chronic sinusitis
Nasopharynx	Anatomic boundary that lies behind nasal cavities and above soft palate	Open space situated just below base of skull behind nasal cavity. Inferior wall is bordered by soft palate, pharyngeal orifice of Eustachian tube, abducens nerve (VI), oculomotor nerve (III), trochlear nerve (IV), optic nerve (II)	Persistent poorly localized frontal headaches; temporal, parietal, orificial pain; decreased hearing, tinnitus; multiple nerve palsies, sensory losses

Continued.

Table 12-1 Cont'd.

Site	Function	Anatomic Relationship	Clinical Features
		Behind Eustachian tube lies internal carotid artery, internal jugular vein, and glossopharyngeal (IX), vagus (X), accessory (XI), and hypoglossal (XII) nerves Lymph node chain that drains these areas: posterior cervical triangles, supraclavicular nodes, jugular chain	Blood in a postnasal drip is very significant Profuse epistaxis is an infrequent presenting symptom
Paranasal sinuses	Air-filled cavities within bones of the skull lined by mucous membranes that drain into nasal cavities	Four pair/maxillary, ethmoid, frontal, sphenoid tumors drain into submaxillary, retropharyngeal, jugular lymph nodes	Chronic sinusitis, bump on hard palate, swelling numbness and/or pain in cheek, swelling gums, toothache, increased lacrimation, visual changes—diplopia exophthalmus

Hypopharynx	Anatomic boundary extending from tip of epiglottis to lower border of cricoid cartilage	Persistent unilateral rhinorrhea—epistaxis
	Structures are important for swallowing, airway protection	Painless enlarged cervical lymph nodes. Odynophagia accompanied by progressive dysphagia and rapid weight loss
	Lower subdivision of oropharynx also called laryngopharynx divided into (1) pyriform sinuses, (2) posterior cricoid area; posterior and lateral pharyngeal walls	Otalgia on same side as tumor
	Pharyngeal constrictions innervated by glossopharyngeal (IX) and vagus (X) nerves	Hoarseness, dysphagia
	Lymphatic drainage—primary along internal jugular vein, retropharyngeal and paratracheal nodes	

Continued.

Table 12-1 Cont'd.

Site	Function	Anatomic Relationship	Clinical Features
Larynx	Serves for speech production, maintaining airway, airway protection	Located directly below hypopharynx; sensory innervation supplied from internal laryngeal branch of superior laryngeal nerve of vagus and recurrent laryngeal nerve. Divided into three anatomic sites: (1) supraglottic, (2) glottic, and (3) subglottic. Lymph drainage to anterior jugular nodes	Persistent hoarseness; change in quality, pitch, voice; pain; hemoptysis; dysphagia; cough; aspiration
Salivary glands	Production of saliva	Divided into major glands—paired parotid, submandibular, sublingual, and minor salivary glands	Painless, rapidly growing mass with or without associated nerve paralysis

| | | | Lymphatic drainage usually to deep jugular or intraglandular or paraglandular lymph nodes; innervation of this area includes mandibular branch of 7th cranial, lingual, and hypoglossal nerve (XII) | Neck pain, tightness or fullness in neck, hoarseness, dysphagia, dyspnea |
| Thyroid gland | Endocrine gland | Highly vascular gland located in anterior and lower part of neck. Composed of an isthmus, the small central part and two lateral lobes; the isthmus covers second, third and fourth tracheal rings; thyroid related medially to esophagus and recurrent laryngeal nerve and laterally to carotid sheath, containing carotid artery, internal jugular vein and vagus nerve. Lymphatic drainage of thyroid gland mainly by lymphatic vessels that accompany arterial blood supply | | |

Diagnosis and Staging

Thorough oral, head and neck examination, specified x-rays, incisional biopsy or triple endoscopy (laryngoscopy, flexible esophagoscopy, and bronchoscopy) with multiple biopsies, are obtained to diagnose the disease. See Chapter 4.

Prior to treatment interventions for surgery and/or radiation therapy, a detailed assessment including pulmonary function, psychosocial and nutritional status, communication and cognitive motor skills, and a thorough dental assessment is essential.

Treatment Modalities

Surgical Procedures

The primary goal of surgery is to remove primary disease and all metastatic lymph nodes to control local disease and prevent recurrent disease. Secondary goals are to preserve structure and function and maximize the cosmetic and functional outcome. Reconstructive surgeries (e.g., skinflaps/grafts) require multiple sequential interventions.

Multiple surgical procedures for head and neck cancers may be selected:

- Laryngectomy (Table 12-3)
- Classic complete radical dissection (Table 12-4)
- Modified neck dissection
- Reconstruction

Moderate-sized defects may require skin grafting or local skin flaps. There are several types of flaps available for reconstruction: (1) tongue flaps are used to cover internal mucosal defects such as floor of mouth, pharyngeal wall, or cheek; (2) skin flaps consist of skin, subcutaneous tissues, and fascia of the underlying muscle; and (3) myocutaneous flaps incorporate an island of desired skin, underlying subcutaneous tissue, and fascia severed from surrounding tissues (Table 12-2).

Side effects related to the above mentioned procedures include:
Surgery
- Potential for structural, functional, or cosmetic loss: e.g., changes in bodily appearance and function (breathing, speaking, swallowing, coughing, and mobility)

- Respiratory distress; hypoxia, airway obstruction, tracheal edema, aspiration; hemorrhage; hematoma; arterial rupture; failure of flap survival; nerve damage

General considerations

- Patients with head and neck cancers receiving multi-modality therapy may experience severe and permanent facial disfigurement and functional loss that resembles what is experienced by burn patients.

Table 12-2 Factors that Affect Surgeon's Choice of Flaps

Tissue Considerations	Physician Considerations
Size of arc	Will flap cover defect?
Vascular supply	Will flap survive?
Accessibility	How close to defect is new tissue?
Donor site	Functional loss/contour of donor site
Sensation	Maintain nerve supply

Radiation Therapy

Treatment planning is based on the nature, size, location, and growth of the tumor, volume of disease, organs to be spared, and purpose of treatment. Radiation energies at or above 1 million V or radioactive isotopes are usually the primary source of treatment in head and neck cancers. Preoperative radiation is usually given for 1 month, followed by a 1-month rest period, which allows time for acute tissue reaction to subside. Radiation treatments are usually given about 3 or 4 weeks after surgery to allow wound healing. Treatment usually lasts 6 to 8 weeks. In addition to external beam radiation, radioactive isotopes and intracavitary implants are sources of radiation that may be applied closely to tumors by hollow containers loaded with radioactive sources.

Complications of Radiation Therapy

- Mucositis
- Infection
- Dermatitis
- Pain
- Fungal infection
- Xerostomia

- Radiation caries
- Trismus

- Osteoradionecrosis
- Dysgeusia

Chemotherapy

Chemotherapeutic drugs that have demonstrated significant activity in head and neck cancer include methotrexate bleomycin, Oncovin, cisplatin, carboplatin, and 5-fluorouracil (5-FU). Chemotherapy sequencing and timing may be given in four ways: induction, concurrent, sandwich (after surgery—before radiotherapy) and maintenance.

Side effects related to these therapies are mucositis, infection, dehydration, weight loss, nausea, vomiting, diarrhea and electrolyte imbalance.

Rehabilitation

Ongoing assessment and evaluation of response to treatment are essential for early diagnosis of disease and validation of health. Routine follow-up of patients should include thorough examination of head and neck with indirect laryngoscopy once a month for the first year, every 2 months during the second year, and every 3 months in the fifth year after treatment. Patients with new symptoms of significant weight loss, dysphagia, chronic soreness, or persistent hoarseness should have an endoscopic examination with biopsy when tumor is not visible by examination.

Recurrent Disease

Recurrent head and neck cancer is a failure to the standard definitive local therapy. Approximately 40% of patients overall will suffer a recurrence; 20% locoregionally, 10% with distant metastasis, and another 10% with both local and distant disease. Many of these patients relapse within 6 to 24 months after treatment and have a median survival rate of 6 months from initial diagnosis to recurrence.

Table 12-3 Functional Loss Associated with Laryngectomy

Procedure	Structures Removed	Structures Remaining	Functions
Total laryngectomy Loss of laryngeal sphincter mechanism may lead to aspiration. Swallowing mechanism must be intact so that when food lands on vocal cords, patient coughs to get it out and swallows instantly	Hyoid bone Entire larynx Epiglottis, false, true cords Cricoid cartilage Two/three rings of trachea	Tongue Pharyngeal walls Lower trachea	Loss of voice (resulting from tracheolaryngectomy Normal swallowing
Supraglottic/horizontal laryngectomy—partial During supraglottic laryngectomy, muscles that elevate larynx are transected, thereby limiting elevation of larynx	Hyoid bone Epiglottis False cords	True cords Cricoid cartilage Trachea	Normal voice Increased risk for aspiration Normal airway

Continued.

Table 12-3 Cont'd.

Procedure	Structures Removed	Structures Remaining	Functions
This, along with loss of supraglottic structures, further downgrades swallowing. Because cough is necessary to clear larynx, patient's pulmonary functions must be adequate			
Hemivertical laryngectomy Interferes very little with swallowing. Removal of arytenoid cartilage may cause aspiration in small percentage of patients. Free or pedicled muscle or submucosal cartilage grafts may prevent aspiration	One true cord, one false cord Arytenoid cartilage One half thyroid cartilage	Epiglottis One true cord, one false cord Cricoid	Hoarse but serviceable voice Normal airway Normal swallowing

If surgical resection extends to base of tongue, swallowing may be affected related to inability to move bolus. Aspiration may occur

Partial laryngectomy laryngo-fissure
Potential to affect predominantly deglutition and phonation

| | One vocal cord | All other structures | Hoarse, but serviceable voice
Normal airway
Normal swallowing |

Table 12-4 Radical Neck Procedures

Procedure	Structures Removed	Advantage	Disadvantage
Classic, Complete, Radical Bilateral or unilateral (Crile, 1906)	Unilateral cervical nodes Submaxillary salivary gland, tail of parotid gland Internal jugular vein Connective tissue of carotid sheath, all lymph nodes, and lymph-bearing tissues of anterior, posterior triangles, and deep jugular chain en bloc Transverse cervical vessels/carotid Spinal accessory nerve and associated lymphatic chain with deep layers of cervical fascia Vagus, hypoglossal, phrenic lingual	Low probability of leaving nodal disease behind	Trapezius muscle dysfunction with shoulder drop; resulting in pain and limitation in motion Mild to moderate neck deformity If bilateral procedure is performed, cerebral edema can persist Painful neuromas can occur Loss of carotid artery

Modified Neck Dissection Approximately six variations (Bocca, 1967)	Selective removal or preservation of spinal accessory nerve (Roy: Bearns) Only lymphatic structures removed Sternocleidomastoid muscle usually saved Carotid sheath opened: internal jugular vein saved	Low incidence of shoulder drop and shoulder disability Carotid artery not sacrificed Cosmetic deformity not as severe as CNN If cervical plexus is preserved, decreased incidence of sensory deficit and painful neuromas	Possible omission of occult positive nodes. Increased risk of hematoma under sternocleidomastoid muscle Increased risk of surgeon cutting into positive nodes and seeding neck

Nursing Management

Nursing Care Guidelines

- Patients undergoing head and neck surgery

Nursing Diagnoses

- *Knowledge deficit related to surgery, preoperative/post-operative procedures*
- *Self-care deficit, related to postoperative treatments*
- *Anxiety related to surgical experience and unpredictable outcome*

Preoperative Interventions

- Review purpose of surgery and rationale (temporary, permanent)
- Explain common terms and procedures, provide written literature (show videos), and show actual equipment
- Discuss potential sequelae of surgery:
    Change in bodily appearance
    Change in bodily function (e.g., breathing, speaking, swallowing, coughing, mobility)
- Explain roles of various medical and nursing personnel and purpose of visits
- Instruct and have patient give verbal return demonstration on all self-care: coughing, deep breathing, ambulation

Postoperative Interventions

- Instruct patient on self-care behaviours
- Discharge patient with written instructions:
    Specific self-care behaviors (e.g., tracheostomy laryngectomy care exercise, wound management, oral dental hygiene)
    Emergency procedures
    Home care referral

Nursing Diagnoses

- *Breathing patterns, altered, related to diversional methods (tracheotomy, laryngectomy)*
- *Airway clearance, ineffective, related to tracheal edema, secretions*
- *Injury, potential for: related hematoma formation between flap and underlying tissue*
- *Tissue perfusion, alteration in: related to arterial erosion rupture around/at surgical site*
- *Skin integrity, impairment of: actual, related to surgery flap reconstruction, flap failure*
- *Swallowing, impaired, related to superior laryngeal nerve injury, loss or weakness of tongue*

Postoperative Interventions

- Monitor signs & symptoms of respiratory distress
- Monitor signs & symptoms of hematoma
- Monitor signs & symptoms of infection: drainage/odor
- Monitor wound and surrounding tissue for signs and symptoms of arterial erosion/rupture:
  Evidence of arterial erosion
  Color (red, pallor, black)
  Vascularity
  Temperature changes
  Edema
  Turgor
- Monitor signs and symptoms of thoracic duct leakage:
  Milky white drainage often mixed with serous fluid in drainage tubes
- Monitor signs and symptoms of fluid and electrolyte imbalance
- Monitor signs and symptoms of nerve injury:
  Superior laryngeal nerve (dysphagia swallowing impairment)
  Recurrent laryngeal nerve
  (bilateral pareses requires immediate tracheostomy)
  Lingual nerve (numbness on ipsilateral tongue can occur if severed)

Hypoglossal nerve (if severed, unilateral tongue paralysis results, causes impairment of speech, mastication)

Glossopharyngeal nerve (altered taste sensation, difficulty in swallowing)

Facial nerve (droop or asymmetry of musculature around the mouth)

Phrenic nerve (if severed, paralysis of diaphragm can result)

Spinal accessory nerve (painful shoulder, droopy atrophy of trapezius muscle)

- Monitor signs and symptoms of infection:
  Tenderness
  Thickness
  Moisture

- Monitor signs and symptoms of flap reconstructive failure:
  Monitor wound, flap, surrounding tissue every 2 hours x 72, then every 4 hours

  Color (redness, pallor, cyanosis), tension, kinking, pressure, hematoma

  Vascularity (presence or absence of blanching)

  Temperature (warm, cool, unilateral)

  Edema (presence or absence)

  Turgor (taut, mobile, shiny, wrinkled)

  Odor (not malodorous)

  "Red Flap"—Appears bright red and, when tested for capillary filling, will feel tense or thick on digital palpation

  "White Flap"—One with limited or no blood supply. Tension, constriction, pressure, or occlusion can cause stop of blood flow. Cool to touch and becomes white.

  "Blue Flap"—Occurs when input of blood exceeds output. Imbalance occurs when arterial pressure remains the same and venous pressure increases. Related to the patient lying on flap, tight pressure dressing, or formation of a clot at venous anastomotic site

Normal tissue/flaps will be warm to touch. Recovers color slowly after testing for blanching. Flaps will have fine wrinkles—indication of minimal edema
Abnormal findings indicate circulatory embarassment, venous congestion. Shiny, taut, reddish. After testing for blanching, flap will recover color quickly

Nursing Care Guidelines

- Patients undergoing radiation therapy for head and neck cancer

Nursing Diagnoses

- *Alteration in oral mucous membrane*
- *Comfort, alteration*
- *Injury, potential for, related to oral hygiene*
- *Potential health maintenance, alteration*

Interventions

- Review purpose of radiation therapy and rationale for treatment
- Explain common terms and procedures, provide written literature, and show actual equipment (light cast molds/bite blocks). Patient will need to be familiar with terminology/equipment. Simulation/dosimetry port films, cobalt/linear accelerator implants
- Discuss potential sequelae of radiation:
    Change in bodily appearance (e.g., skin)
    Change in bodily function (e.g., mucositis, xerostomia, swallowing)
    Potential for infection
    Potential for radiation caries
    Potential for soft tissue and osteoradionecrosis
    Nutritional stomatitis and taste loss
    Trismus
- Explain roles of various medical, nursing personnel, technicians, doismetrists, and purpose of visits
- Instruct and have patient give verbal/return demonstration on all self-care:
    Oral hygiene (for dentulous and edentulous patients)

- Provide instructions for dentulous patients
- Provide instructions for edentulous patients
- Instruct dentulous and edentulous patients to rinse mouth often
- Instruct patient to report to physician/nurse/dentist as early as possible, regarding clinical problems related to:

  Xerostomia   Infection

  Loss of taste   Pain

  Inability to maintain nutritional intake or hydration
- Monitor signs and symptoms for infections and trisomas, tissue necrosis, mucositis, xerostomia, radiation caries

Geriatric Consideration

- *Age-related losses* such as vision, hearing, communication, fine motor skills (writing), and swallowing/eating functions will be further compromised by effects of surgery/radiation therapy and/or chemotherapy
- *Nutritional and dental assessment* with appropriate interventions will need to be adapted to age-related changes (diet history-likes/dislikes; dentures and/or lack of due to age or finances)
- *Pretreatment evaluation*: psychosocial, cardiopulmonary, health history will require age-related adjustments and appropriate interventions
- *Treatment-related factors*: surgery, radiation therapy, chemotherapy, and rehabilitation will require age-related adjustments and appropriate interventions. Patients with chronic diseases such as hypertension, cardiopulmonary insufficiency, diabetes, chronic obstructive pulmonary disease, arthritis, and chronic renal disease will require medical treatment adjustments

  Surgery: potential for longer recovery and rehabilitation period

  Radiation therapy: treatment schedule may require adjustment for recovery of side effects; fatigue/immunosuppression, weight loss, stomatitis, and infection

  Chemotherapy: drug dosage, frequency of infusion, and monitoring of blood count will require adjustment

(drug toxicities may increase related to aforementioned chronic disease)
- Transportation, financial, family resources, and home care responsibilities will require assessment and intervention based on deficits and/or availability

---

Bibliography

1. Aaronson NK and Beckman J: *The quality of life for cancer patients*, New York, 1987, Raven Press.
2. Baker SR, editor: *Microsurgical reconstruction of the head and neck*, New York, 1989, Churchill Livingstone.
3. Belcher AE: *Nursing aspects of quality of life enhancement in cancer patients*, Oncol 4(5):197-199, 1990.
4. Cook TA and others: *Cervical rotation flaps for midface resurfacing*, Arch Otolaryngol Head Neck Surg 117:77-82, 1991.
5. DeSanto L and Beahrs OH: The modified and radical neck dissection for squamous cell carcinoma of the upper aerodigestive system. In Jacobs J and others, editors: *Scientific and clinical perspective of head and neck cancer management strategies for cure*, New York, 1987, Elsevier.
6. Dudas S and Carlson CE: *Cancer rehabilitation,* Oncol Nurs Forum 15:183, 1988.
7. Elias EG: Surgical management of head and neck neoplasia. In Peterson DE and others, editors: *Head and neck management of the cancer patient*, Boston, 1986, Martinus Nijhoff.
8. Germino B: Cancer and the family. In Baird SB, McCorkle R, and Grant M, editors: *Cancer nursing: A comprehensive textbook*, Philadelphia, 1991, WB Saunders.
9. Giunta JL: Pathology of malignancy. In Peterson DE and others, editors: *Head and neck management of the cancer patient,* Boston, 1986, Martinus Nijhoff.
10. Gotay C: Research in cancer rehabilitation. In McGarvey C, editor: *Physical therapy for the cancer patient,* New York, 1990, Churchill Livingstone.

11. Hooper JA and Sigler BA: Nursing care of the head and neck cancer patient. In Myers EN and Suen JY, editors: *Cancer of the head and neck*, New York, 1988, Churchill Livingstone.

12. Johnston JL and Lane CA: Helping families respond to cancer. In Baird SB, McCorkle R, and Grant M, editors: *Cancer nursing: a comprehensive text book*, Philadelphia, 1991, WB Saunders.

13. Kramer S and others: *Combined radiation therapy and surgery in the management of advanced head and neck cancer: final report of Study 73-03 of the Radiation Therapy Oncology Group,* Head Neck Surg:19, 1987.

14. Mendenhall W, Parson SJ, Mendenhall N, and Million R: *Brachy therapy in head and neck cancer: Selection criteria and results at the University of Florida*, Oncology 5(1):87-93, 1991.

15. Mendenhall W and others: T*he role of radiation therapy in laryngeal cancer,* CA 40(3):150-165, 1990.

16. Muldooney JB, Cohen JJ, Porto DD and Maisel RH: *Oral cavity reconstruction using the free arm radial flap,* Arch Otolaryngol Head Neck Surg 13:1219-1224, 1987.

17. Netterville JL and Wood DE: *The lower trapezius flap vascular anatomy and surgical technique,* Arch Otolaryngol Head Neck Surg 117:73, 1991.

18. Rirken M and others: *Rectus abdominis free flap in head and neck reconstruction.* Arch Otolaryngol Head Neck Surg 117:857-866, 1991.

19. Sigler BA: Nursing care for head and neck tumor patients. In Thrawley SE and Panye WR, editors: *Comprehensive management of head and neck tumors,* Philadelphia, 1987, WB Saunders.

20. Sonis ST: Oral complication of cancer therapy. In DeVita VT, Hellman S, Rosenberg SA, editors: *Cancer: principles and practice of Oncology,* ed 4, Philadelphia, 1993, JB Lippincott.

21. Taylor I, Graeme D, Miller M, and Ham F: *Free vascularized bone graft: plastic and reconstruction of patients with oral cancer,* Oral Surg Oral Med Path 68(4):449-504, 1992.

22. Urken MD and others: *Rectus abdommis free flap in head and neck reconstruction*, Arch Otolaryngol Head Neck Surg 117:501-511, 1991.
23. Welch-McCaffery D and others: *Surviving adult cancers: Part 2—psychosocial implications,* Ann Intern Med 111:517-524, 1989.
24. Wells R: Rehabilitation: *Making the most of time,* Oncol Nurs Forum 17:503-507, 1990.
25. Weing B and Keller AJ: *Microvascular free flap reconstruction for head and neck defects,* Arch Otolaryngol Head Neck Surg 115:118-120, 1989.

HIV and Related Cancers

13

Human Immunodeficiency Virus (HIV)

Epidemiology

HIV infection has occurred in approximately 3 million Americans and progressed to AIDS in 339,250. This epidemic has killed 204,390 Americans, and the numbers increase daily. Throughout the world, more than 12 million people are infected with HIV and nearly 2 million have progressed to an AIDS diagnosis. It is estimated that greater than one million people have died of AIDS worldwide. Estimates of worldwide infection rates suggest approximately 40 million infections by the year 2000.[3,4,8]

Etiology and Risk Factors

The causative agent of AIDS is infection with HIV. HIV is a human retrovirus and belongs to the lentivirus subfamily. Currently, five human retroviruses have been identified: HTLV-1, HTLV-2, HTLV-5, HIV-1, and HIV-2. HTLV-2 has not been conclusively associated with human disease. HTLV-1 and HTLV-5 have been associated with human T-cell leukemia and lymphoma, conditions characterized by proliferation of CD4+ (T4) helper cells. HIV-1 and HIV-2 both cause depletion of T4 helper cells, resulting in loss of cellular immunity, characterized by AIDS. HIV-1 is the predominant cause of AIDS in the United States, accounting for greater than 95% of AIDS cases. HIV-2 seems to be limited to geographic distribution and is most prevalent in West Africa.

The routes for transmission of HIV are well documented: (1) intimate sexual contact; (2) parenteral exposure to blood, blood-containing body fluids and blood products; and (3) from mother to child during the perinatal period. Transmission has also been associated with breast milk. The natural history of HIV infection is associated with an unpredictable course of disease progression. Most patients undergo a prolonged period of clinically silent infection, often lasting for more than 10 years.

Opportunistic infections associated with the disease include a wide variety of organisms such as viruses (herpes simplex, Epstein-Barr, cytomegalovirus), protozoans *(Pneumocystis carinii,* toxoplasma), mycobacteria (tuberculosis and avium complex), and fungi (histoplasma, cryptococci). The profound immune dysfunction also allows for the development of several neoplasms including non-Hodgkin's lymphoma, Kaposi's sarcoma, and cervical carcinomas.[1,4,9]

Prevention, Screening, and Detection

Safe Sex Counseling

Any exchange of blood, semen, or vaginal secretions can potentially put an individual at risk for HIV disease. Common sexual practices that are risky behaviors include vaginal or anal penetration without a condom and possibly oral sexual practices. Use of barrier products such as latex condoms while engaging in these behaviors markedly reduces the likelihood of exposure to potentially infectious blood, semen, or vaginal secretions. Minimizing the number of sexual partners and engaging in a mutually monogamous sexual relationship also reduces one's risk.[17]

Intravenous Risk Reduction

The use of contaminated needles for subcutaneous, intramuscular, or intravenous injection represents a serious risk for HIV infection.

Perinatal Transmission

Women who are HIV-infected may pass the virus on to their newborns via three potential routes: during gestation, during delivery, and via breastfeeding.

Public Health Measures

Currently, each unit of donated blood is tested for HIV infection as well as several other blood-borne infections such as hepatitis. Because HIV screening of blood products has been conducted since 1985 in the United States, only recipients of transfusions prior to this time are at significant risk of infection via the blood supply.

Screening

The most common form of screening for HIV disease is the use of the antibody test with the enzyme-linked immunosorbent assay (ELISA) technique and with the Western blot technique. The ELISA is highly sensitive and specific with a sensitivity of 98.4 to 99.6%. A positive ELISA test must be confirmed by the Western blot technique. Since newborn infants maintain maternal antibodies for as long as 18 months, antibody testing is unreliable until the infant is 18 months of age. A newer test, the polymerase chain reaction (PCR) is now available.[5,14]

Clinical Features

- Viral syndrome resembling mononucleosis or influenza
- Persistent generalized lymphadenopathy
- Dermatologic manifestations—seborrhea
- Opportunistic infections, malignancies
- Unexplained weight loss greater than 10%
- Persistent fever, diarrhea, or night sweats

Table 13-1 lists specific clinical features of various opportunistic infections.

Diagnosis and Staging

The CDC Classification System for HIV infection in adults is currently the most widely used staging system. See Chapter 4.

Metastasis

HIV disease is a chronic, systemic infection of lymphocytes, monocytes and macrophages, and possible muscle and nerve cells. As the disease progresses, nearly every organ system is affected by one or more of the opportunisitic infections that occur secondarily to the profound immune deficiency resulting from the original HIV infection. The majority of patients experience illness affecting the skin and mucous membranes, the respiratory tract, the gastrointestinal tract, and the central nervous system.[5]

Table 13-1 Opportunistic Infections

Opportunistic Infection	Clinical Features
Bacterial Infections	
Mycobacterium avium	General: persistent fever, night sweats, fatigue, weight loss, abdominal pain, weakness, lymphadenopathy, hepatosplenomegaly
Fungal Infections	
Candidiasis	Oral: white patches on tongue or buccal mucosa
	Vaginal: vulvar pruritus, vaginal discharge
Cryptococcosis	Meningitis: headache, fever, progressive malaise, altered mental status, seizures
	Pneumonia: fever, shortness of breath, cough
Histoplasmosis	Fever, weight loss, shortness of breath, lymphadenopathy
Protozoal Infections	
Cryptosporidiosis	Diarrhea, abdominal cramping, nausea, vomiting, fatigue, weight loss, dehydration
Pneumocystis	Pneumonia: fever, nonproductive cough, shortness of breath, weight loss, night sweats, fatigue
Toxoplasmosis	Encephalitis: altered mental status, seizures, fever, coma
Viral Infections	
Cytomegalovirus	Retinitis: unilateral visual deficit or change
	Gastrointestinal: dysphagia, wasting, nausea, fever, diarrhea
Herpes simplex	Painful blisters or ulcers

Treatment Modalities

Chemotherapy

Because of the variabality of the disease progression, immune system surveillance on a regular basis is an important component of HIV treatment. It is recommended that patients with stable T4 helper counts above 500/mm^3 undergo a physical examination and laboratory evaluation every 3 to 6 months. Currently, the T4 helper count is the single most important indicator in tracking progressive deterioration of immune system function in HIV infected individuals. If the T4 helper cell count falls below 500 cells/mm^3, initiation of antiretroviral therapy is indicated. Zidovudine (also called Retrovir or AZT) was the first drug approved to treat HIV infection and remains the first choice of therapy for patients with less than 500/mm^3 T4 helper cells. If patients fail to tolerate zidovudine, or the disease progresses despite zidovudine therapy, two other similar drugs are now available: Didanosine (also called ddI or Videx) and Zalcitabine (also called ddC or Hivid).[5,7,15]

Biotherapy

Use of colony stimulating factors (CSFs) such as granulocyte and granulocyte-monocyte colony stimulating factors (G-CSF and GM-CSF) have proven useful in decreasing myelotoxity.[11]

Prognosis

Although HIV disease appears to be a universally fatal illness, the time to progression of profound immune deficiency varies widely among patients. Mortality rates in the United States currently approach 80% within 2 years of an AIDS diagnosis, and may be even higher in undeveloped countries where treatment is virtually nonexistent.[9]

HIV-Related Cancers

Kaposi's Sarcoma

Kaposi's sarcoma (KS) remains the most common neoplasm in HIV-infected patients.

Epidemiology, Etiology and Risk Factors

Although all types of patients with AIDS have been found to have KS (heterosexual, homosexual, and IVDU), the incidence is greatest among homosexual HIV positive men. KS is a multifocal neoplasm, capable of arising simultaneously at multiple sites. It is suspected that AIDS-KS may not be secondary to infection with HIV disease itself, but may, in fact, be another sexually transmitted infection. Cytomegalovirus has long been suspectred as a possible etiology. Other immunodeficient states such as iatrogencially induced immunosuppression, as seen in renal transplant patients, have also been the setting for KS.[12]

Prevention, Screening and Detection

As with the prevention of HIV disease, prevention of KS must involve barrier protection such as condoms and avoidance of potentially infectious body fluids, including blood, semen, and vaginal secretions. Since HIV-infected patients are at a significant risk for AIDS-KS, all HIV patients should be screened routinely for potential signs and symptoms of KS.

Classification

AIDS-KS (also called epidemic KS) is usually characterized by multifocal, widespread lesions at the onset of the illness. It has a wide range of virulence in patients with HIV disease, ranging from limited stable involvement to fulminant disease with rapid, continuous development of new lesions. AIDS-KS is usually classified based on the site of lesions. Nodular KS is characterized by subcutaneous nodular lesions that vary in size from several millimeters to several centimeters in diameter. Lymphadeno-pathic KS primarily affects the peripheral lymph nodes. Oral KS lesions can produce bleeding, tooth displacement, and pain. Visceral KS most commonly affects the lungs and gastrointestinal tract.

Clinical Features

Most patients present with skin lesions appearing as flat or raised plaques ranging in size from a few millimeters to several centimeters. Colors range from blue-purple to red-brown. Although lymph node involvement occurs frequently, it is often difficult to distinguish from HIV-associated lymphadenopathy. Other clinical features include: diarrhea, blood loss, weight loss, cough, dyspnea, and fever.

Diagnosis and Staging

AIDS-KS is generally diagnosed by examining biopsies of skin or mucous membrane lesions. AIDS-KS involving the lungs or gastrointestinal tract is usually diagnosed by endoscopic examination. Critical elements include: extent of the tumor, status of the immune system, and presence or absence of other HIV-related disease manifestations. See Chapter 4.

Metastasis

A rapid course with short survival is seen in patients with opportunistic infections, systemic symptoms, and low T4 helper cell counts. This rapid course is typically associated with aggressive, disseminated disease involving the lungs and visceral organs.

Treatment Modalities

Curative therapy for AIDS-KS does not exist. AIDS-KS, however, is rarely life-threatening. Most patients with AIDS-KS ultimately die of opportunistic infections related to the profound immunodeficiency produced by HIV infection. Treatment of AIDS-KS is, therefore, usually instituted for the relief of symptoms and to eliminate or reduce cosmetically unacceptable lesions. Local modalities include surgical excision, electrodesiccation, and radiation therapy.

KS is generally very responsive to radiation therapy, and good palliation can usually be obtained. Excellent responses can be obtained in treatment of cutaneous KS using whole-body electron beam therapy, fractionated focal x-ray therapy, or single dose treatments. Radiation therapy is particularly useful when a prompt local response is desired.

Chemotherapy is most appropriate for patients who have relatively limited disease and for those with relatively intact immune function. Single agent chemotherapy can produce cosmetic and symptomatic improvement with little toxicity or significant immune impairment. Single agent chemotherapy regimens may employ vinblastine, bleomycin, VP-16, or doxorubicin. Combination regimens may include: vinblastine and vincristine; vinblastine and bleomycin; doxorubicin, bleomycin, and vinblastine; doxorubicin, bleomycin, and vincristine; or vinblastine, vincristine and methotrexate.[5,7,14]

Prognosis

Although curative therapy for AIDS-KS does not yet exist, KS is rarely life threatening. Most patients with AIDS-KS ultimately die of opportunistic infections resulting from the profound immunodefiency that develops secondary to HIV infection.

Non-Hodgkin's Lymphoma (NHL)

Epidemiology

It has been estimated that of the approximately 45,000 cases of NHL to be diagnosed in 1994, up to 30% will occur in individuals infected with HIV. The incidence of NHL among the population with advanced HIV infection has been estimated at 2%. The median age of diagnosis in HIV-related NHL ranges from 26 to 40 years; the median age among HIV negative patients is 56. Clearly, immune suppression as a result of HIV infection is a risk factor in the development of NHL.[3,7]

Etiology and Risk Factors

Pathogenesis of many of these lymphomas has been linked to latent infection of B lymphocytes with the Epstein-Barr virus (EBV). EBV is present in approximately 50% of tumors with monoclonal origins, but not in those of polyclonal origin. In both EBV positive and negative tumors, however, the onset of disease appears related to the degree of immune suppression in the patient created by the original HIV infection.

Prevention, Screening, and Detection

Clinicians should be suspicious toward a NHL diagnosis in any HIV-infected patient who presents with a history of a lump or other masses. A complete blood count is usually normal, although anemia may be present and lymphopenia can occur in as many as 50% of cases. Erthrocyte sedimentation rate and lactic acid dehydrogenase may be elevated.

Classification

NHL in HIV-infected patients are classified similarly to those occurring in noninfected patients. See Chapter 4.

Clinical Features

The most common symptom of NHL is painless lymphadenopathy that may involve the abdominal nodes. Patients may present with systemic B symptoms such as fever, chills, and weight loss. Since extranodal sites such as the gastrointestinal tract, bone marrow, spleen, and liver may be affected, patients may present with symptoms of vague abdominal discomfort, back pain, gastrointestinal complaints, or ascites.

Diagnosis and Staging

A complete physical examination, blood count, and chemistries should be obtained. Abnormal liver function tests may suggest involvement of the hepatic system, and liver biopsy may be indicated. Bone marrow involvement is common in HIV-associated NHL, and bone marrow aspiraton and biposy should be performed early in the diagnostic work-up. Chest x-ray, CAT scan, and MRI may also be ordered.

Metastasis

Most patients present with stage IV disease, which is further complicated by frequent involvement of the bone marrow and central nervous system. In addition, the immunodeficiency and possible history of previous opportunisitic infections may potentiate the aggressive course of the disease. Widely disseminated disease is diagnosed at the time of initial presentation in greater than two thirds of patients.

Treatment Modalities

Standard chemotheraphy doses should be given to patients with T4 helper counts greater than 200/mm^3. Growth factor support is also recommended in this population. For patients with more compromised immune function (with T4 helper cell counts below 200/mm³), reduced dosage chemotherapy regimens are advised, since these patients are less likely to tolerate cytotoxic therapy. The most commonly used regimen is that of mBACOD, which includes methotrexate, bleomycin, doxorubicin, cyclophosphamide, vincristine, dexamethasone, and folinic acid. For patients who are profoundly ill with significantly compromised immune status, the option of only palliative therapy should be considered.[5,15,18]

Prognosis

The prognosis for patients with HIV-associated NHL is poor. Median survival for patients with peripheral NHL treated with a variety of standard chemotherapeutic regimens ranges from 4 to 7 months. For those with CNS involvement, the prognosis is even poorer, with median survival of approximately 2.5 months.

Other HIV Related Malignancies

Primary CNS Lymphoma

Primary CNS lymphoma is of B-cell origin in the majority of reported cases. HIV-infected individuals demonstrate an increased frequency of primary CNS lymphoma, and it is now estimated that its incidence is approaching 6% of all cases of AIDS. Presenting signs and symptoms may include confusion, lethargy, memory loss, hemiparesis or dysphasia, seizures, or headaches. Computer-assisted tomographic brain scanning is usually nonspecific for CNS lymphoma, and lumbar puncture is rarely diagnostic. Open brain biopsy is technically required to confirm the diagnosis. The current treatment approach includes combination radiation therapy and corticosteroids. The prognosis for these individuals remains poor with long-term survival of only a few months.[5,9]

Cervical Cancer

Genital warts in HIV-infected women may exist as multiple small lesions or as unusually large and profuse lesions. External warts often extend to adjacent, moist epithelium, including the vagina, cervix, urethra, and rectum. Cervical dysplasia, the premalignant changes noted on Pap smear screening, can result from HPV infection and can progress to cervical cancer. Cervical dysplasia occurs at an unusually high rate in HIV-infected women at 5 to 10 times the expected rate. Cervical cancer caused by HPV is potentially fatal and is the most serious gynecologic disease for HIV-infected women. In addition, cervical dysplasia and cancer may be more aggressive and persistent among HIV-positive women than among uninfected women. The presence and severity of cervical neoplasia correlates with both absolute number and function of T4 helper cells. Women with more profound immunodeficiency are more likely to have high-grade lesions than are asymptomatic HIV-positive women. Lymph node involvement is common, although markedly enlarged nodes may also result from HIV disease. Women with HIV disease also have higher recurrence and death rates with shorter intervals to recurrence.

For patients with early disease, radical hysterectomy and pelvic lymphadenectomy may be performed safely. In patients with advanced or systemic disease, chemotherapy may be used along with radiation therapy, although careful monitoring of hematologic toxicities must be performed. Drugs that are relatively sparing of the bone marrow, such as cisplatin, bleomycin, and vincristine, may be used.[10,16]

Anal Carcinoma

Anal carcinoma in HIV-infected men is similar to cervical carcinoma in HIV-infected women. Increasing numbers of men with concurrent HIV and HPV infection are now showing signs of intra-anal cytologic abnormalities. Greater than 50% of patients with abnormal anal cytology have been shown to have HPV DNA on specimen. AIN and early stages of anal cancer are usually not associated with any symptoms. Some individuals may notice rapid growth of an external anal lesion or may develop new onset of anal pruritus or other changes in bowel habits. In advanced disease, anal cancer may be associated with weight loss, pelvic pain, and even obstruction of the anal canal. Although the optimal forms of treatment have not been identified, fulguration or cryotherapy of anal lesions through the use of a proctoscope or sigmoidoscope seems reasonable. If the lesion has progressed to anal carcinoma, chemotherapy and possibly radiation therapy may be considered.[13]

Nursing Management

Nursing Diagnosis
- *Potential for infection*[6,17,18]

Interventions
- Carefully monitor vital signs and laboratory results for signs of possible infection
- Institute a low microbial diet for patients with an absolute neutrophil count below 500 cell/cm^3. Patients should receive only pasteurized dairy products and no fresh fruits or vegetables
- Perform appropriate physical assessment including careful examination of skin integrity and respiratory and gastrointestinal status
- Perform appropriate mental status examinations
- Maintain asepsis when caring for patient, including appropriate handwashing, limiting of infectious visitors
- Educate patient in protective strategies such as handwashing, diet precautions such as thorough cooking of meat products, pet care precautions, avoiding rectal thermometers and suppositories

Nursing Diagnosis
- *Self-concept disturbance related to cancerous lesions*

Interventions
- Establish a therapeutic nursing relationship based on acceptance and encouraging open sharing of feelings.
- Identify sources of threats to self-concept
- Educate the patient in the use of self-affirmation techniques
- Facilitate incorporation of past adaptive coping behaviors
- Involve family and significant others in support of the patient
- Utilize multidisciplinary group such as dermatology, psychology, social work, and support groups

- Educate patient in techniques to reduce visibility of lesions
- Assess skin surfaces at least every 8 hours for erythema, breakdown, excessive moisture, or other changes
- Keep skin clean and dry; provide skin care at least every 4 hours
- Provide appropriate beds, mattresses, or other appliances for pressure relief
- Maintain adequate hydration and nutrition
- Utilize multidisciplinary teams including dermatology, and skin care speciality nurses

Patient Teaching Priorities

- Risk Reduction Techniques: Minimize the number of sexual partners and engage in a mutually monogamous sexual relationship
- Safe Sex Counseling: Any exchange of blood, semen, or vaginal secretions can potentially put an individual at risk for HIV disease
- Intravenous Risk Reduction: The use of contaminated needles for any injection represents a serious risk for HIV infection
- Signs and Symptoms of Infectious Process: These include fever, chills, shortness of breath, cough, pain, diarrhea, nausea, vomiting, skin breakdown, weight loss, and a sense of mental confusion
- Self-Help Care Strategies: Know where and when to seek medical, psychosocial, and financial assistance

Bibliography

1. Abrams DI: *Acquired immunodefiency syndrome and related malignancies: A topical overview*, Semin Oncol 18(5):41-45, 1991.
2. ACOG: *Human immunodeficiency virus infections*, ACOG Tech Bull 165:1-11, 1992.
3. American Foundation for AIDS Research: *Statistics*, AIDS Clin Care 4(6):1, 1992.

4. Centers for Disease Control: *Update: Acquired immun-odeficiency syndrome: United States, 1991,* Morbid Mortal Weekly Report 41(16):308-309, 1993.

5. Errante D and others: *Management of AIDS and its neo-plastic complications,* Eur J Cancer 27(3):389-399, 1991.

6. Gee G: AIDS: *Concepts in nursing practice,* Baltimore, 1988, Williams & Wilkins.

7. Kaplan L: *HIV-associated lymphoma,* AIDS File 6(1):6-8, 1992.

8. Lucey D: *The first decade of human retroviruses: A no-menclature for the clinician,* Military Med 156(10):555-557, 1991.

9. Lusso P and Gallo R: *Pathogenesis of AIDS,* J Pharmaceut Pharmacol 44(suppl 1):160-164, 1992.

10. Marte C and Allen M: *HIV-related gynecologic condi-tions: Overlooked complications.* Focus: A Guide to AIDS Research and Counseling 7(1):1-4, 1991.

11. McPhedran P: *Using hematopoietic hormones in HIV dis-ease,* Aids Clin Care 4(6):43-44, 1992.

12. Northfelt D: *AIDS-associated Kaposi's sarcoma,* AIDS File 6(1):1-4, 1992.

13. Palefsky J: *Anal cancer among HIV-positive men,* AIDS File 6(1):9-10,1992.

14. Schwartz J, Dias B, and Safai B: *HIV-related malignan-cies,* Dermatol Clin 9(3):503-515, 1991.

15. Thompson D: *Invincible AIDS,* Time August 3:30-37, 1992.

16. Tinkle M, Amaya M, and Tamayo O: *HIV disease and pregnancy,* JOGNN 21(2):86-92, 1992.

17. Volberding P: *Management of HIV infection: Treatment team workshop handbook,* New York, 1991, World Health Communications.

18. Wright M: *Guide to opportunistic infections,* Project In-form Perspective Oct:11-13, 1991.

Leukemia

14

Acute Lymphocytic Leukemia (ALL)

Epidemiology and Etiology

Radiation, chemicals, drugs, viruses, and genetic abnormalities have been implicated in the etiology of this disease. A causal relationship between the human T-cell leukemia virus-I (HTLV-I) and T-cell leukemias and lymphoma is suspected, but not proven. ALL leukemia in adults usually occurs in the third decade of life. This disease is seen less often in adults than acute myelocytic leukemia. ALL is more common in children; 85 % of all cases of ALL occur in children. This disease comprises 20 % of adult leukemia.[1,2,16,25]

Clinical Features

- Fatigue
- Anorexia
- Malaise
- Weight loss
- Bleeding
- Infection
- Headache or visual disturbances
- Adenopathy
- Gingival hypertrophy
- Splenomegaly
- Hepatomegaly
- Bone or joint pain

Diagnosis

The diagnosis of ALL is often indicated by the peripheral blood smear; and, a bone marrow evaluation is essential to finalize the diagnosis and provide specimens for further subclassification studies. The bone marrow aspirate is hypercellular. The white blood cell (WBC) count is normal to high in the majority of

ALL patients. Platelet counts in most cases of ALL are normal to moderately decreased and only 30% of patients present with less than 50,000/mm^3 platelets. Most patients will have hematocrits in the 30% to 35% range. Lymphoblasts comprise at least 50% of the marrow cells in ALL.[7,17,23]

Classification

The French-American-British (FAB) classification system, based on cellular morphology and histochemical staining of blast cells, is used.

The three FAB classes of acute lymphocytic leukemia are L_1, L_2, and L_3. The L1 classification is most common in childhood leukemias. The common adult form of ALL is the L_2 classification. The L_3 classification is very rare and resembles Burkitt's lymphoma. Cell surface marker studies are performed on the blast cells of a patient with ALL to identify leukemia associated antigens. These groups are: common ALL (CALLA), Pre-B ALL, Pre-T ALL, null cell ALL, B-cell, and T-cell.[1,7]

Prognosis

Approximately 75% of adults treated for acute lymphocytic leukemia will achieve complete remission, and 40% will be cured. Patients who do not achieve complete remission have a median survival of less than 6 months.

Treatment Modalities

Induction Therapy

The purpose of induction therapy is to induce a complete response (CR). A CR is documented by a bone marrow aspirate containing <5% lymphoblasts and the elimination of extramedullary disease. The primary chemotherapeutic agents used to induce remission are vincristine, prednisone, and danorubicin. Some induction regimens use additional drugs: L-asparaginase, cyclophosphamide, methotrexate, 6-mercaptopurine, cytosine arabinoside.[7]

Central Nervous System Treatment

Leukemic involvement in the CSF at the time of diagnosis is more common in children than in adults, where it is detected 5% to 10% of the time. Repeated treatments with intrathecal methotrexate via Ommaya reservoir or lumbar puncture is the standard preventative therapy.

Postremission Therapy

Consolidated/Intensification Therapy

The regimens may include high-dose chemotherapy or may repeat the drugs used in induction therapy.

Maintenance Therapy

An extended program of low-dose maintenance therapy using weekly 6-mercaptopurine and methotrexate is effective in preventing relapse and improving survival in children.

Recurrent Disease Therapy

Patients with resistant disease who fail to achieve a first remission may respond to treatment with intermediate to high-dose methotrexate and leukovorin rescue or 1-asparaginase. Bone marrow transplantation may allow long-term survival for up to 50% of patients after second relapse and 10% to 20% of patients after third relapse.[17,20]

Acute Myelogenous Leukemia (AML)

Epidemiology and Etiology

People with certain genetic disorders, such as Downs syndrome (trisomy 21), Bloom's syndrome, Klinefelter's syndrome, and Fanconi's anemia, are at increased risk to develop AML. Exposure to the hydrocarbon benzene also increases the risk of disease development. Leukemia has been associated with exposure to ionizing radiation from nuclear reactions and from exposure to therapeutic and occupational radiation. The incidence of therapy-related acute nonlymphocytic leukemias (T-AML) has increased dramatically over the past decade. The median interval of occurence of T-AML is 4 to 6 years after the original cancer treatment and is usually preceded by a preleukemic state detectable for 6 months.

Alkylating agents, especially prolonged use of melphalan in ovarian cancer, multiple myeloma and breast cancer, and nitrogen mustard for Hodgkin's disease are strongly implicated. Chlorambucil, busulfan, and thiotepa are also associated with an increased risk of developing a later malignancy. The incidence of AML is 3 cases per 100,000 population with approximately 11,000 new cases each year in the United States. The median age at diagnosis is about 50 years.[2,7,20]

Clinical Features

As with ALL, AML symptoms are related to the rapidly expanding leukemic cell population:

- Anemia
- Recurrent infection
- Bruisability
- Bone or joint pain
- Osteolycitic lesions
- Visual disturbances
- Hepatomegaly

- Epistaxis
- Gingival bleeding
- Headache, vomiting
- Dysphagia
- Papilledema
- Menorrhagia
- Adenopathy

Diagnosis

A diagnosis of AML is highly suspect when the examination of peripheral blood smears shows an increased number of immature blast cells associated with anemia and thrombocytopenia. The presence of Auer bodies (rods) suggests a diagnosis of AML before other diagnostic results are available. The total white blood cell count in AML may be normal, decreased, or increased. Platelet counts of less than 20,000/mm^3 are common in AML. A bone marrow aspirate is used to obtain the differential count, and the biopsy is used to establish the percentage cellularity.[20]

Classification

AML is classified morphologically according to the FAB criteria by the degree of differentiation along different cell lines and the extent of cell maturation. The FAB classification for AML is described in Table 14-1.

Table 14-1 Classification of Acute Myelogenous Leukemias, French-American-British System (FAB)

FAB Type/Bone Marrow Morphology		Clinical Features/Prognosis
M_0	Myeloid lineage cannot be determined by conventional morphologic or cytochemical analysis; can be identified by immunophenotyping	
M_1; Myeloblastic	Without maturation > 90% blasts Auer bodies present	M_1, M_2 are the most common adult AML diagnoses
M_2; Myeloblastic	With maturation Blast + promyelocytes > 50% Auer bodies and/or granules	
M_3; Promyelocytic (APL)	Majority of cells are abnormal promyelocytes Cells filled with large granules; may be microgranular	10% of adult AML, disseminated intravascular coagulation present in 80% of patients: may occur after treatment initiation

Continued.

Table 14-1 Cont'd.

FAB Type	Bone Marrow Morphology	Clinical Features/Prognosis
	Nucleus varies in size and shape Bundles of Auer bodies 15:17 chromosome translocation	Granules are released as blasts which die and initiate coagulation cascade Good duration of remission
M_3 variant (M_3V)	Granules detected only on electron microscopy (microgranular variant)	
M_4: Myelomonocytic	Promonoblasts and monoblasts > 20%, myeloblasts plus promyelocytes > 20% of cells	Organomegaly Lymphadenopathy Gingival hyperplasias Soft tissue infiltration CNS leukemia
M_4E	Variable number of morphologically abnormal eosinophils present; associated abnormalities of chromosome 16	

M₅: Monocytic
Subtype A—
poorly differentiated:

Monocytic cells exceed 80%
Granulocytic component
rarely exceeds 10%

Organomegaly
Lymphadenopathy
Gingival hyperplasia

Subtype B—
differentiated: pro-
monocytes predominant

Few cells may have Auer bodies

Soft tissue infiltration
CNS leukemia

M₆: Erythroleukemia
(Di Guglielmo syndrome)

Erythropoietic component exceeds
50% of marrow cells
Blasts have bizarre morphology
Myeloblasts and promyelocytes > 30%
of erythroid cells

Occurs in <5% AML
Prolonged prodromal period
May present with rheumatic disorder;
75% have positive Coombs' test;
30% have rheumatoid factor
Almost always progresses to M_1, M_2, M_4

M₇: Megakaryocytic

Reticulin and collagen fibrosis;
blasts resemble immature
megakeryocytes or may be
quite undifferentiated

Rare variant
Marrow difficult to aspirate
Increased LDH
Intense myelofibrosis
Very poor prognosis

Prognosis

Patients presenting with a WBC count $> 100,000/mm^3$ have significantly more deaths during the first week of therapy, die more frequently of CNS hemorrhage, and have shorter overall remissions and survival than those presenting with lower white cell counts. The worst prognostic factor in AML patients is prior treatment with chemotherapy or ratiation therapy. This group includes patients with a treatment-related secondary leukemia and AML patients with recurring or resistant disease.[20]

A preexisting hematologic disorder, serious infection at diagnosis, CNS leukemia, organomegaly, and lymphadenopathy are clinical features indicative of poor prognosis. Laboratory findings predictive of poor response include anemia, high peripheral blast count, thrombocytopenia, elevated BUN and creatinine, increased LDH, or increased fibrogen. Specific chromosomal abnormalitites are also associated with a poorer prognosis.

Treatment Modalities

A complete remission in AML is defined as less than 5% marrow blasts and less than 5% progranulocytes in a normocellular marrow. Peripheral blood counts must return to normal, and preexisting adenopathy or organomegaly must be absent.

Induction Chemotherapy

Cytarabine with an anthracycline, either daunorubicin or doxorubicin, are the most effective induction agents, and result in complete remission 65% of the time. Newer anthracyclines, mitoxantrone and Idarubicin have been approved for AML if used in combination with other approved drugs.

A bone marrow examination is repeated the second week after treatment to assess for antileukemic response. A positive response is indicated by a hypocellular, aplastic marrow. The marrow examination is repeated as the peripheral counts begin to recover. If evidence of leukemia persists 3 to 4 weeks after the start of induction and the marrow cellularity is recovered, the patient is reinduced with the same drugs and doses.[7,17,20]

Bone Marrow Transplant

Bone marrow transplant may be the treatment of choice in certain AML patients in first remission. See Chapter 24 for more information on transplant options in AML patients.

Recurrent Disease Therapy

Retreatment with ara-C and daunorubicin in patients treated with this regimen initially have a 30% to 50% chance of attaining a second remission. High-dose ara-C with or without daunorubicin, L-asparaginase, amsacrine, or mitoxantrone has been used with some success in resistant AML.

Chronic Myelogenous Leukemia

Chronic myelogenous leukemia (CML) is a myeloproliferative disorder characterized by proliferation of the granulocyte cell series. Chronic leukemias differ from acute leukemias in that the malignant white cells are mature-appearing and well-differentiated.[2]

Epidemiology and Etiology

The incidence of CML increases with exposure to radiation but is not clearly associated with alkylating agents or hereditary factors. The chemical benzene is also associated with chronic myelogenous leukemia. The annual incidence of CML is 1.4 per 100,000 44; chronic myelogenous leukemia is less common than chronic lymphocytic leukemia and is one fourth as common as acute leukemia. This disease is most frequently encountered between the ages of 20 and 60 with the peak incidence between 50 and 60 years.[11]

Philadelphia Chromosome

The hallmark of CML is the presence of a Philadelphia chromosome (Ph[1]). Chromosome 22 is missing part of its long arm, which is translocated to the long arm of chromosome 9. Although this translocation is identified in nearly 95% of CML patients, controversy exists as to whether all malignant cells are Ph[1]-positive, or if the acquisition of the Ph[1] chromosome is the initial oncogenic event.[7,9]

Clinical Features and Diagnoses

Chronic Phase

Diagnosis of CML is established by hematologic evaluation. The following results on a complete blood cell count are characteristic of CML: WBC > 100,000/mm^3, mature and immature granulocytes, myelocytes > metamyelocytes, increased eosinophils and basophils, and normal or increased platelets. A bone marrow evaluation is required to assess cellularity, detect fibrosis, and to obtain a specimen for cytogenetic analysis.

Accelerated Stage

Progression to accelerated phase is characteristic of all patients with CML. The time of progression to accelerated phase is variable and greatly impacts length of survival. The leukocyte doubling time (LDT) shortens to 20 days or less during this stage. (Box 14-1).

Blastic Phase

Patients with CML inevitably enter the blastic stage, an aggressive, rapidly terminal phase, which is refractory to treatment. Criteria include:
- Blasts > 20% in peripheral blood or marrow
- Blasts plus promyelocytes > 30% in peripheral blood
- Blasts plus promyelocytes > 50% in marrow
- Extramedullary blastic infiltrates
- Leukemic tumor masses

The blastic stage resembles a disease similar to acute myelogenous leukemia or acute lymphocytic leukemia.[8]

Treatment Modalities

Chemotherapy

Busulfan and hydroxyurea are used in the treatment of chronic phase CML. Intensive multidrug regimens are the treatment of choice for the blastic transformation phase of CML in patients who are not BMT candidates. These regimens include ara-C, programs with anthracyclines, amsarcine (m-AMSA), 6-thioguanine (6TG), and hydroxyurea.[11,14]

Box 14-1

Comparison of Clinical Features in Chronic Phase CML
and Accelerated Phase/Blastic Transformation

Chronic phase	*Accelerated phase/blastic transformation*
Fatigue	Increased fatigue
Pallor	Increasing anemia
Dyspnea	Recurrence of splenomegaly
Anemia	Thrombocytopenia
Anorexia	Fever of unknown origin
Weight loss	Lymphadenopathy
Sternal tenderness	Hepatomegaly
Splenomegaly	Thrombocytosis/ thrombocytopenia

Interferon

Interferon is capable of slowing the leukocyte doubling time and prolonging busulfan-induced remissions. Findings suggest that alpha-2b interferon can partially suppress the expression of Ph.[1]

Bone Marrow Transplantation and Prognosis

Bone marrow transplantation following high-dose chemotherapy and radiation is the only potentially curative treatment for CML. Best results occur when the transplant is performed early in the chronic phase of the disease. The 5-year survival for chronic phase patients is 60%, compared to 22% in accelerated phase, and 13% in blast phase.[27]

Chronic Lymphocytic Leukemia

Chronic lymphocytic leukemia (CLL) is a malignant hematologic disorder characterized by proliferation and accumulation of relatively normal appearing lymphocytes. The majority of cases (95%) are B-cell lymphoproliferative disorders with a single clone of B-cell lymphocytes undergoing malignant transformation. The remaining 5% of cases are T-cell lymphoproliferative disorders.[9,13]

Epidemiology and Etiology

A familial tendency has been suggested and there is a strong correlation between CLL and autoimmune diseases such as systemic lupus erythematosus, Sjögren's syndrome, and autoimmune hemolytic anemia.

CLL is the most common leukemia in the United States, accounting for 30% of all newly diagnosed leukemias. The median age of CLL patients is 60 years. The disease affects twice as many males as females.[2,24]

Clinical Features

- Skin and respiratory infections
- Fatigue
- Lymphadenopathy
- Thrombocytopenia
- Malaise
- Anorexia
- Splenomegaly
- Anemia

Diagnosis and Staging

The *RAI Clinical Staging System* is used for diagnosis and staging:

Stage 0   Lymphocytosis only, in blood (>15,000/mm^3)
              and bone marrow (>40%).
              Median survival = 12+ years.
Stage I   Lymphocytosis with lymphadenopathy.
              Median survival = 8+ years.
Stage II   Lymphocytosis + splenomegaly ± hepatomegaly.
              Median survival rate = 6 years.
Stage III   Lymphocytosis + anemia (Hbg < 11 g%).
              Median survival = 1.5 years.
Stage IV   Lymphocytosis + thrombocytopenia
              (platelets < 100,000/mm^3).
              Survival = 1.5 years.

Treatment Modalities

Indications for Treatment

- *Disease related symptoms*—fevers, sweats, weight loss, fatigue, or mechanical problems related to lymphadenopathy or organomegaly

- *Progressive cytopenias:* symptomatic anemias or progressive thrombocytopenia with transfusion requirements
- *Repeated infections:* systemic or disseminated bacterial, viral, or fungal infections requiring antibiotics or localized infections poorly responsive to conventional anitbiotic therapy.[11,13]

Chemotherapy

Chlorambucil, cyclophophosphamide, prednisone, and fludarabine are used as single agents. Combination chemotherapy with doxorubicin, cyclosphosphamide, vincristine, and prednisone has been used.

Splenectomy

Splenectomy has no influence on survival in CLL but may be indicated for autoimmune anemia or thrombocytopenia refractory to systemic therapy, or persistent symptomatic splenomegaly in a patient responding to chemotherapy.

Radiation Therapy

- A total of 300 to 800 cGy in 150 cGy fractions may benefit cases of hypersplenism, progressive splenomegaly, or lymphocytosis. Splenic radiation alone results in a partial remission rate of 70%, but the resulting neutropenia, thrombocytopenia, and short remission duration limit the utility of this treatment.[9]
- Nodal radiation may be employed to palliate symptoms or relieve organ dysfunction caused by abdominal adenopathy, such as biliary tract or urinary tract obstruction.[19]
- Total body radiation is infrequently used because it is less effective at controlling disease than chlorambucil and induces more profound cytopenias.

Prognosis

The clinical course and prognosis of B-cell CLL is quite variable and depends on the disease stage at the time of diagnosis. Patients with early stage disease may live 10 years or longer without treatment; patients with a more aggressive, advanced stage at diagnosis usually die within 2 years.

Hairy Cell Leukemia

Epidemiology and Etiology

Hairy cell leukemia (HCL) is a rare chronic lymphoproliferative disorder of unknown etiology. There does not seem to be an aassociation with ionizing radiation or other environmental factors. The disease is usually diagnosed in middle-aged patients and is quite rare, representing less than 2% of adult leukemias.

Clinical Features

- Weakness
- Fatigue
- Lethargy
- Splenomegaly

Diagnosis

The hallmark of HCL is the presence in the blood, bone marrow, and reticuloendothelial organs of the peculiar hairy cell. This cell is characterized morphologically by its hair-like projections. Patients are diagnosed based on the presence of cytopenias, hairy cells in peripheral blood, splenomegaly, and bone marrow aspiration biopsy.[1,19]

Treatment

Alpha-interferon, deoxycoformycin, and leustatin are the treatments of choice.[5,12,28]

Myelodysplastic Syndromes

Epidemiology, Etiology, and Classification

The myelodysplastic syndromes (MDS) are a heterogenous group of disorders previously referred to as oligoblastic leukemia, smoldering acute leukemia, or preleukemia. The syndrome is classified into five distinct pathologic entities: (1) refractory anemia (RA), (2) refractory anemia with ringed sideroblasts (RARS), (3) chronic myelomonocytic leukemia (CMML),

(4) refractory anemia with excess blasts (RAEB), and (5) refractory anemia with excess blases in transition (RAEB-T). Myelodysplasia is a disease of the elderly and most commonly affects people over 60 years of age and is rarely seen in people under the age of 30. Some studies have implicated exposure to benzene, radiation, chemotherapy, and alkylating agents in particular as initiating factors in the development of myelodysplasia.[4]

Clinical Features

Patients with MDS usually present with severe cytopenias or pancytopenia. Infections, particularly respiratory or gram-negative septicemias, are frequently the presenting symptom. Bleeding may be present as a result of either thrombocytopenia or poorly-functioning circulating platelets.

Diagnosis and Treatment

The diagnosis is established by bone marrow aspiration and biopsy. Chromosomal studies are also performed as approximately half of all MDS patients display karyotypic abnormalities. Chemotherapy for the myelodysplastic syndromes has ranged from single agent to low doses of multi-agent regimens, to conventional antileukemia programs. Many patients die during treatment with complications related to marrow hypoplasia and a significant number show clinical drug resistence. Allogeneic bone marrow transplantation is the only curative approach currently available, but unfortunately this disease most commonly occurs in people too old for transplantation.[6,10]

Nursing Management

Nursing Diagnosis

- *Anxiety related to new diagnosis, uncertain outcome of potentially fatal disease, loss of control in hospital environment, alteration in body image, alteration in interpersonal relationships.*

Interventions

- Perform psychosocial assessment of patient, family; identify strengths, weaknesses, coping skills.
- Recognize increased anxiety levels that may occur while awaiting an official diagnosis, before painful or frightening procedures, before major treatments, upon learning of relapse, and on anniversary dates.
- Administer antianxiety medications as ordered, assess effectiveness.
- Use guided imagery, relaxation training, and cognitive distraction to alleviate anxiety before painful or stressful procedures.
- Assist patient and family to set realistic goals concerning level of activity, work schedule, and self-care activities.[30]
- Encourage patient/family to verbalize questions, fears, concerns.
- Involve chaplaincy services, social workers, support volunteers as needed.
- Inform patient/family of available community resources: Leukemia Society of America and American Cancer Society.

Nursing Diagnosis

- *Infection, potential for, related to alteration in immune function secondary to leukemia and immunosuppressive chemotherapy.*

Interventions

- Teach patient/family the purpose and importance of neutropenic precautions.
- If appropriate, encourage patient to keep a chart of daily blood counts.
- Monitor temperature and vital signs every shift. Assess for changes in blood pressure, urine output, mental status that may be early signs of septic shock.
- Avoid fresh fruits and vegetables.
- No fresh flowers in patient's room.
- No rectal manipulation.

- Consistent handwashing by all people entering patient's room.
- Limit number of visitors to two at a time. No visitors with colds, influenza, herpes, or recent vaccinations.
- Avoid trauma to skin and mucous membranes.

Nursing Diagnosis

- *Injury, potential for bleeding related to alteration in clotting factors, thrombocytopenia secondary to leukemia and/ or treatment.*

Interventions

- Teach patient/family the significance of platelet function, bleeding precautions.
- Check platelet count at least every other day during immunosuppressive leukemia therapies.
- Monitor results of coagulation studies; assess for signs and symptoms of disseminated intravascular coagulation.
- Assess for petechiae, bruising, epistaxis, hematuria, hematochezia, oral, rectal, or vaginal bleeding.
- Monitor platelet transfusions.
- No intramuscular or subcutaneous injections or rectal manipulation.
- Use Water-pik® on lowest setting or toothettes for oral care.
- No aspirin-containing medications.
- Ensure safe environment: no sharp objects, bed rails up, ambulate with assistance.
- Prevent trauma to skin and mucous membranes.

Disease-Related Complications

Leukostasis

This occurs most commonly in the brain because of its vascularity and limited space. Intrapulmonary bleeding can also result; complications are associated with significant morbidity and mortality; medical emergency necessitates immediate reduction of the circulating leukocytes.

Interventions

- Monitor for changes in level of consciousness; perform neurologic examinations as ordered.
- Monitor respiratory status.
- Administer high-dose chemotherapy as ordered.
- Monitor leukapheresis process.
- Monitor absolute blast counts after interventions.

Disseminated Intravascular Coagulation

A complex syndrome characterized by activation of coagulation and formation of fibrin within the general circulation. Patients with promyelocytic leukemia (M_3) are at high risk of developing DIC after the intiation of chemotherapy, as granules from promyelocytes are released and initiate the coagulation cascade.

Interventions

- Ensure systematic assessment for occult, overt, or sudden massive bleeding.
- Initiate antileukemia therapy to correct underlying disease pathology.
- Administer antibiotics for sepsis.
- Administer blood products (platelets, fresh-frozen plasma) as ordered.
- Apply pressure to venipuncture sites.
- Administer heparin if ordered.

Typhilits

Inflammation of the cecum is related to *Clostridia* sepsis or other bacteria including *Pseudomonas, Escherichia coli,* or *Klebsiella.* This diagnosis should be considered in the neutropenic patient who develops severe abdominal pain. Bloody diarrhea, absence of bowel sounds, rebound tenderness, and fever may accompany the pain. The pathologic diagnosis is established by stool culture, abdominal x-ray (dilated colon), and the identified pathogen is treated with appropriate antibiotics.

Interventions

- Maintain intravenous fluids.
- Assess fluid and electrolyte balance.
- Ensure patient has no oral intake.
- Administer and evaluate analgesics.

Renal Failure

Renal failure in leukemia patients may result from urate nephropathy, aminoglycoside toxicity, sepsis, or leukemic infiltration of the kidneys.

Interventions

- Monitor BUN and creatinine values.
- Record accurate intake and output.
- Monitor vital signs, mental status.
- Assess for signs of alteration in tissue perfusion.

Geriatric Considerations

- Cardiovascular evaluation including radionucleotide ventriculogram to assess left ventricle ejection fraction.
- Modify doses of daunorubicin and high-dose cytosine arabinoside for patients over 60 years old.
- Monitor for signs and symptoms of fluid overload.
- Maintain a safe environment: bed rails, call light within reach, assistance with ambulation.
- Assess potential barriers to learning: decreased visual acuity, poor hearing, decreased concentration.

Bibliography

1. Alkire K and Collingwood J: *Physiology of blood and bone marrow,* Semin Oncol Nurs 6:99, 1990.
2. American Cancer Society: *Facts and figures—1994,* Atlanta, 1994, American Cancer Society.

3. Bishop JF and others: *Etoposide in acute nonlymphocytic leukemia,* Blood 75:27, 1990.

4. Cain J and others: *Myelodysplastic syndromes: a review for nurses,* Oncol Nurs Forum 18(1):113, 1991.

5. Cassileth PA and others: *Pentostatin induces durable remissions in HCL,* J Clin Oncol 9:243, 1991.

6. Cheson BD: *The myelodysplastic syndromes: current approaches to therapy,* Ann Intern Med 112:932, 1990.

7. Cheson BD: The acute leukemias. In Wittes RE, editor: *Manual of oncology therapeutics,* Philadelphia, 1989/1990, JB Lippincott.

8. Cheson BD: Chronic leukemias. In Wittes RE, editor: *Manual of oncology therapeutics,* Philadelphia, 1989/1990, JB Lippincott.

9. Clarkson B: The chronic leukemias. In Wyngaarden JB and Smith LJ, editors: *Cecil textbook of medicine,* ed 19, Philadelphia, 1988, WB Saunders.

10. Dang CV: *Myelodysplastic syndrome,* JAMA 267 (15): 2077, 1992.

11. Deisseroth AB and others: Chronic leukemias. In DeVita VT, Hellman S, and Rosenberg SA, editors: *Cancer: principles and practice of oncology,* ed 3, Philadelphia, 1993, JB Lippincott.

12. Estey EH and others: *Treatment of hairy cell leukemia with 2-chlorodeoxyadenosine (2-CdA),* Blood 79:882, 1992.

13. Foon KA and Gale RP: *Biology of chronic lymphocyte leukemia,* Semin Hematol 24(4):209, 1987.

14. Foon KA and Gale RP: *Staging and therapy of chronic lymphocytic leukemia,* Semin Hematol 24(4):264, 1987.

15. Golomb HM and Ellis E: *Treatment options for hairy cell leukemia,* Semin Oncol 18(suppl 7): 1991.

16. Heath CW: Epidemiology and hereditary aspects of acute leukemia. In Wiernik P, editor: *Neoplastic diseases of the blood,* New York, 1985, Churchill Livingstone.

17. Jacobs AD and Gale RP: Acute lymphoblastic leukemia in adults. In Gale RP, editor: *Acute leukemia,* Boston, 1986, Blackwell Scientific Publications.

Leukemia   **275**

18. Johnson BL: Leukemias. In Groenwald SL, editor: *Cancer nursing: practice and principles,* ed 3, Boston, 1993, Jones & Bartlett.
19. Kantarjian HM, Schachner J, and Keating MJ: *Fludarabine therapy in hairy cell leukemia,* Cancer 67:1291, 1991.
20. Keating MJ and others: Acute leukemia. In DeVita VT, Hellman S, and Rosenberg SA, editors: *Cancer principles and practice,* ed 4, Philadelphia, 1993, JB Lippincott.
21. Levenson JA and Lesko LM: *Psychiatric aspects of adult leukemia,* Semin Oncol Nurs 6:76, 1990.
22. List AF and others: *The myelodysplastic syndromes: biology and implications for management.* J Clin Oncol S: 1424, 1990.
23. Maguire-Eisen M: *Diagnosis and treatment of adult acute leukemia,* Semin Oncol Nurs 6:17, 1990.
24. Rai KR and Montserrat E: *Prognostic factors in chronic lymphocytic leukemia.* Semin Hematol 24(4):252, 1987.
25. Rinsky RA and others: *Benzene and leukemia,* N Engl J Med 316:1044, 1987.
26. Saven A and Piro LD: *Treatment of hairy cell leukemia,* Blood 79:1111, 1992.
27. Silver RT: *Chronic myeloid leukemia; a perspective of the clinical and biological issues of the chronic phase,* Hematol Oncol Clin N Am 4:319, 1990.
28. Smith JW and others: *Prolonged continuous treatment of hairy cell leukemia patients with recombinant interferon-alpha 2a,* Blood 78:1664, 1991.
29. Wujick D: *Options for postremission therapy in acute leukemia,* Semin Oncol Nurs 6:25, 1990.

Lung Cancer

15

Epidemiology

It is estimated that there will be 172,000 new cases of lung cancer in the United States in 1994 and 153,000 deaths.[2] More men than women develop lung cancer, but the gap is narrowing. Lung cancer mortality among women has skyrocketed over 400% during the past 30 years. Although not the most common cancer in either sex, lung cancer will continue to be the leading cause of cancer death for both men (33%) and women (23%) in 1994.[1,27]

Etiology and Risk Factors

Smoking

Observers note that lung cancer mortality rates in people who have smoked two packs per day for ten years (twenty pack years) are fifteen to twenty-five times higher than in nonsmokers.[14,25] It is estimated that 85% of lung cancer deaths are related to smoking. The latency period between initiation of smoking and the development of lung cancer is about fifteen to twenty years.[14,25]

Race and Socioeconomics

Lung cancer mortality is higher among nonwhites than whites and may be related to the increased smoking and use of nonfilter cigarettes by blacks. Unconfirmed studies suggest, that there is an increased risk of squamous cell and small cell lung cancers in men with diets low in vitamin A.

Geography

Geographic clustering of lung cancer among males has been noted along the Gulf of Mexico and the southeastern Atlantic coast. Mortality rates are lowest in farming areas and lower in rural versus urban counties.

Industry

Industrial exposure to the following agents is believed to place persons at greater risk of getting lung cancer: mustard gas, radon, asbestos, radioisotopes, polycyclic aromatic hydrocarbons (present in crude petroleum, coal tars, combustion products of most organic materials), nickel, chromium, haloethers, iron ore, inorganic arsenic, wood dust, and isopropyl oil.

Family and Health History

The risk of lung cancer is increased in persons with a prior history of lung disease or a family history of lung cancer. A specific gene that predisposes to early age onset of lung cancer may account for up to 47% of cases by age 60.

Prevention, Screening, and Detection

Primary lung cancer prevention focuses on decreasing the number of new smokers and helping present smokers to quit. It may involve decreasing the hazards of smoking through use of low tar and filtered cigarettes for those who continue to smoke. Secondary prevention is aimed at early diagnosis of lung cancer in populations at high risk. Populations considered at high risk generally include persons more than forty-five years of age who have smoked heavily, that is, one or more packs per day.

Teach these persons:

- Avoid use of tobacco
- Know environmental carcinogens that increase risk
- Personal and family history risk factors[14,29]

Classification

Squamous cell carcinoma is the most common type (30% to 64% of all lung cancers). Small cell anaplastic carcinoma (19% to 25%), large cell carcinoma (9% to 20%), and all other types (1% to 3%) occur less often. Some 2% to 4% may be an adenosquamous hybrid.[20]

Small Cell Lung Cancer

Small cell anaplastic carcinoma behaves biologically and clinically so differently from all other cell types that the latter are referred to as non-small cell lung cancers (NSCLC). Although usually metastatic at the time of diagnosis because of its rapid growth and aggressive nature, small cell lung cancer (SCLC) is the most sensitive of all lung cancers to chemotherapy and radiation therapy. Because it most often arises in the central part of the chest, postobstructive pneumonia and atelectasis are common. Frequent sites of distant metastasis are brain, liver, and bone marrow. SCLC has sometimes been referred to as oat cell carcinoma due to its microscopic resemblance to oats.[9,27,31]

Non-Small Cell Lung Cancer

Squamous cell carcinoma

- Is moderately, or poorly differentiated, arises in the central portion of the lung, may present as Pancoast's tumor and have sudden onset of hypercalcemia

Adenocarcinoma

- Is often recognized microscopically by its glandular appearance and mucin production, and includes acinar, papillary, solid, and bronchioalveolar types
- Patients may present with or develop brain, liver, adrenal, or bone metastasis

Large cell anaplastic carcinoma

- Appears microscopically as large cells lacking any distinguishing features. Clinical signs and symptoms and pain from pleural or chest wall invasion and lung abscesses

Mixed Cell Types

- Multiple cell lines are found in 10% to 20% of lung tissure specimens

Clinical Features

Most common symptoms at presentation

- A change in cough
- Recurrent bronchitis or pneumonia unresponsive to antibiotics
- Hemoptysis
- Chest pain
- Wheezes
- Weight loss
- Dysphagia
- Fatigue

Symptoms of regional tumor spread

- Superior vena cava syndrome
- Phrenic nerve paralysis with an elevated hemidiaphragm and dyspnea
- Horner's syndrome
- Tracheal or esophageal obstruction
- Pleural effusion
- Hypoxia and dyspnea related to lymphangitic spread
- Hoarseness as a result of recurrent laryngeal nerve paralysis
- Pancoast's syndrome (shoulder pain radiating down an arm along ulnar nerve distribution)
- Pericardial effusion and tamponade

Evidence of metastatic disease or a paraneoplastic syndrome

- Headaches, mental status changes
- Bone pain related to bone involvement
- Other paraneoplastic syndromes[15,18]
- Abdominal discomfort, elevated liver function tests
- Pancytopenia secondary to bone marrow involvement

Diagnosis

Diagnostic procedures for lung cancer include:

- History and physical exam
- Chest x-ray
- Complete blood count and blood chemistries
- Fiberoptic bronchoscopy with biopsy or bronchial brushings or washings for cytology
- Percutaneous transthoracic needle aspiration
- Biopsy of supraclavicular or scalene lymph nodes
- Mediastinoscopy
- Biopsy of accessible metastatic sites

- Thoracentesis for cytology or pleural biopsy
- Thoracotomy
- Bone scan
- CT scan of the abdomen or liver
- CT or MRI study of the head
- Liver or bone marrow biopsy
- Plain films of bone[15]

Staging

Because two-thirds of SCLC patients have metastatic disease, initial staging will routinely include:

- Bone scan
- CT scan of the abdomen
- Liver biopsy
- Bone marrow biopsy
- MRI study of the head

If the cancer is deemed resectable, pulmonary function and blood gas studies are required to determine if the patient is able to undergo pneumonectomy or pulmonary resection. See Chapter 4. Non-small cell lung cancer is also staged by using the following criteria:

- Limited—Disease restricted to one hemithorax with regional lymph node metastases including hilar, ipsilateral and contralteral mediastinal and/or supraclavicular nodes, and including ipsilateral pleural effusion regardless of cytology.
- Extensive—Disease beyond the above definition and which may involve metastasis to liver, bone, bone marrow, brain, adrenals, and lymph nodes.

Metastasis

Cancers of the lung find many distant sanctuaries including bone marrow, pericardium and heart, kidney, and adrenal gland. The most common sites of metastasis of lung cancer are the other lung and pleura, brain, bone, liver, and lymph nodes.

Treatment Modalities

Non-small Cell Lung Cancer

Surgery

Surgery is the treatment of choice for stages I and II NSCLC. Pneumonectomy for stage I & II patients may be required unless precluded by preexisting cardiopulmonary disease. Lobectomy with regional lymph node dissection is most optimal for early stage disease whenever possible. Complications for these procedures include pneumothorax, pulmonary embolus, pneumonia, hemorrhage and infection.[2,9]

Radiation Therapy

Optimal doses of external beam radiation for NSCLC are now believed to be around 60 Gy. Best tumor control occurs with five treatments per week over six to seven weeks without interruption. Side effects related to this therapy are: erythema, esophagitis, dysphagia, pneumonitis, pericarditis, myelosuppression and fatigue.[19,21]

Brachytherapy

This technology allows for careful placement of catheters close to the tumor. Then, via computerized remote control, HDR iridium (^{192}IR) is introduced into the catheter. Within a few minutes, while caregivers are safe from exposure, a very high dose of radiation (5 to 10 Gy/session) can be delivered to select tissue without injury to adjacent healthy tissue, especially critical at this anatomic site. Sessions may be repeated every 1 to 2 weeks for a cumulative dose in the range of 20 to 43.6 Gy.[19,21,31]

Chemotherapy

The most active single agents in NSCLC include mitomycin-C, vindesine, vinblastine, etoposide, ifosfamide, cisplatin, carboplatin, cyclophosphamide, vincristine, doxorubicin, bleomycin, and pacilitaxel. Current combination chemotherapy regimens are cisplatin, etoposide, ifosfamide, and carboplatin.[6,31]

Small Cell Lung Cancer

Surgery

The current recommended treatment of SCLC presenting as a single pulmonary nodule is surgery, followed by adjuvant chemotherpay and prophylactic cranial irradiation with or without radiation to the chest.[2,8]

Radiation Therapy

In limited disease (LD) SCLC, trials combining chest radiation and chemotherapy have now shown improved long-term survival rates and a decrease in local recurrences.[9,19]

Chemotherapy

Single agents include cyclophosphamide, doxorubicin, vincristine, methotrexate, nitrogen mustard, hexamethylmelamine, and lomustine. Combination chemotherapy regimens are lomustine, methotrexate, cyclophosphamide, doxorubicin, vincristine, cisplatin, carboplatin, and etoposide.[17]

Treatment of Metastasis

Brain Metastasis

Treatment should be palliative to correct the patient's neurologic deficits, which in turn enhances quality of life. For acute management of increased intracranial pressure, large doses of corticosteroids or triamcinolone can be administered, followed by radiation therapy to the whole brain (20 to 40 Gy). Certain patients can benefit from surgical resection of solitary lesions followed by a course of radiation therapy.[31,33]

Bone Metastasis

Narcotic medications, local nonsteroidal antiinflammatory drugs, and radiation therapy are commonly and successfully used to promote comfort and increase ambulation and mobility. Orthopedic management can be attempted to promote spinal stabilization and prevent cord compression. Prophylactic fixation or metastatic lesions in the long bones with rods or implants can prevent pathologic fractures and ensure ambulation or upper extremity control. Combination chemotherapy may also help alleviate or modify this painful process.[31]

Liver Metastasis

Systemic chemotherapy may be somewhat effective for a brief period of symptom control, however liver metastasis is part of the malignant process that often leads to early death. Patients with painful liver involvement can usually be made comfortable with narcotics and celiac plexus blocks.

Cardiac Metastasis

Treatment is generally conservative and consists of pericardio-centesis, systemic chemotherapy, or intrapericardial administration of various other agents. Cardiac tamponade can be treated successfully and easily with a cardiac window done under local anesthetic.

Pleural Effusions

Various methods of treatment for pleural effusion are available, including repeated thoracentesis, intrapleural instillation of chemotherapy, intracavitary radioactive colloids, via chest tubes, and pleurectomy. See chapter 19.[7,12,13]

Prognosis

Prognostic Factors

The survival rate for patients with localized disease is 37%, however, survival at 5 years is 13% for all patients regardless of stage at diagnosis. Prognosis is best for patients with well-differentiated squamous cell lung cancer, and those with small cell cancer have the poorest survival rate. Patients who are ambulatory tolerate treatment better than those who are not fully ambulatory, but are out of bed 50% of the time.[15,29]

Correlation with Histologic Cell Type and Stage

Non-small Cell Lung Cancer (NSCLC)

Patients with squamous cell cancer survive longer than do those with adenocarcinoma and large cell undifferentiated carcinoma. Stage I squamous cell cancers do significantly better than those with stage II and III tumors. For stage IIIa patients, survival ranges from 18% to 40%.

Small Cell Lung Cancer (SCLC)

Patients with limited stage disease who are treated with combination chemotherapy experience a 12- to 16-month median survival time, and a 15% to 20%, two-year disease free survival rate.

Nursing Management

Nursing diagnoses related to lung cancer listed below are followed by nursing interventions for various treatments and rehabilitation.

Principal Nursing Diagnoses

- *Knowledge deficit related to prevention of lung cancer*
- *Impaired gas exchange related to decreased passage of gases between the alveoli of the lungs and the vascular system (actual or potential)*
- *Knowledge deficit related to a new medical condition, new treatments, surgical procedures (preoperative and postoperative), and medications*
- *Alteration in comfort related to liver and/or bone metastasis (actual or potential)*
- *Alteration in thought processes related to brain metastasis (actual or potential)*
- *Fatigue related to treatment and treatment sequelae*

Secondary Nursing Diagnoses

- *Anxiety related to dyspnea*
- *Powerlessness related to hospitalization and feelings of lack of control*
- *Grieving related to loss of function of body system*

- *Coping, ineffective individual/family related to rapidly progessive disease process*

Surgery

Interventions

Preoperative

- Describe the type of procedure to be done (wedge resection, lobectomy, pneumonectomy).
- Discuss the need for optimal ventilation (stop smoking, cough, and take deep breaths immediately after surgery).
- Explain the need for leg and arm exercises.
- Discuss different methods of pain relief (IM, IV, epidural) with the patient. Encourage the patient to ask for medication when needed.
- Explain the postoperative routine and that the patient will most likely have a chest tube in place.[23]

Postoperative

- Reinforce the need for early ambulation despite the chest tube, and also the need to cough and breathe deeply.
- Review surgical results with the patient and ensure proper follow-up.
- Explore with the patient the implications of altered body image:
  - Changes in lifestyle[29,32]
  - Changes in relationships
  - Problems with sexuality
- Educate about strategies for dyspnea (Box 15-1).

Box 15-1

Strategies for Managing Dyspnea	
Breathing	
Teach new breathing pattern	Take slow, deep breaths
	Use diaphragm
	Exhale through pursed lips
	Exhale longer than inhale

Continued.

Box 15-1 Cont'd.

Positioning

Have patient assume comfortable position

Sit on bedside, fold arms over pillow on bedside table

Sit on chair, feet wide apart, elbows resting on knees

Lean on wall, feet apart, shoulders relaxed and bent forward

Elevate head of bed

Emotional support

Do not leave patient in distress alone

Observe patient frequently

Place frequent phone calls to patient on home care

Teach coaching and support to family or caregiver

Relaxation

Relaxation conserves oxygen

Place hands on patient's shoulders and press downward

Dangle arms and rotate shoulders

Planned activity

Have patient conserve energy and get adequate rest

Assess normal life-style and activities of daily living

Plan chores around rest period

Establish support for household activities, recreation

Oxygen therapy

Provide oxygen supply and implement safety precautions

Provide instruction regarding smoking, storage, heat, and use of equipment

Pharmacologic agents

Some agents relieve dyspnea, especially in patients who are terminally ill

Sedatives, narcotics, steroids, scopolamine

Reprinted with permission from Haylock P: *Breathing difficulty: changes in respiratory function,* Semin Oncol Nurs 3:293, 1987.

Radiation

Radiation to the brain can lead to hair loss, but the severity of hair loss is usually dose-dependent. At doses of 15 to 30 Gy, the degree of hair loss is variable. At a dose of 45 Gy or more, permanent loss is likely. During brain irradiation, patients are placed on dexamethasone to reduce resultant edema of brain tissue. However, symptoms of neurologic impairment related to edema should be monitored and could include irritability, confusion, restlessness, headaches, memory loss, a change in personality or mental status, nausea, unequal or decreased pupil reactivity to light, elevated blood pressure, sensory or motor changes, or a drop in pulse rate. Cerebral edema can lead to obstruction of the eustachian tube with resultant local ear pain or infection. Late effects of whole brain irradiation can include memory loss, problems in judgment, parkinsonian symptoms, weakness, confusion, depression, dizziness, organic brain syndrome, abnormal gait, ataxia, intention tremors, inability to concentrate, and cerebral atrophy.[10,19]

Interventions

General side effects of radiation therapy

- Explain measures to limit, as necessary, the patient's activities during treatment to conserve energy
- Discuss measures to maintain adequate nutritional intake
- Discuss reasons for and measures to deal with sexuality concerns[30]

Site-specific side effects

- Describe signs and symptoms of pneumonitis, esophagitis, and cough
- Discuss measures to maintain adequate oxygenation
- Consider forcing fluids to loosen thick secretions
- Administer antiemetics for nausea/vomiting
- Caution patient to avoid tobacco and alcohol

Emotional support

- Educate patient/family regarding radiation therapy procedures to decrease anxiety
- Explain that side effects may last for 2 to 4 weeks after treatment completion

■ Ensure understanding of anxiety or grief process because of illness and reassure patient that this is normal response

Combined Radiation and Chemotherapy

The severity of the toxicity depends on the drug and its dose, the radiation dose, and the timing of each in relation to the other. Damage to the target organ may be short-term, permanent and life-changing, or fatal. Because radiation therapy ports for lung cancer patients can involve the heart, the lungs, the brain, and other contents of the mediastinum, the potential severity of any synergistic drug-radiation toxicity is great. Specifically, esophagitis can lead to a stricture, CNS damage can include leukoencephalopathy or necrosis, or fatal interstitial fibrosis of large lung volumes can occur.[6]

Bibliography

1. American Cancer Society: *Cancer facts & figures, 1994,* Atlanta, GA, 1994.
2. Baker R and others: *The role of surgery in the management of selected patients with small cell cancer of the lung,* J Clin Oncol 5:697, 1987.
3. Bernhard J and Ganz P: *Psychosocial issues in lung cancer patients* (Part I), Chest 90:216, 1991.
4. Bernhard J and Ganz P: *Psychosocial issues in lung cancer patients* (Part II), Chest 90:480, 1991.
5. Boring CC, Squires TS, and Tong T Mongomerys: *Cancer Statistics, 1994*, CA 44(1):7, 1994.
6. Burke MB and others: *Cancer chemotherapy: a nursing process approach,* Boston, 1991, Jones and Bartlett.
7. Chernecky C and Krech R: Complications of advanced disease. In Baird S, McCorkle R, and Grant M, editors: *Cancer nursing: a comprehensive textbook*, Philadelphia, 1991, WB Saunders.
8. Comis R and Marstin G: *Small cell carcinoma of the lung: an overview,* Semin Oncol Nurs 3:174, 1987.
9. Diggs CH and others: *Small cell carcinoma of the lung: treatment in the community,* Cancer 69:2075, 1992.

10. Dow K and Hilderly L: *Nursing care in radiation oncology,* Philadelphia, 1992, WB Saunders.

11. Engelking C: *Comfort issues in geriatric oncology,* Semin Oncol Nurs 4:198, 1988.

12. Erickson R: *Mastering the in's and out's of chest drainage (Part I),* Nursing '89 19:36, 1989.

13. Erickson R: *Mastering the in's and out's of chest drainage (Part II),* Nursing '89 19:46, 1989.

14. Garfinkel L and Silverberg E: *Lung cancer and smoking trends in the United States over the past 25 years,* CA 41:137, 1991.

15. Ginskey RJ and others: Cancer of the lung. In DeVita V and others, editors: *Cancer: principles and practice of oncology,* ed 4, Philadelphia, 1993, JB Lippincott.

16. Green MR: *New directions in chemotherapy for non-small cell lung cancer,* Educa Session, Proc Am Soc Clin Oncol, May, 1992.

17. Hansen HH and Kristjansen PE: *Chemotherapy of small cell lung cancer,* Eur J Cancer 27:342, 1991.

18. Haque AK: *Pathology of carcinoma of the lung: an update on current concepts.* J Thorac Imaging 7:9, 1991.

19. Hilderly L and Dow K: Radiation oncology. In Baird S, McCorkle R, and Grant M, editors: *Cancer nursing: a comprehensive textbook,* Philadelphia, 1991, WB Saunders.

20. Ihde DC and Minna JD: *Non-small cell lung cancer: Part I: biology, diagnosis and staging,* Curr Prob Cancer 15:61, 1991.

21. Ihde DC and Minna JD: *Non-small lung cancer, Part II: treatment,* Curr Prob Cancer 15:105, 1991.

22. Lind J: Lung cancer. In Clark JC and McGee RF, editors: *Core curriculum for oncology nursing,* Philadelphia, 1992, WB Saunders.

23. Miaskowski C: Knowledge deficit related to surgery. In McNally J and others, editors: *Guidelines for cancer nursing practice,* ed 2, Philadelphia, 1991, WB Saunders.

24. Mountain CF: *Surgical treatment of lung cancer,* Crit Rev Oncol Hematol 11:179, 1991.

25. National Cancer Institiute: *Self-guided strategies for smoking cessation: a program planner's guide,* Bethesda, MD, US Department of Health and Human Services, 1990, NIH Pub. No. 91-3104.

26. Neuberger JS: *Residential radon exposure and lung cancer: an overview of published studies,* Cancer Detect Prev 15:435, 1991.

27. Oleske D: *The epidemiology of lung cancer: an overview,* Semin Oncol Nurs 3:165, 1987.

28. Rubin SA: *Lung cancer: past, present, and future,* J Thorac Imaging 7:1, 1991.

29. Ryan L: *Lung cancer: psychosocial implications,* Semin Oncol Nurs 3:222, 1987.

30. Shell J: Knowledge deficit related to radiation therapy. In McNally J, Sommerville E, Miaskowski C, and Rostad M, editors: *Guidelines for cancer nursing practice,* ed 2, Philadlephia, 1991, WB Saunders.

31. Splinter TA: *Management of non-small cell and small cell lung cancer,* Curr Opin Oncol 3:312, 1991.

32. White E: *Home care of the patient with advanced lung cancer,* Semin Oncol Nurs 3:216, 1987.

33. Wright D, Delaney T, and Buckner JC: Treatment of metastatic cancer to the brain. In DeVita and others, editors: *Cancer: principles and practice of oncology,* ed 4, Philadelphia, 1993, JB Lippincott.

Malignant Lymphoma

16

Hodgkin's Disease

Epidemiology and Etiology

Each year, there are an estimated 7,900 new cases of Hodgkin's disease and an estimated 1,600 deaths. Hodgkin's disease is the most common cancer of young adults. Incidence peaks in the second and third decades then gradually declines until age 45. Clinical manifestations and epidemiologic studies have suggested a viral etiology or disturbance of the immune system. The infectious agent most frequently implicated is the Epstein-Barr virus (EBV). Genetic and occupational (e.g., woodworking) predispositions for Hodgkin's disease may also exist.[2,8,14]

Prevention, Screening, and Detection

Prevention of Hodgkin's disease is not applicable because there are no identified preventable risks. Early detection is important but may be hampered by the vagueness of the common symptoms.

Classification

Since the identification of Reed-Sternberg cells (giant multinucleated transformed lymphocytes) as the diagnostic hallmark of Hodgkin's disease, histologic subtypes have been recognized. The Rye histopathologic classification identifies four subtypes of Hodgkin's disease based primarily on the microscopic features of the involved tissues. The identified characteristics help to distinguish Hodgkin's disease from other disorders. The characteristics of the four subtypes are: lymphocyte predominance, nodular sclerosing, mixed cellularity, lymphocyte depleted.

Clinical Features

Hodgkin's disease
- Painless lymphadenopathy
- Fever
- Night sweats
- Weight loss
- Pruritus
- Alcohol-induced pain

Non-Hodgkin's lymphoma
- Generalized painless lymphadenopathy
- Vague abdominal discomfort
- Back pain
- Gastrointestinal complaints

Diagnosis and Staging

After a tissue diagnosis of Hodgkin's disease has been established, the extent of disease involvement must be determined. See Chapter 4. To stage the extent of the disease accurately, the following procedures may be used.[3,10,12]

- Detailed history and physical examination
- Laboratory tests; CBC platelet count, ESR, liver, renal function, and cytogenetic studies.
- Radiology; chest x-ray, CT scans, MRI, and lymph-angiogram.
- Bilateral bone marrow biopsy and aspirate.
- Percutaneous liver biopsy
- Exploratory laparotomy and splenectomy

Metastasis

Involvement of retroperitoneal nodes, liver, spleen, and bone marrow usually occur after the disease is generalized. Mesenteric lymph nodes and any organ can be involved in advanced disease cases.

Treatment Modalities

The appropriate use of radiotherapy and chemotherapy is required for effective treatment of Hodgkin's disease. Radiation therapy is generally given to nodal areas (Figure 16-1). A total dose of 4000 to 4400 cGy (rads) to the involved nodal areas is usually well tolerated and curative. The most common chemotherapy regimens are MOPP and ABVD. Both regimens are given in 28-day cycles for a minimum of six cycles. Chemotherapy is generally continued for two cycles after complete remission is achieved. Staging is the most important factor in determining if radiotherapy alone, chemotherapy alone, or a combination of both is the treatment of choice (Table 16-1).[3,4,7,15]

Prognosis

Patients who achieve remission after second-line therapy have a wide range of reported long-term survival—20% to 80%. Patients who have residual disease or who relapse after second-line therapy have diseases that are difficult to control.

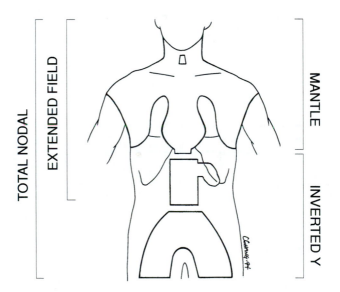

Figure 16-1. Standard radiation fields for Hodgkin's disease. *Mantle*, from mandible and diaphragm. Lungs, heart, spinal cord and humeral heads are shielded. *Inverted Y*, from diaphragm to ischial tuberosities, including the spleen if not removed; spinal cord, kidneys, bladder, rectum, and gonads are shielded. *Extended field*, involves mantle zone and uppermost inverted Y zone, does not include the pelvic, inguinal, or femoral nodes. *Total nodal*, mantle zone and complete inverted Y zone.

Table 16-1 Treatment for Hodgkin's Disease

Stage	Common Treatment	Prognosis
IA and IIA without bulky disease	Radiation to nodal areas of known and suspected disease	70%-85% 10-year DFS*
IB and IIB without bulky disease	Radiation to nodal areas of known and suspected disease; no clear evidence that addition of chemotherapy increases DFS	40% 10-year DFS
IIA and B with bulky disease	Chemotherapy followed by radiation to bulky disease	75% 10-year DFS
IIIA and B	Optimal treatment unresolved Possibilities: Chemotherapy alone Chemotherapy with radiation to bulky disease Chemotherapy with total nodal radiation	No long-term results available
IVA and B	Chemotherapy (MOPP alternating with ABVD)	70% 8-year DFS

*DFS, disease free survival.
Data from Bonadonna G and others: *Treatment strategies for Hodgkin's disease*, Semin Hematol 25(suppl 2):51, 1988.

Non-Hodgkin's Lymphoma

Epidemiology and Etiology

In 1994, there were an estimated 45,000 new cases of NHL and 24,200 deaths attributed to NHL. Men are at slightly higher risk than women, and whites are at higher risk than blacks. There is a preadolescent peak of incidence, then a later teenage drop off followed by a steady increase of incidence with age. The etiology of NHL remains unknown. There is increased incidence of NHL with age, in patients on long-term immunosuppression (e.g., organ transplant recipients), and in patients with autoimmune diseases, primary immunodeficiency, or acquired immunodeficiency. Patients who are HIV positive have four times greater risk of developing NHL. Viruses may also be etiologic factors by virtue of contributing to the chronic stimulation of the immune system. Two viruses linked to NHL are the Epstein-Barr virus and the human T-cell leukemia virus-I (HTLV-I). EBV is most commonly associated with the Burkitt's NHL; HTLV-I is implicated in the etiology of adult T-cell NHL.[2,4,6]

Prevention, Screening, and Detection

Prevention of NHL is not applicable because there are no identified preventable risks. Early detection is important but may be hampered by the vagueness of common symptoms.

Classification

The lymphomas are divided into histologic grades based on the aggressiveness of the cell type and the observed growth pattern. The histologic grades—low, intermediate, and high—generally correspond with the expected clinical course. For example, diseases with a low-grade histology are the least aggressive, and survival is measured in years.

Clinical Features

The most common symptom of NHL unrelated to AIDS is a painless, enlarged, discrete lymph node in the neck (lymphadenopathy) similar to that of Hodgkin's disease.

Symptoms of vague abdominal discomfort, back pain, gastrointestinal complaints, and ascites may be present and are usually indicative of abdominal node or gastrointestinal involvement. The "B" symptoms (fever, night sweats, and weight loss) occur 20% to 30% of the time. Other possible signs and symptoms depend on the location and extent of involvement. Cough, dyspnea, and chest pain occur about 20% of the time and are indicative of lung involvement. Superior vena cava syndrome may occur. Skin lesions that appear as isolated nodules or papules and frequently ulcerate, occur in about 20% of cases and are most common in diseases of a T-cell origin, specifically cutaneous T-cell lymphoma.[4,6]

Diagnosis and Staging

The recommended staging procedures for NHL may include:

- Detailed history and complete physical examination with close examination of all peripheral node regions
- Laboratory tests, CBC, platelet count, ESR, liver function tests, renal function tests, uric acid, calcium, alkaline phosphatase, LDH, serum immunoglobulins, and serologic tests
- Radiology, chest x-ray, CT scan, MRI
- Bilateral posterior iliac crest bone marrow aspirate and biopsy
- Diagnostic lumbar puncture
- Endoscopy or gastroscopy
- Diagnostic thoracentesis or paracentesis
- Lymphangiogram, liver biopsy, laparotomy

See Chapter 4

Metastasis

The metastatic process varies with the type of lymphoma. The follicular type has bone marrow involvement and the diffuse type disseminates rapidly and involves areas such as the central nervous system, bone, and gastrointestinal tract.

Treatment Modalities and Prognosis

The histologic type, extent of the disease, and patient's performance status are the most important factors in determining the
treatment approach to NHL. Indolent (low-grade) lymphomas
have a natural histroy that can be measured in years, aggressive
(intermediate-grade) lymphomas have a natural history measured
in months, and highly aggressive (high-grade) lymphomas natural history which can be measured in weeks. The treatment of
primary lymphomas in extra nodal sites is the exception to determining treatment by histologic type. Surgery, chemotherapy,
and radiation therapy may all be used to treat primary lymphoma
involving the gastrointestinal tract. Surgery alone is curative only
in patients with truly localized disease. The addition of either
radiation or chemotherapy postoperatively has improved survival.[4,5,10,12]

Indolent Non-Hodgkin's Lymphoma

Localized (stage I or II) indolent NHL is rare and easily treated.
Radiation therapy to the involved field or total nodal radiation
produces 60% to 80% 5-year disease-free survival. The role of
chemotherapy in the treatment of localized indolent lymphoma
has not been greatly explored and is, therefore, unclear. Treatment may be deferred until symptoms become bothersome or
the disease has evolved into a more aggressive type of lymphoma.
Patients whose histology converts to an aggressive type are then
treated with curative therapy appropriate for the more aggressive histology.

Aggressive Non-Hodgkin's Lymphoma

Localized disease occurs in less than 20% of aggressive lymphomas. Radiation to the site of disease is the treatment of choice.
However, the addition of chemotherapy to radiation regimens
seems to improve results because it decreases the risk of relapse
in unirradiated sites. Patients with disseminated disease and those
with local disease that have one or more poor prognastic features, are considered to have advanced aggressive lymphoma.
Combination chemotherapy is the treatment of choice.

Patients with advanced aggressive lymphoma are more readily cured than those with indolent lymphomas, and more than 60% of these patients are being cured.[5,22,23]

Highly Aggressive and Non-Hodgkin's Lymphoma

The treatment of highly aggressive lymphomas requires an intense chemotherapy regimen similar to those used to treate acute leukemia. The treatment regimen should include induction, consolidation, and maintenance phases and provide prophylactic treatment to the central nervous system.[5]

Drugs used in combination therapies for advanced aggressive lymphoma include:

- Cyclophosphamide
- Etoposide
- Bleomycin
- Methotrexate
- Cotrimoxazole
- Procarbazine
- Doxorubicin
- Cytarabine
- Vincristine
- Prednisone
- Nitrogen mustard

Nursing Management[11,14]

Nursing Diagnosis

- *Coping, ineffective, individual:*
  Related to new diagnosis
  Related to potential life-style changes

Interventions

- Assess patient's level of distress and anxiety
- Assess for signs of maladaptive or risky behaviours that interfere with responsible health practices
- Identify patient's support system, resources, and communication patterns
- Assess patient's problem solving capabilities
- Assess patient's level of knowledge regarding recurrence, development of secondary malignancy, and long-term effects of treatment

- Listen attentively and provide support
- Encourage verbalization of fears and concerns
- Assist patient to recognize stressors and assist with problem solving
- Provide reassurance that anxieties or distress about health are common feelings among cancer survivors
- Initiate referrals to social work, psychology, or community resources

Nursing Diagnosis

- *Sensory alteration, potential for:*
  Related to CNS involvement

Interventions

- Assess patient for level of orientation and level of activity
- Orient patient to all three spheres as needed
- Provide meaningful sensory input (e.g., clock, calendar, familiar objects)
- Explain all activities and request patient's perception of situation
- If patient becomes confused, direct back to reality

Patient Teaching Priorities

Signs and symptoms of disease
- Fever, night sweats, weight loss, painless lymphadenopathy, generalized vague gastrointestinal discomfort, and back pain

Signs and symptoms of infection
- Fever, chills, cough, erythema, and malaise

Sexual dysfunction
- Infertility, sterility, discuss options for contraception and ovary and sperm banking

Discuss treatment options
- Chemotherapy, radiation therapy, surgery, bone marrow transplant: purpose, schedule, simulation plan for radiation therapy, monitoring weekly blood counts, chemotherapy drug side effects and schedule, bone marrow transplant types (allogenic/autologus), pre-, during, and post-transplant care components.

Geriatric Considerations

Chemotherapy dose and schedule may be altered related to compromised cardiac, hepatic, renal, respiratory, and or neuromuscular function. Radiation therapy side effects: skin-excessive dryness, and early skin reactions; increased fatigue; medication dose adjustment to minimize side effects; consider facilitation with transportation. Financial consideration: Fixed income—consider consultation with social services regarding housing, meals on wheels, medication prescriptions, self-care needs.

Bibliography

1. Acker B and others: *Histologic conversion in the non-Hodgkin's lymphomas,* J Clin Oncol 1:11, 1983.
2. American Cancer Society: *Cancer facts and figures—1994,* Atlanta, 1994, American Cancer Society.
3. *Hodgkin's disease,* Semin Hematol 25(Suppl 2):51, 1988.
4. DeVita VT, Hellman S, and Rosenberg SA: *Cancer: principles and practice of oncology,* ed 4, Philadelphia, 1993, JB Lippincott.
5. DeVita VT and others: *The role of chemotherapy in diffuse aggressive lymphomas,* Semin Hematol 25:2, 1988.
6. Guyton AC: *Textbook of medical physiology,* ed 7, Philadelphia, 1986, WB Saunders.
7. Jottis GS and Bonadonna G: *Prognostic factors in Hodgkin's disease: implications for modern treatment (review),* Anticancer Res 8:749, 1989.
8. Lacher MJ: *Hodgkin's disease and infectious mononucleosis: is there a casual association?* CA 31:359, 1981.
9. Liang R and others: *Chemotherapy for early-stage gastrointestinal lymphoma,* Cancer Chemother Pharmacol 27:385, 1991.
10. List AF and others: *Non-Hodgkin's lymphoma of the gastrointestinal tract: an analysis of clinical and pathologic features affecting outcome,* J Clin Oncol 6:1125, 1988.
11. McNally JC, Miaskowski C, Rostad M, Sommerville ET, editors: *Guidelines for oncology nursing practice,* Philadelphia, ed 2, 1991, WB Saunders.

12. Miller TP and others: *Southwest Oncology Group clinical trials for intermediate- and high-grade non-Hodgkin's lymphomas,* Semin Hematol 25(suppl 2):17, 1988.

13. Silverberg E, Boring CC, and Squires TS: *Cancer statistics,* 1994 44(1):7,1994.

14. Stanley H, Fluetch-Bloom M, and Bunce-Clyma M: *HIV-related non-Hodgkin's lymphoma,* Oncol Nurs Forum 18:875, 1991.

15. Vose JM, Bierman PJ, and Armitage JO: *Hodgkin's disease: the role of bone marrow transplantation,* Semin Oncol 17:749, 1990.

Multiple Myeloma

17

Epidemiology, Etiology and Risk Factors

Multiple myeloma is a rare malignancy of plasma cells that accounts for only 1% of all hematologic malignancies diagnosed in the United States. The disease accounts for an estimated 12,700 new cases and 9,800 deaths each year. An increase in the incidence rate over the past decades is partially attributable to an improvement in diagnostic techniques.

Multiple myeloma is diagnosed in an equal number of men and women and occurs 14 times more frequently in blacks than whites, and occurs primarily in individuals over 40 years of age with a peak incidence at about 60 years of age.[1,8] The etiology of multiple myeloma is not completely understood. Host factors, such as increasing age, race, and occupational exposure to petroleum products, asbestos, and radiation, may contribute to increasing risk for the disease.

Prevention, Screening, and Detection

Detection of multiple myeloma in symptomatic individuals is based on a thorough history, physical examination, laboratory, and radiographic studies.

Clinical Features

- Anorexia
- Weight loss
- Recurrent infections
- Fatigue
- Back and bone pain
- Urinary pattern
- Changes in cognitive, sensory, and motor function (Figure 17-1)

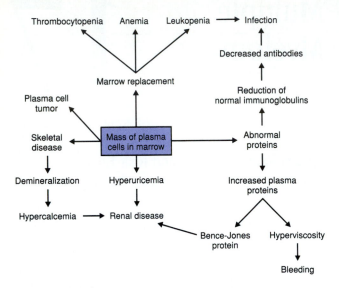

Figure 17-1. *Pathogenesis of multiple myeloma.* (From Megliola B: Multiple myeloma, Cancer Nursing 3(3):221, 1980.)

Diagnosis and Staging

Serum and urine electrophoretic and immunologic studies reveal elevation in IgG, IgA, and/or light chain levels. Additional laboratory studies include BUN, creatinine, and Bence-Jones urine protein levels. Radiographic studies include skeletal x-rays, bone surveys, and MRI.[2,3]

For a diagnosis of multiple myeloma to be made, one or more of the following criteria must be met: (1) plasma cell infiltration of the bone marrow of at least 10%, (2) a monoclonal spike on serum or urine electrophoresis, (3) radiographic confirmation of osteoporosis and osteolytic lesions, and (4) soft tissue plasma cell tumors. See Chapter 4.

Treatment Modalities

Treatment for multiple myeloma in the early stages of the disease consists of observation if patients are asymptomatic. Patients are monitored with interval clinical examinations, laboratory, and radiographic studies for signs of progressive disease such as severe anemia, thromboctyopenia and leukopenia, bone pain, osteolysis, or renal failure. Once progression of disease is documented, active treatment with antineoplastic agents or radiation therapy is initiated.[2,3]

Chemotherapy

Chemotherapy most commonly consists of intermittent melphalan and prednisone. Clinicians have used combinations of prednisone, high-dose melphalan, vincristine, BCNU, cyclophosphamide, and doxorubicin as salvage therapy with limited success. The use of biologic therapy, alpha interferon and interleukin-2, has shown some potential when used in combination with antineoplastic agents.[8]

Radiation Therapy

Radiation therapy may be used to treat patients with chemotherapy-resistant disease, to relieve bone pain, and to treat spinal cord compression.

Bone Marrow Transplantation

The role of autologous bone marrow transplantation in the treatment of patients with multiple myeloma has been explored. Success has been limited by the inability to eradicate the malignant plasma cell clone. However, researchers continue to evaluate the effectiveness of high-dose antineoplastic therapy, followed by an autologous transplant with marrow that has been purged with an antibody specific for plasma cells.[8]

Prognosis

Prognosis for patients with multiple myeloma is determined by the severity of organ involvement at the time of diagnosis and response to active treatment. Asymptomatic patients may live with the disease for months to years without active treatment. For symptomatic patients requiring treatment, a pattern of response has been described. During the initial 2 to 3 years of treatment, patients respond well to antineoplastic therapy. A plateau phase follows when the disease remains stable but does not respond as well as in the initial phase. During the third phase, the disease becomes resistant to the antineoplastic therapy and progresses at a rapid rate.[2,3,5]

Nursing Management

Nursing Diagnosis

- *Potential for injury related to bony destruction by plasma cell tumors.*[4,6,7,9]

Interventions

- Consult physical therapy for instruction in proper body mechanics, transfer techniques, positioning, and use of assistive devices, for development of an exercise program to maintain muscle strength and range of motion without jeopardizing risk of pathologic fractures.
- Arrange the hospital room environment to decrease the risks to safety: phone, call light, and personal articles within easy reach, clear pathway to the bathroom.
- Refer to home health agency to evaluate home environment for safety risk factors and recommended modifications prior to discharge.
- Encourage the patient to ask for assistance from health care team or significant others as needed, with ambulation or activities of daily living. The nurse also assumes responsibility to monitor for complications of multiple myeloma.

Complication	Nursing Assessments
■ Renal Insufficiency	• Monitor BUN, creatinine, uric acid, calcium, potassium, glucose, and phosphorus levels as ordered by the physician • Assess for changes in the character of the urine: volume, color, and odor
■ Hyperviscosity Syndrome	• Monitor for intermittent claudication and changes in the skin color of the extremities • Assess for neurologic changes such as headache or visual disturbances

	• Monitor for changes in mental status such as irritability, drowsiness, confusion, or coma
	• Assess for signs and symptoms of congestive heart failure
■ Dehydration	• Monitor intake and output every 8 hours
	• Assess skin turgor each day
	• Evaluate subjective symptoms by patient such as thirst, dryness of skin

Geriatric Considerations

- ■ Peak incidence of disease 60 years of age
- ■ Issues regarding occupation and potential for early retirement
- ■ Social and recreational activities may need adjustment to conserve energy and minimize injury risks
- ■ Potential for mental status changes
- ■ Consider environmental safety factors and abilities to meet self-care needs for hygiene, nutrition, elimination, and comfort[4,7]

Bibliography

1. American Cancer Society: *Cancer facts and figures—1994.* Atlanta, 1994, American Cancer Society.
2. Anderson MG: The lymphomas and multiple myeloma. In Baird SB, Donehower MG, Stalsbroten VL, and Ades TB, editors: *A cancer source book for nurses,* ed 6, Atlanta, 1991, American Cancer Society.
3. Bubley GJ and Schnipper LE: Multiple myeloma. In Holleb AI, Fink DJ, and Murphy GP, editors: *American Cancer Society textbook of clinical oncology,* Atlanta, 1991, American Cancer Society.
4. Clark JC, McGee RF, and Preston R: Nursing management of responses to the cancer experience. In Clark JC and McGee RF, editors: *Core curriculum for oncology nursing,* ed 2, Philadelphia, 1992, WB Saunders.
5. Cook MB: Multiple myeloma. In Groenwald SL, Frogge MH, Goodman M, and Yarbo CH, editors: *Cancer nursing: principles and practice,* ed 2, 1990, Boston, Jones and Bartlett.
6. Finley JP: Nursing care of patients with metabolic and physiological oncological emergencies. In Clark JC and McGee RF, editors: *Core curriculum for oncology nursing,* ed 2, Philadelphia, 1992, WB Saunders.
7. North Central New Jersey Local Chapter. Mobility, impaired physical, related to primary bone malignancy or metastatic bone disease. In McNally JC, Stair JC, and Somerville ET, editors: *Guidelines for cancer nursing practice,* Orlando, FL, 1985, Grune & Stratton.
8. Salmon SE and Cassady JR: Plasma cell neoplasms. In DeVita VT Jr., Hellman S, Rosenberg SA, editors: *Cancer: principles and practice of oncology,* ed 4, Philadelphia, 1993, JB Lippincott.
9. Willoughby S: Pain. In McNally JC, Stair JC, and Somerville ET, editors: *Guidelines for cancer nursing practice,* Orlando, FL, 1985, Grune & Stratton.

Skin Cancers

18

Nonmelanoma Skin Cancers

Basal Cell Carcinoma

Epidemiology

Basal cell carcinoma is the most commonly occurring skin cancer and malignant tumor found in humans; it largely affects whites and rarely occurs in dark-skinned persons. Basal cell carcinoma is two times more common in men than women and is usually seen in people after the age of 40.[1]

Etiology and Risk Factors

Ultraviolet radiation, primarily chronic exposure to the sun, appears to be the most important environmental risk factor.[7,8] Other environmental factors in basal cell carcinoma may include exposure to coal tar, pitch, creosote, and arsenic and chronic ingestion of inorganic arsenicals. Genetic factors such as basal cell nevus syndrome, fair skin, and light-colored hair have been associated with the development of basal cell carcinoma. An increased risk of developing basal cell carcinoma is present in people who have received a deep burn.[1,2,11]

Prevention, Screening, and Detection

Prevention of skin cancer measures
- Avoid excessive sun exposure, particularly the hours between 10:00 AM and 3:00 PM
- Wear sunscreen and lip balm with a sun protection factor of 15 or greater

- Use available shade
- Wear protective clothing
- Refrain from using manufactured tanning devices[5,13]

Skin cancer screening and detection
- Perform monthly self-examination of skin
- With good lighting, use two mirrors to visualize the abdomen, perineal area, and back
- Use blow hairdryer and mirror to visualize the scalp
- Observe each body part carefully, especially hidden areas such as between the toes and folds of skin
- Use of body chart will facilitate documentation of changes and suspected lesions to report
- Persons with two or more family members with a history of malignant melanoma should be examined by a dermatologist every 6 months
- Recognize and report symptoms or changes in skin characteristics promptly to the physician such as:[1,5,13]

    A = Asymmetry of shape
    B = Border irregularity
    C = Color variegation
        (black, brown, white, blue, and red)
    D = Diameter larger than 5 mm

Classification and Clinical Features

Basal cell carcinoma is classified according to clinical and histologic differences.[3]

- Nodular basal cell carcinoma
- Superficial basal cell carcinoma
- Pigmented basal carcinoma
- Morphea-form or sclerotic basal cell carcinoma
- Keratonic basal cell carcinoma

Diagnosis and Staging

Clinical diagnosis of skin cancers must be confirmed by histologic studies. A shave biopsy (top of lesion into depth of mid-dermis) is performed using local anesthesia. Punch biopsy (sharp, small circular "punch," similar to a cookie cutter approach) is used if the tumor is suspected to be in the deeper layers of the skin. The tissue sample is examined to determine the clinical diagnosis and identifying features of the various classifications. Upon determination of the clinical diagnosis, classification, and histopathologic grading, specific treatment modalities are recommended. See Chapter 4.[3]

Metastasis

Basal cell cancer metastasizes via the lymphatics or blood and is a rare occurrence. The most common predisposing factors are size of primary tumor and response to surgery and radiotherapy.

Treatment Modalities

Surgery

Surgical intervention is used to treat about 90% of basal cell carcinoma. The goal is the complete removal of the tumor.[20]

Excisional Surgery

Excisional surgery is usually performed with a 4 mm margin. This is the treatment of choice in large tumors or those with poorly defined margins on cheeks, forehead, trunk, and legs.

Cryosurgery

Cryosurgery involves tissue destruction by freezing. Liquid nitrogen is administered by a spray or the use of cryoprobes. Rapid freezing results in intracellular and extracellular ice crystallization. Cell destruction is potentiated by a rapid freeze and slow thaw cycle. This method is useful in small to large nodular and superficial basal cell carcinomas, but is not indicated for deeply invasive tumors.[18]

Electrodesiccation and Curettage

This surgical method uses heat to destroy tissue. After the tumor is marked and anesthetized, a debulking process is used to scrape away abnormal tissue within 1 to 2 mm. The base of the tumor is then electrodesiccated. Curettage of the base is performed using a large and tiny curet to track any extension of the tumor. The procedure is repeated as necessary until a normal plane of tissue is reached.

Moh's Chemosurgery

Moh's chemosurgery involves surgical removal of the tumor, layer by layer until all margins are free of the tumor on microscopic examination.

Radiation Therapy

Tissue conservation is a benefit of radiation therapy, especially when dealing with lesions on the nose, eyelid, or lips. Cosmetic results are good with this type of treatment because surgical scars and skin grafting are eliminated. A combined approach of preoperative and postoperative radiation and surgery may be indicated for extensive tumors. Radiation is fractionated over multiple treatment sessions (usually 450 Gy/3 weeks in 300 cGy daily fractions) to reduce radiation-induced side effects. Radiation therapy is not recommended for tumors located on the trunk, extremities, dorsum of the hands, tumors of the scalp, those arising in sweat and sebaceous glands and for morphea-form basal cell, verrucous squamous cell, tumors over 8 cm in size, and/or those tumors located on the upper lip growing into the nostril.[18]

Chemotherapy and Biotherapy

Topical 5-fluorouracil (5-FU) may be used in nevoid basal cell carcinoma syndrome but is contraindicated in treating any of the other types of basal cell carcinoma. Biologic response modifiers (BRM), especially alpha-interferon, has produced a 50% objective response rate in clinical testing. Intralesional alpha-interferon has produced an even greater response rate of 77%. Other agents, specifically retinoids, have also shown some activity against basal cell carcinoma.[3]

Metastasis

Metastatic disease is rarely seen with basal cell carcinoma, even though it tends to be a locally aggressive tumor. If left untreated, the tumor will locally invade vital structures such as blood vessels, lymph nodes, nerve sheaths, cartilage, bone, lungs, and the dura mater.

Prognosis

Basal cell carcinoma is highly curable with early detection and treatment. Cure rates are close to 100% in persons with lesion less than 1 cm. The overall 5-year survival rate is approximately 95% when surgical intervention or radiation therapy is used.

Squamous Cell Carcinoma

Epidemiology

Squamous cell carcinoma occurs more frequently in persons with light complexions, is more common in men, and the incidence increases with advancing age. The average age of onset for squamous cell carcinoma is approximately 60 years.[1,8]

Etiology and Risk Factors

Squamous cell carcinoma is most often found in sun-damaged skin previously affected by actinic keratoses. All of the predisposing risk factors mentioned in regards to basal cell carcinoma have also been associated with the development of squamous cell carcinoma.

Prevention, Screening and Detection

Prevention and detection methods are similar for both squamous cell and basal cell carcinoma. The avoidance of ultraviolet light and the use of sunscreens and protective clothing are important. In addition to the head and neck area, sunscreen should also be liberally applied to the hands and forearms. See Prevention and Detection section for basal cell carcinoma earlier in this chapter.

Classification and Clinical Features

Squamous cell carcinoma has a more indiscriminate method of classification. Because of the varying general characteristics and the source of tissue presentation, it is classified by presenting symptoms, tissue source, and histologic difference.[13]

Clinical Features of Squamous Cell Carcinoma

General characteristics

- Occurs anywhere on sun-damaged skin and/or on mucous membrane with squamous epithelium
- Appears as a round to irregular shape, with a plaque-like or nodular character covered by a warty scale, indistinct margins, firm erythematous dome-shaped nodule with a corelike center that ulcerates
- Dull red in color
- Grows by expansion and infiltration as well as by tracking along various tissue planes
- Invades below the level of the sweat gland and has a higher degree of malignant potential[13]

Classifications

- Ishemic ulceration
- Bowen's disease
- Actinic chelitis
- Verrucous

Diagnosis and Staging

Diagnosis and staging for squamous cell carcinomas are the same as for basal cell described in Chapter 4.

Metastasis

Metastasis occurs late via the lymphatics (within 2 years) after the tumor has invaded the subcutaneous lymph nodes and the lymphatics of the deeper structure.

Treatment Modalities

Surgery

Squamous cell carcinoma can be treated by procedures similar to those used with basal cell carcinoma.

Chemotherapy

Topical 5-FU is recommended for treatment of premalignant actinic keratosis. In advanced squamous cell carcinoma, systemic retinoids have produced response rates greater than 70%.[12]

Radiation Therapy

Radiation therapy is used for primary squamous cell carcinoma using a variety of fractionation regimens ranging from 22 Gy in a single fraction to 70 Gy in multiple fractions.

Prognosis

Of the two nonmelanoma skin cancers, metastasis is seen more often on squamous cell carcinoma. Squamous cell carcinoma also has high cure rates (75% to 80%) when either surgery or radiation therapy is used. Because this lesion has the ability to metastasize as well as recur, it is generally considered a higher risk skin cancer.

Malignant Melanoma

Epidemiology

Melanoma, a relatively uncommon tumor, affects approximately 32,000 persons in the United States each year. The incidence of melanoma is increasing at the rate of 4% annually. Estimates are that, by the year 2000, 1 in 100 persons will develop a primary malignant melanoma during their lifetime. Incidence among white males has increased 5.1% each year, 93.3% overall, while in females it has increased only 3.8% per year, 67.7% overall.[1,7]

Malignant melanoma most frequently affects whites. The most common site of occurrence in dark-skinned persons are palms, soles, nailbeds, fingers, toes, and mucous membranes. Unlike basal and squamous cell carcinomas, melanoma may occur in person in their teens and early twenties and thirties. Figure 18-1 depicts the sites of most common occurrence.

Etiology and Risk Factors

Genetic risk factors, such as fair complexion and blond or red hair color, are similar for the development of both nonmelanoma skin cancers and malignant melanoma. A person's ability to tan seems to be a factor; persons who burn easily and are poor tanners have an increased risk. Persons who experience intermittent heavy sun exposure are also at higher risk. In addition, a personal or family history of melanoma, dysplastic nevus syndrome, or

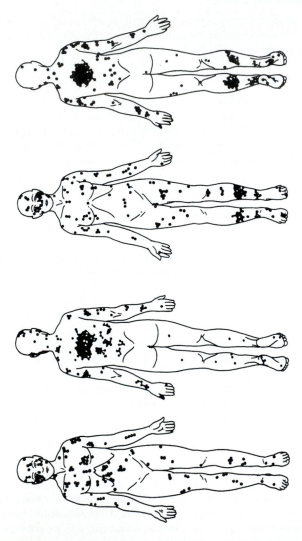

Figure 18-1. Anatomic distribution of malignant melanoma in men and women. (From Becker J, Goldberg L, and Tschen J: *Differential diagnosis of malignant melanoma,* Am Fam Physician 39(5), 1989.)

congenital nevi also increases one's risks. First-degree relatives of patients with melanoma are roughly two to eight times more likely than the general public to be diagnosed with melanoma.[1,6,7]

Prevention, Screening, and Detection

Prevention methods for nonmelanoma skin cancers and malignant melanoma are similar. Avoiding intense sun exposure and using protective clothing and sunscreens are important. Children should also be protected from sunburns because there is an increased risk of melanoma in persons who have experienced traumatic sunburns as children.[10]

Classification and Clinical Features

Clinical characteristics of dysplastic nevus (DN) are compared and contrasted with common acquired nevus (CAN) in Table 18-1. Four types of malignant melanoma exist: superficial, spreading, nodular lentigo maligna, and acral lentiginous.[3]

Common Benign Pigmented Lesions:

- Simple lentigo
- Junctional nevi
- Compound nevus
- Solar lentigo
- Seborrheic keratosis

Malignant Melanoma Pigmented Lesions:

- Superficial spreading melanoma
- Nodular melanoma
- Lentigo malignant melanoma
- Acral lentiginous melanoma

Diagnosis and Staging

When a lesion is suspected to be melanoma, a biopsy should be performed. The technique of choice is a total excisional biopsy with narrow margins. The biopsy procedure is accompanied by a thorough history and a complete physical examination. The skin should be carefully inspected and palpated for intracutaneous metastasis. Further diagnostic evaluation includes routine labora-

Table 18-1 Comparison of Common Acquired Nevus and Dysplastic Nevus

Characteristic	Common Acquired Nevus	Dysplastic Nevus
Color	Uniformly tan or brown; one mole looks much like another	Variegated, mottled, mixture of tan, red/pink, brown, within a single nevus; nevi look very different from each other
Shape	Round; sharp, clear-cut borders between nevus and surrounding skin; may be flat or elevated	Irregular, notched border; borders may fade off into surrounding skin; always have a macular or flat component
Size	Usually <5 mm diameter (smaller than the size of a pencil)	Usually >5 mm diameter
Number	Average adult has 20 to 40 scattered over body	Typically 100, although some people may have only a few nevi
Location	Usually on sun-exposed surfaces of body above waist; scalp, breast, and buttocks rarely involved	Back is most common site; may occur below waist and on scalp, breast, buttocks and genitals

Modified from Lawler PE and Schreiber S: *Cutaneous malignant melanoma: nursing's role in prevention and early detection,* Oncol Nurs Forum 16(3):348, 1989.

tory tests (CBC, LDH, BUN, PTT), liver enzyme studies, urine analysis, serum creatinine, blood chemistries, and a chest x-ray. Histopathologic grading for melanoma is identical to the grading system used for basal and squamous cell carcinoma.[4,16]

See Chapter 4.

Metastasis

Malignant melanoma may spread to any organ or remote viscera. Common sites for disseminated disease are the skin, bone, brain, liver, and lung.

Treatment Modalities

Surgery

Elective Regional Node Dissection (ERLAND)

The rationale for performing ERLAND is based on the hypothesis that melanoma metastasizes sequentially first to the regional lymph nodes and later from the nodes to distant sites. ERLAND improves survival rates for intermediate thickness (1.5 to 4 mm); for melanomas 0.76 to 1.5 mm thick there is no significant difference in survival; and ERLAND has no advantage for patients with melanomas less than 0.75 mm or more than 4 mm in thickness.[9,14,16]

Radiation Therapy

Melanoma has traditionally been considered relatively radio-resistant. Experimental radiation therapy endeavors include radiosensitizers such as Misonidiazole, and the use of fast neutrons.

Chemotherapy

Dacarbazine (DTIC) is the most extensively studied and regarded as the most effective single agent. Other cytotoxic agents reported to demonstrate some efficacy include carmustine, semustine (methyl CCNU), vindesine, and cisplatin. Combination chemotherapy includes: DTIC, BCNU, cisplatin, tamoxifen, bleomycin, eldesin, CCNU, and vincristine.

Hyperthermic Regional Perfusion

Hyperthermic regional perfusion or isolated limb perfusion is being used for intransit metastasis and as an adjuvant therapy. This form of therapy allows a large dose of chemotherapy to be delivered to a malignant melanoma affected extremity with minimal systemic toxicity. The limb is usually perfused for 1 hour with a high concentration of melphalan at 39 to 41°C with a perfusion pump and extracorporeal circulator. The hyperthermia enhances the cytotoxic effect so that the total dose of drug may be reduced. This procedure should only be performed by experts. Complications include arterial and venous thrombosis, tissue necrosis, nerve and muscle damage, and, rarely, loss of the extremity.[16]

Biotherapy

High-dose recombinant interleukin-2 has been used to treat distant metastasis with some success. BCG has shown tumor regressions when injected intralesionally.[11,13]

Hormonal Therapy

Hormonal therapy for malignant melanoma is under investigation. Currently tamoxifen and diethylstilbestrol are being explored.[16]

Prognosis

The overall 5-year survival rate for melanoma is 80%. The difference in 5-year survival rates of localized (90%) versus regional disease (50%), and distant (14%) validates the importance of early diagnosis and prompt treatment to ensure high cure rates.

Nursing Management

Nursing Diagnosis

- *Knowledge deficit related to prevention and early detection of skin cancer.*[5,13]

Interventions

- Define and describe risk factors: fair complexion, sunburn easily, red or blond hair, reside in geographic region that receives high levels of ultraviolet radiation, history of nonmelanoma/melanoma skin cancer[16]
- Describe and discuss methods to minimize sun exposure: wear lip balm/sunscreen with SPF of 15 or more; avoid exposure to sun between hours of 10:00 A.M. and 3:00 P.M.; wear protective clothing, maximize use of available shade, keep infants and children out of the sun, and teach and practice sun protection measures early in children's growth and developmental process
- Discuss importance of and procedure for routine skin self-examination: Cover entire skin in a methodic fashion, use good lighting, use mirrors, blow hairdryer, and a buddy system to examine difficult-to-see areas (scalp, perineum, back), document and report promptly any changes and/or new conditions

Nursing Diagnosis

- *Knowledge deficit regarding home care management of surgical wound.*

Interventions

- Demonstrate dressing change with return demonstration of procedure, patient/family states place for purchase of supplies, resources to contact for assistance and/or report symptoms, signs and symptoms that may indicate infection, knows procedure and can demonstrate proper body mechanics for mobility purposes, limitations and/or restrictions for elevation of extremity and/or general hygiene[13]

Nursing Diagnosis

- *Impaired physical mobility, potential for, related to surgical treatment and possible skin graft.*

Interventions

- Discuss and teach proper body mechanics when transferring to/from bed/chair/commode; and/or walking
- Discuss and demonstrate restriction and limitations for affected extremity
- Discuss/demonstrate rationale for body position changes if immobilized in bed
- Discuss/demonstrate body mechanics for daily hygiene; any restrictions on shower/tub bath[13]

Geriatric Considerations

- Geriatric population has the greatest incidence of precancerous and cancerous skin legions
- Average age of onset for squamous cell, lentigo malignant melanoma, and acral lentiginous melanoma is 60 years
- Age-related sensory and muscle deficits require assistance of buddy for monthly self-skin examination
- Age-related changes in skin characteristics include fair skin, easily bruised superficial tissue
- Limited access to health care system, and limited health care resources that may inhibit preventative care
- Target senior citizen centers to reach those who participate in organized activities

Bibliography

1. American Cancer Society: *Cancer facts and figures—1994*, Atlanta, 1994, American Cancer Society.
2. Amron DM and Moy RL: *Stratospheric ozone depletion and its relationship to skin cancer,* J Dermatol Surg Oncol 17:370, 1991.
3. Arnold HL and others: Epidermal nevi, neoplasms, and cysts. In Arnold HL, Odom RB, and James WD, editors: *Andrew's diseases of the skin, clinical dermatology,* ed 8, Philadelphia, 1990, WB Saunders.

4. Becker JK, Goldberg LH, and Tschen JA: *Differential diagnosis of malignant melanoma,* Am Fam Physician 39(5):203, 1989.

5. Berwick M and others: *The role of the nurse in skin cancer prevention, screening, and early detection,* Semin Oncol Nurs 7(1):64, 1991.

6. Crijins MB and others: *Dysplastic nevi occurrence in first- and second-degree relatives of patients with 'sporadic' dysplastic nevus syndrome,* Arch Dermatol 127(9):1346, 1991.

7. Fraser MC and others: *Melanoma and nonmelanoma skin cancer: epidemiology and risk factors,* Semin Oncol Nurs 7(1):2, 1991.

8. Glass AG and Hoover RN: *The emerging epidemic of melanoma and squamous cell skin cancer,* JAMA 262:2097, 1989.

9. Ho VC and Sober AJ: *Therapy for cutaneous melanoma: an update,* J Am Acad Dermatol 22:159, 1990.

10. Lawler PE and Schreiber S: *Cutaneous malignant melanoma: nursing's role in prevention and early detection,* Oncol Nurs Forum 16(3):345, 1989.

11. Lawler PE: *Cutaneous malignant melanoma,* Semin Oncol Nurs 7(1):26, 1991.

12. Loescher LJ and Meyskens FL, Jr: *Chemoprevention of human skin cancers,* Semin Oncol Nurs 7(1):45, 1991.

13. Longman A: Skin cancer. In Clark JC and McGee RF, editors: *Core curriculum for oncology nursing,* ed 2, Philadelphia, 1992, WB Saunders.

14. McFadden ME: *Cutaneous T-cell lymphoma,* Semin Oncol Nurs 7(1):36, 1991.

15. Rigel DS and others: *Dysplastic nevi-markers for increased risk for melanoma,* Cancer 63:386, 1989.

16. Shapiro PE: Malignant melanoma. In Schein PS, editor: *Decision making in oncology,* Philadelphia, 1989, BC Decker.

17. Shimm DS and Wilder RB: *Radiation therapy for squamous cell carcinoma,* AM J Clin Oncol 14(5):383, 1991.

18. Vargo NL: *Basal and squamous cell carcinomas: an overview,* Semin Oncol Nurs 7(1):13, 1991.

19. Volker DL: Standards of oncology practice and standards of oncology education; patient, family, and public. In Clark JC and McGee RF, editors: *Core curriculum for oncology nursing,* ed 2, Philadelphia, 1992, WB Saunders.

20. Wolf DJ and Zitelli JA: *Surgical margins for basal cell carcinomas,* Arch Dermatol 123:340, 1987.

Oncologic Complications

19

Management of an oncologic complication is dependent upon many important factors related to the patient and the underlying disease (symptoms and signs, natural history of the primary tumor, efficacy of available treatment and treatment goals). These factors must be given consideration prior to interventions. Additional concepts are the identification of patients at risk for developing an oncologic complication and secondly, the involvement of the family and significant other(s).

Disseminated Intravascular Coagulation

Disseminated intravascular coagulation (DIC) is a bleeding disorder; and alteration in the blood clotting mechanism, with abnormal acceleration of the coagulation cascade in which both thrombosis and hemorrhage may occur simultaneously.[1,23]

Etiology and Risk Factors

Shock or trauma, infections, obstetric complications, malignancies (APML, AML, melanoma, cancers of the lung, colon, breast, stomach, pancreas, ovary, and prostate), blood vessel injuries, infectious vasculitis, vascular disorders, and intravascular hemolysis.

Pathophysiology

DIC is a disruption of body hemostasis. One of the triggering mechanisms from the underlying pathology initiates the process (Figure 19-1), which results in the formation of thrombin and fibrinolysin (plasmin). Thrombin acts to convert fibrinogen to fibrin to form clots. At the same time fibrinolysin degrades some of the fibrin into a soluble monomer form; this initiates clot dissolution. The remaining portion of fibrin is an insoluble polymer, which continues to form clots. These clots may be deposited in the extremities or in organs such as the lungs, kidneys, and brain. Capillary clots result in tissue ischemia, hypoxia, necrosis, and thrombocytopenia. Fibrin degradation products are produced which lead to capillary hemorrhage.

Clinical Features

- Signs of bleeding: menstrual, gastrointestinal, intracerebral, hematuria, hematemesis, scleral changes, and bleeding from injection or injury sites

Diagnosis

Laboratory findings substantiate a diagnosis of DIC (Table 19-1).

Treatment Modalities

The goal of therapy is to eliminate or alter the triggering event. Common examples are the treatment of sepsis with antibiotics and treatment of cancer with surgery, chemotherapy, and radiation therapy. When bleeding is severe, blood component therapy is necessary to achieve hemostasis.[11]

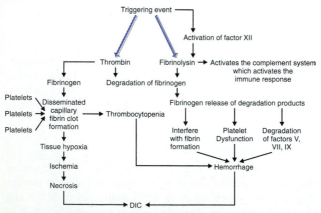

Figure 19-1. Pathophysiology of disseminated intravascular coagulation.

Table 19-1 DIC Laboratory Profile

Diagnostic Test	Normal Value	Expected Value in DIC
Prothrombin time	10-13 sec	Prolonged
Partial thromboplastin time	39-48 sec	Usually prolonged
Thrombin time	10-13 sec	Usually prolonged
Fibrinogen level	200-400 mg/100 ml	Decreased
Platelet level	150,000 - 400,000/mm^3	Decreased
Factor assay (II, V, VII, VIII, IX, X, XI, XII)		Decreased levels of factors VI, VIII, and IX
Fibrinogen/fibrin degradation products	< 10	Increased
Protamine sulfate test (soluble fibrin monomer)	Negative	Strongly Positive
Antithrombin III levels (AT-III) (used to monitor response to therapy)	89%-120%	Decreased

From Yasko JM and Schafer SL: *Disseminated intravascular coagulation.* In Yasko JM, editor: *Guidelines for cancer care: symptom management,* Reston, Va, 1983, Reston Publishing Co, p 327.

Common blood products used in treating DIC are as follows:
- Platelets
- Fresh frozen plasma (FFP)
- Packed red blood cells (PRBCs)
- Cryoprecipitate

Heparin therapy, which inhibits thrombin formation, interferes with thrombin and stops the conversion of fibrinogen to fibrin, which prevents clot formation. Usual doses of heparin are from 2,500 to 5,000 U subcutaneously every 8 to 12 hours, 50 U/kg by IV bolus every 4 to 6 hours, or 100 to 200 U/kg every 24 hours by IV infusion.

Prognosis

The prognosis of DIC is dependent upon the underlying cause, the degree of disruption of the coagulation system, and the effects of bleeding and clotting. The estimated mortality rate for DIC is 54% to 68%. Increasing age, severity of laboratory abnormalities, and number of clinical manifestations increase the mortality from DIC.

Hypercalcemia

Hypercalcemia occurs when the serum calcium level rises above the normal level of 9 to 11 mg/100 mL.

Etiology and Risk Factors

Common malignancies associated with this condition include cancers of the breast and kidney, squamous cell cancers of the lung, head, neck, or esophagus, lymphoma, leukemia, and multiple myeloma.

Other causes include: primary hyperparathyroidism, thyrotoxicosis, prolonged immobilization, renal failure, and diuretic therapy with thiazide preparations.[2]

Pathophysiology

Hypercalcemia resulting from malignancies occurs through several different mechanisms, depending upon the location and action of the cancer cells, as follows:[6,33]
- Direct bony destruction by tumor cells
- Prolonged immobilization

- Ectopic parathyroid hormone production by tumor cells
- Metabolic substances produced by the tumor

Clinical Features

- Lethargy
- Change in mental status
- Constipation
- Arrhythmias
- Polyuria, Polydipsia
- ECG changes
- Renal calculi and failure

Diagnosis

Laboratory tests to determine serum calcium level, urinary calcium level, phosphorous alkaline phospatose, BUN, creatinine, electrolytes, and PTH; chest x-ray, CT scan, and electrocardiograms.

Treatment Modalities

Hydration

Large volumes of isotonic saline (Table 19-2) restores plasma volume and promotes urinary calcium excretion through sodium diuresis. Calcium loss follows sodium loss. Fluid volume in the range of about 5 to 8 L/day is common for the first 24 hours followed by 3L/day thereafter.[27]

Mobilization

Immobilization should be avoided since it will increase resorption of calcium from the bones.

Dialysis

Dialysis removes both excess calcium and phospate. Serum phospate levels should be measured and phosphates replaced as necessary.

Dietary Manipulation

Excessive volumes of milk and dairy products should be discouraged.

Pharmacologic Therapy

Chemotherapeutic agents used to treat hypercalcemia are: diuretics (furosemide, ethacrynic acid phosphates) and oral and IV phosphates (Table 19-2).

Prognosis

Hypercalcemia is reversibe in 80% of episodes if it is recognized and prompt aggressive therapy is initiated. Without prompt treatment, it is associated with a 50% mortality rate.

Malignant Pleural Effusion

Etiology and Risk Factors

Benign causes of pleural effusion include congestive heart failure, pericarditis, respiratory infections (pneumonia, tuberculosis), superior vena cava syndrome, mediastinal irradiation, ascites, hypoalbuminemia, and nephrosis.

Malignant pleural effusion is the result of metastatic disease of the pleura or mediastinal lymph nodes, lung, breast, ovary, lymphomas, and leukemias.

Pathophysiology

Equilibrium of pleural fluid movement is regulated by five dynamic forces: capillary permeability, hydrostatic pressure (capillary and interstitial), colloidal osmotic pressure (plasma protein and interstitial protein), negative intrapleural pressure, and lymphatic drainage. The lymphatic channels regulate fluid and protein reabsorption. It is estimated that 5 to 10 L of fluid pass through the pleural space in 24 hours, yet only 5 to 10 mL remain in the space at any give time. Abnormal fluid accumulation occurs when there is a disruption of the regulating forces, causing excessive fluid production or decreased fluid reabsorption.[22]

Clinical Features

- Labored breathing, desire to lie on affected side
- Tachypnea
- Restricted chest wall expansion; Egophony
- Dullness or flatness to percussion of the affected side

Table 19-2 Therapy for Hypercalcemia of Malignancy

Therapy	Dosage	Comments
Saline; add loop diuretics such as furosemide	5-8 L IV during the first 24 hr, then 3 L/day of normal saline. Diuretic dose 20 mg q 4-6 hr. Calciuretic dose 80-100 mg q 1-2 hr.	Restores plasma volume, increases glomerular filtration rate and promotes renal calcium excretion. Loop diuretics block calcium radsorption in the loop of Henle. Especially important when hypercalcemia is severe and the patient is dehydrated. Should not be used as sole therapy.
Pamidronate disodium (Aredia)	60-90 mg IV infusion over 4-24 hours for 1 day	Interferes with osteoclast activity by absorbing to calcium crystals in bone blocking dissolution of calcium. This inhibits bone resorption. Safe in patients with renal failure.
Gallium nitrate (Gallium)	200 mg/m^2/d IV 24 hr infusion for 4-5 days	Inhibits bone resorption without compromising bone strength. Nephrotoxicity is a potential toxicity. Discontinue this drug if serum creatinine exceeds 2.5 mg/dL.

Continued.

Table 19-2 Cont'd.

Therapy	Dosage	Comments
Etidronate (Didronel, Didronel IV)	7.5 mg/kg/day IV infusion over 2 hours for 4-5 days, then 10 mg/kg/day orally for up to 3 mo	Inhibits bone resorption. Limits calcium absorption from gut. Promotes soft tissue and skeletal calcification. Returns serum calcium level to normal within 3 to 5 days. Contraindicated in patients with renal failure. Give with saline hydration.
Calcitonin-salmon* (Calcimar, Miacalcin) plus a glucocorticoid	Calcitonin-salmon, 200 MRC U every 12 hr subcutaneously; hydrocortisone, 100 mg IV every 6 hr	Impairs bone resorption and increases renal calcium excretion. Especially effective in patients with hematologic malignancies. Safe in patients with renal or cardiac failure.
Plicamycin (Mithracin)	15-25 ug/kg/day by slow IV infusion over 4 hr for 1 day	Inhibits bone resorption by direct injury to osteoclasts. Calcium-lowering effects not seen for 24-48 hr. Potentially dangerous in patients with renal or hepatic failure.

| Phosphate | Up to 0.5 g orally 4 times daily | Reciprocal relationship between calcium and phosphorus. Useful when hypercalcemia is associated with low serum phosphorus level. Diarrhea may be a problem. Contraindicated in patients with renal failure or serum phosphorus levels >3.8 mg/dL. Often used as maintenance therapy. |

*Calcitonin–human (Cibacalcin) has not yet been approved for use in hypercalcemia but is expected to be as effective as calcitonin-salmon for this condition.
Adapted from Mundy G: *Options for correcting hypercalcemia of malignancy*, Hospital Therapy, Feb 1988; and Zimberg M and Mahon S: *Understanding delirium: an impediment to quality of life*, Quality of Life—A Nursing Challenge 1(1).

- Decreased diaphragmatic excursion with percussion
- Diminished or absent breath sounds
- Anxiety malaise
- Dry-non-productive cough
- Pleuritic rub over the affected area during auscultation
- If the effusion is large, additional signs could include:
  Bulging of the intercostal spaces on the affected side
  Splinting of the chest on the affected side
  Cyanosis, chest tenderness
  Tracheal deviation to the unaffected side

Diagnosis

Pleural effusion is usually detected by chest x-ray, ultrasound of the chest, CT, scan of the thorax, or a thoracentesis.[24,28,29]

Treatment Modalities

Treatment modalities of malignant pleural effusion are as follows: (Figure 19-2)

- Systemic Therapy—Chemotherapy
- Local Therapy—Radiation Therapy
- Pleurodesis (Chemical Sclerosing)
- Surgery—Pleurectomy (Mechanical Pleurodesis)
- Pleuroperitoneal Shunts
- Long-term thoracotomy access and drainage

Prognosis

Survival rates vary from 3 months to 4 years, with the longest survival in patients with lymphoma.

Neoplastic Cardiac Tamponade

Neoplastic cardiac tamponade is the compression of the cardiac muscle by pathologic fluid accumulation under pressure within the pericardial sac. Compression of the myocardium interferes with dilatation of the heart chambers, which prevents adequate cardiac filling during diastole, reduces blood flow to the ventricles and reduces stroke volume, which results in decreased cardiac output.[33]

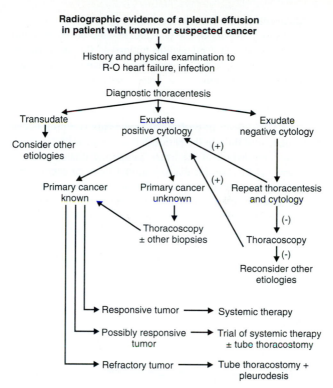

Figure 19-2. Clinical algorithm for prompt diagnosis and management of malignant pleural effusions. R-O, rule out; (+), positive; (–), negative. (From Ruckdeschel JC: *Management of malignant pleural effusion: an overview,* Semin Oncol 15(suppl 3):27, 1988.)

Etiology and Risk Factors

- Heart surgery, chest trauma, aneurysm
- Bacterial, fungal, viral, or tubercular infections
- Systemic lupus erythematosus, scleroderma, rheumatoid disease
- Myxedema
- Uremia
- Pharmacologic therapy (anthracyclines, anticoagulants, hydralazine, procainamide)

Malignant causes include the following:

- Primary tumors of the pericardium (mesotheliomas and sarcomas); and metastatic tumors of the pericardium (lung, breast, leukemia, lymphoma, melanoma, sarcomas)
- Radiation therapy

Pathophysiology

The pathophysiology of pericardial tamponade is a progressive accumulation of fluid in the pericardial sac (Figure 19-3), which leads to compression of the heart, hampering dilatation of its chambers and thus limiting diastolic atrial filling: intrapericardial pressure rises and bilateral ventricular stroke volume decreases.

The severity of cardiac tamponade depends on the amount of fluid in the pericardium, the rate of accumulation, and the degree of pericardial and organic compromise. Usually there will be no change in cardiac activity with the addition of 50 mL or less of fluid in the pericardial space. However, 100 to 200 mL of fluid may cause severe cardiac impairment if the accumulation occurs rapidly.[4,18]

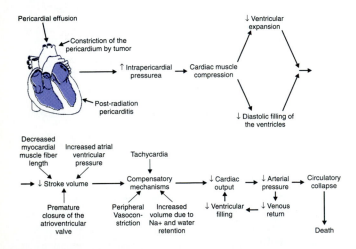

Figure 19-3. Development of neoplastic pericardial tamponade. (From Yasko JM and Schafer SL: *Neoplastic pericardial tamponade*. In Yasko JM, editor: *Guidelines for cancer care: symptom management*, Reston, Va, 1983, Reston Publishing Co.)

Clinical Features

- Tachycardia
- Vasoconstriction
- Increased CVP
- Arterial hypotension
- Cardiomegaly
- Engorged neck veins
- Ascites
- Hepatojugular reflux
- Distant weak heart sounds
- Tachypnea
- Hypotension
- Distant weak heart sounds
- Pericardial friction rub
- Peripheral edema
- Oliguria
- Hepatomegaly
- Anxiety, clouded sensorium
- Thready diminished pulse pressure or pulsus paradoxus

Diagnosis

Tests ordered will include a chest x-ray, ECG, echocardiogram, transesophageal echo, stress echo, intraarterial echo, cardiac catheterization, and laboratory blood work.[3]

Treatment Modalities

Neoplastic cardiac tamponade is a life-threatening situation that requires immediate medical intervention as soon as the diagnosis is confirmed. The immediate goal of treatment is the removal of pericardial fluid to relieve impending circulatory collapse. Following symptomatic relief of tamponade, the longer-range goal is management of the underlying disease.

- Pharmacologic Therapy[24]
  Corticosteroids, Diuretics, Vasoactive Drugs
  Blood products and intravenuous fluids infusions
- Pericardiocentesis
- Surgery
  Pericardial "window" or total pericardiectomy
- Radiation Therapy
- Chemotherapy

Prognosis

Survival of the patient with neoplastic cardiac tamponade depends upon the cause of the primary malignancy, the stage of cancer at the time of intervention, tumor responsiveness to radiation therapy or chemotherapy, the hemodynamic significance of the tamponade, the effectiveness of therapy, and the general

medical condition of the patient. Response rate with local therapies is 50%, with duration of remission approximately 4 to 6
months.

Septic Shock

Shock comprises a group of diverse life-threatening syndromes
that result from different pathophysiologic circumstances (decreased cardiac function, hemorrhage, trauma, antigen/antibody
reaction, and sepsis). There are three major classifications of
shock: hypovolemic, cardiogenic, and distributive or vasogenic.
Hypovolemic shock is a result of decreased intravascular volume. Cardiogenic shock results from the impaired ability of the
heart to adequately pump blood. Distributive or vasogenic shock
is the result of an abnormality in the vascular system. Included
under distributive shock is neurogenic, anaphylactic, and septic
shock.

Etiology, Risk Factors, and Pathophysiology

Septic shock is a complex interaction of hemodynamic, humoral,
cellular, and metabolic abnormalities. This is a result of the effects of the proliferation of gram-negative bacteria and/or the
release of endotoxins by those bacteria (Figure 19-4). Endot-
oxin is a component of the cellular wall of gram-negative bacteria and, when released, it activates the coagulation complement
and kinin systems. This toxin-induced reaction activates the humoral cellular and immunologic defense mechanisms leading to
a generalized inflammatory response. Evidence of this response
is the production of various chemical mediators such as pros-
taglandins, endorphins, and kinins, which modulate the variety
of multisystem alterations seen in septic shock.[10,25]

The abnormalities seen in septic shock are summarized as
follows:

- Hemodynamic Instability
  - hemolysis—cardiovascular alteration
- Humoral/Cellular Alterations
  - vasodilation/vasoconstriction—fluid shift to interstitial
    space
- Metabolic Dysfunction
  - metabolic acidosis—septic shock cell death

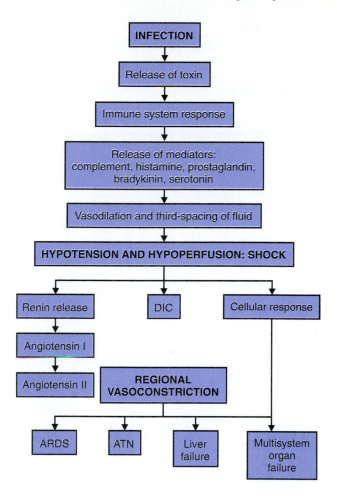

Figure 19-4. The pathophysiology of septic shock. (From McMorrow ME and Cooney-Daniello M: *When to support septic shock*, RN 54(10):32, 1991.)

Clinical Features

The clinical features associated with a three stage classification of shock are as follows:

Stage One: hyperdynamic stage (early shock, warm shock)
Decreased tissue perfusion—10% reduction in blood volume
Usually lasts less than 24 hours

- Feelings of anxiety, apprehension, nervousness
- Altered mental status, restlessness, irritability, disorientation, or inappropriate euphoria
- Temperature normal, below normal, or above normal
- Skin warm and flushed because of arteriole dilatation
- Peripheral cyanosis
- Tachycardia and bounding peripheral pulses
- Normal or slightly elevated blood pressure with a widening pulse pressure
- Tachypnea and/or hyperventilation
- Rales and decreased breath sounds
- Respiratory alkalosis—decreased PO^2
- Renal output normal or elevated (polyuria)
- BUN and creatinine may be slowly increasing
- Hyperglycemia
- Glycosuria

Stage Two: normodynamic stage (intermediate shock, cool shock)
Decreased tissue perfusion—15% to 20% reduction in blood volume
Usually lasts a few hours

- Complaints of thirst, tachycardia
- Altered mental status—lethargy, confusion
- Skin pale, cool, and clammy because of peripheral vasoconstriction and diversion of blood to vital organs
- Peripheral edema may be present because of increased secretion of ADH and aldosterone leading to sodium and water retention
- Temperature normal or subnormal
- Blood pressure decreases with a narrow pulse pressure because of decrease in cardiac output
- Respirations slow and shallow
- Respiratory acidosis
- Renal output decreased

- Urine specific gravity elevated
- Abdominal distention because of air swallowing and decreased peristalsis
- Hemorrhagic lesions may be apparent

Stage Three: hypodynamic stage (late shock, refractory shock, irreversible shock, cold shock, "classic" shock)
Decreased cardiac output, decrease in blood volume

- Altered mental status, stupor, coma
- Skin cold, possible cyanosis of digits and mottling
- Temperature subnormal
- Tachycardia, hypotension
- Weak or absent pulses because of decreased myocardial contractility—"pump failure"
- Respiratory depression
- Pulmonary edema, or "shock lung," because of decreased PO_2 and decreased pulmonary microcirculatory ARDS
- Metabolic acidosis because of anaerobic metabolism and increased levels of lactic acid
- Hypoglycemia
- No renal output
- Renal failure—ATN
- Hemorrhagic lesions

Diagnosis

- Various culture and sensitivity (blood, urine, wound, sputum)
- Chest x-ray, EKG, WBC and Platelet count
- Urine analysis
- Coagulation profile, arterial bloodgases
- Cardiac and liver enzymes
- Serum glucose and lactate

Treatment Modalities

Treatment modalities for septic shock include:
- Antibiotic therapy
- Invasive hemodynamic monitoring
- Blood volume replacement
- Vasoactive drugs
- Inotropic agents
- Oxygen and respiratory therapy

- Mechanical ventilation
- Maintain fluid and electrolyte balance
- Steroid therapy
- Administer hematopoietic growth factors[24]

Prognosis

Survival is contingent upon preventing or reversing the process of shock and on the status of the underlying disease (nonfatal, ultimately fatal, rapidly fatal); 60% of all patients survive warm shock, and 40% survive cool or cold shock.

Spinal Cord Compression

A malignant tumor in the epidural space can encroach upon the spinal cord or cauda equina and result in spinal cord compression (SCC), a medical emergency requiring early detection and prompt treatment.

Etiology and Risk Factors

Bone metastases are second only to pulmonary metastases in frequency of occurence followed by cancers of the lung, breast, prostate, lymphoma, and myeloma.[5] The location of epidural metastasis and cord compression is related to the origin of the primary cancer and influenced by vascular supply and venous drainage. The ribs, sternum, humerus, femur, and skull are also common areas of disease spread.

Pathophysiology

Bone metastasis involves the vertebral column and invades the epidural space (Figure 19-5). It is estimated that 95% of SCC are due to tumor in the epidural space or outside the spinal cord. The destruction taking place in the bone is one of two types: osteolytic or osteoblastic.[8] The epidural space is invaded by tumor by one of three mechanisms:

- Direct extension of the tumor into the space following bony erosion of the vertebral body
- Lymph node growth through the foramina into the epidural space
- Hematogenous spread by means of an embolic process

Neurologic deficits result from these three mechanisms of metastases by three different processes:

- Direct compression of the spinal cord or cauda equina by the tumor itself
- Interruption of the vascular supply to neural structure by the tumor
- Compression due to vertebral collapse resulting from pathologic fracture or dislocation

Clinical Features

- Muscle weakness
- Sensory impairment (paralysis, loss of bowel and bladder control, paraplegia)
- Pain—radicular in nature; intense persistent and progressive
- Tingling and/or numbness in extremities
- Diminished pain and temperature sensation
- Sexual dysfunction

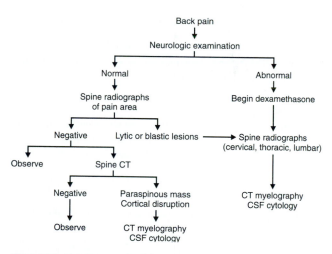

Figure 19-5. Algorithm of epidural spinal cord compression. (From Gilbert MR: *Epidural spinal cord compression and carcinomectous meningitis.* In Johnson RT, editor: *Current therapy in neurologic disease,* 3rd ed, St Louis, 1990, Mosby.)

Diagnosis

A diagnosis should be confirmed immediately because of the potential for rapid progression and possible permanent neurologic dysfunction. A good history and physical examination should be accompanied by neurologic testing, x-ray films, radioisotope bone scan, a lumbar puncture, myelography, and MRI.[16]

Treatment Modalities

The choice of treatment for patients with SCC is dependent on the primary tumor, the rapidity of onset of the compression and the level, severity, and duration of the blockage. The two most frequent treatment modalities for SCC are surgery and radiation therapy. Laminectomy, with decompression of the spinal cord and nerve roots, bone grafting and/or stabilization with hardware, is the most common treatment.[9,12,15] Following surgery, postoperative radiation therapy is administered to treat the remaining tumor. Portal size depends on residual tumor and extends one to two vertebrae above and below the level of involvement to assure an adequate dosage and field. Irradiation may be initiated a few days after surgery and continued for 2 weeks. The use of steroids is advocated to decrease edema, relieve symptoms, and control pain. Chemotherapy may be given concomitantly or following radiation therapy as systemic treatment for the primary underlying malignancy.

Prognosis

Response to therapy for SCC depends on the severity and rapidity of onset of symptoms more than on their duration. Patients with intramedullary metastasis usually have a rapid progression of dysfunction and therefore a poorer prognosis. If patients are ambulatory at the initiation of therapy, 80% will retain the ability to walk after treatment, whereas only 30% to 40% of patients with pretreatment motor dysfunction are ambulatory after treatment.

Superior Vena Cava Syndrome (SVCS)

Obstruction of the venous flow through the superior vena cava results in impaired venous drainage with engorgement of the vessels from the head and upper body torso.

Etiology and Risk Factors

Cancer is responsible for more than 97% of all cases of SVCS. Three fourths of all malignant cases of SVCS are caused by bronchogenic cancer, particularly oat cell carcinoma of the lung. Hodgkin's disease and non-Hodgkin's lymphoma, Kaposi's sarcoma, adenocarcinoma of the breast, thymomas, and primary or metastatic seminoma and other germ cell tumors are some of these cancers. Other causes are related to venous thrombosis (indwelling central venous catheters) and radiation therapy.

Pathophysiology

Obstruction of the superior vena cava can be a consequence of three physiologic events:

- External compression by an extrinsic mass, solid tumor, or enlarged lymph node
- Intravascular obstruction by tumor or thrombosis
- Intraluminal reaction to tumor invasion or inflammation

Impairment of the venous circulation through the superior vena cava reduces blood flow to the right atrium, which results in venous hypertension with venous stasis and a decrease in cardiac output. If untreated, the progression is from vascular congestion to thrombosis, cerebral edema, pulmonary complications, and death.[7]

Clinical Features

- Edema of the face, neck, upper thorax and breasts and upper extremities
- Periorbital edema and/or edema of the conjunctivae, with or without protrusion of the eye
- Horner's syndrome
- Respiratory compromise
- Increased pressure of the jugular veins

■ Dilatation and prominence of collateral vessels in upper thorax and neck
■ Telangiectasis
■ Compensatory tachycardia

Diagnosis

The diagnostic evaluation of a patient with SVCS is highly dependent on the patient's physical condition. SVCS may be considered one of the rare occasions when treatment can be started even before a tissue diagnosis is confirmed. Diagnostic tests include: chest radiography, tissue biopsy, CT scan, MRI, sputum for cytology, bone marrow biopsy, bronchoscopy, mediastinoscopy, thoracotomy, or supraclavicular lymph node biopsy.[33,34]

Treatment Modalities

The choice of treatment depends on the rate of onset, the causative process (benign or malignant), and the type of mass (intraluminal or extraluminal).[14]

Radiation Therapy

Radiation therapy is the treatment of choice for SVCS because of its local therapeutic response and minimal toxicities. Treatment is begun immediately in acute and life-threatening situations. The total dose, dose fractionation, and size and type of the field depend on tumor histology, patient condition, radiologic response, and symptom relief.

Chemotherapy

The use of chemotherapy to treat SVCS is an effective primary treatment when the cause is small cell lung cancer lymphoma or a germ cell tumor. The choice of chemotherapeutic agents is based on the malignant cause of SVCS.

Surgery

Specific surgical approaches to SVCS include superior vena cava bypass or stent placement. Bypass surgery is indicated when the tumor could be completely removed if the superior vena cava were excised with it; where venous return is inadequate in spite of collateral circulation; and when the obstruction is due to venous thrombosis or fibrosis.

Pharmacologic Therapy

Anticoagulation therapy is indicated for SVCS because of venous stasis. It may be used alone to resolve thrombus obstruction secondary to a central venous catheter or following initial fibrinolytic therapy. It is also used as a maintenance treatment to reduce the extent of the thrombus and prevent its progression. Removal of the central venous catheter should also be followed by anticoagulation to avoid embolization.

Prognosis

The prognosis of patients with SVCS strongly correlates with the prognosis of the underlying disease. The best responses are seen in patients with lymphoma and small cell lung cancer. Other types of lung cancer have fewer long-term responses. Only 10% to 20% of all patients are alive 2 years after therapy. Of patients with lymphoma, 45% have survived to 30 months, compared to 10% of patients with lung cancers.

Syndrome of Inappropriate Antidiuretic Hormone Secretion

The syndrome of inappropriate antidiuretic hormone secretion (SIADH) is a disorder of water balance and is characterized by elevated serum blood levels of antidiuretic hormone (ADH), excessive water retention, and hyponatremia.

Etiology and Risk Factors

Approximately two thirds of patients with documented SIADH have a neoplasm. The most common malignant disease associated with this syndrome is lung cancer (oat cell), cancer of the duodenum and pancreas, lymphoma, thymoma, and mesothelioma. Several chemotherapeutic agents, cisplatin, cyclophosphamide, vinblastine, and vincristine have demonstrated the inappropriate release of ADH.[21] Nonmalignant conditions are central nervous system disorders, pumonary infections, asthma, hypoadrenalcorticism, lupus erythematosus, and acute intermittent porphyria.

Pathophysiology

A variety of conditions can disrupt the body fluid regulating system and cause the inappropriate secretion of ADH. Three pathophysiologic mechanisms are responsible for SIADH:[23]

- Inappropriate secretion of ADH from the supraoptic-hypophyseal system. This mechanism results from CNS disorders such as head trauma, stroke, meningitis, brain abscess, CNS hemorrhage and tumors, encephalitis, and Guillain-Barré syndrome. Patients in shock, experiencing status asthmaticus, pain, or high stress levels, or on positive pressure breathing may also experience SIADH.
- ADH or an ADH-like substance is secreted by cells outside of the supraoptic-hypophyseal system, referred to as ectopic secretion (e.g., infections).
- The action of ADH on the renal distal tubules is enhanced. Various drugs can stimulate or potentiate the release of ADH. These include narcotics such as nicotine, tranquilizers, barbiturates, general anesthetics, potassium supplements, thiazide diuretics, hypoglycemia agents, acetaminophen, isoproterenol, and four antineoplastic: cisplatin, cyclophosphamide, vinblastine, and vincristine.[33]

Clinical Features

- Hyponatremia
- Decreased osmolality of serum and extracellular fluid
- Excessive water retention
- Urine osmolarity greater than appropriate for plasma osmolarity, producing less than maximally dilute urine
- Continued urinary excretion of sodium
- Absence of fluid volume depletion
- Suppression of plasma renin
- Normal renal, adrenal, and thyroid function

The symptomatology experienced by the patient with SIADH depends on the degree of duration of water retention and

hyponatremia. Serum osmolality levels and serum, BUN, creatinine, Na^+, K^+, and Cl^- levels are obtained, and a water loading
test may be ordered.

Treatment Modalities

The primary treatment of choice for SIADH is to treat or eliminate the underlying cause. Other medical orders would include:

- Discontinue any medications that might cause SIADH
- Restrict fluids to 500 to 1000 mL/24 hr
- Administer pharmacologic agents that interfere with the
  action of ADH on the renal tubules and induce polyuria,
  such as lithium carbonate or demeclocycline
- If symptoms of water intoxication are severe, administer
  hypertonic (5% NaCl) solution with or without furosemide
  (Lasix) via volumetric pump

Prognosis

The rapidity and duration of response is highly dependent on the
underlying cause. SIADH usually resolves with tumor regression but it can persist despite control of the tumor. Neurologic
impairment from water intoxication is usually reversible and does
not require long-term rehabilitation.

Nursing Management

Disseminated Intravascular Coagulation

Nursing Diagnosis

- *Potential for injury (bleeding and/or thrombosis) related
  to:*
  - *Fibrous clot formation in the microcirculation*
  - *Clotting factor consumption and decreased platelets*
  - *Fibrinolysis or clot dissolution*

Interventions

Observation for signs of bleeding and thrombosis

- Assess organ systems for evidence of bleeding and
  thrombosis:

- Monitor vital signs
- Test all excreta for blood
- Assess for fatigue, lethargy, muscle weakness, and pain
- Monitor laboratory values

Hypercalcemia

Nursing Diagnoses

- *Potential for fluid volume deficit related to:*
    Effects of the disease
    Effects of treatment
- *Potential for fluid volume excess related to effects of treatment (hydration)*

Interventions

- Assess for signs and symptoms of alterations in fluid volume: Excess or Deficit
- Auscultate lungs for breath sounds every 4 hours
- Monitor intake and output closely
- Obtain daily weight
- Monitor laboratory values
- Administer diuretics
- Obtain urine pH

Malignant Pleural Effusion

Nursing Diagnoses

- *Ineffective breathing patterns related to limited lung expansion secondary to pleural effusion*
- *Potential for impaired gas exchange related to ineffective breathing patterns and pleural effusion*

Interventions

- Determine current respiratory status
- Assist with breathing and pulmonary toilet
- Provide oxygen therapy
- Administer respiratory medications

- Provide mechanical ventilation
- Teach measures to maintain optimal respiratory abilities
- Make referrals to other health care professionals
- Monitor chest tube drainage if indicated
- Assist with pleurodesis if ordered

Neoplastic Cardiac Tamponade

Nursing Diagnoses
- *Decreased cardiac output related to diastolic filling of the ventricles due to compression of the heart*
- *Alteration in tissue perfusion related to decreased cardiac output*

Interventions
- Assess hemodynamic status
- Monitor laboratory values and test results
- Reposition patient to enhance circulation
- Perform measures to reduce the work load of the heart
- Administer vasoactive drugs
- Be prepared for cardiac arrest and emergency resuscitation

Nursing Diagnosis
- *Potential for impaired gas exchange related to decreased circulation and pulmonary congestion*

Interventions
- Monitor respiratory status
- Assist with breathing and pulmonary toilet
- Administer oxygen therapy and mechanical ventilation
- Monitor respiratory status closely
- Observe monitoring equipment frequently for changes
- Assess all catheters for patency and drainage

Septic Shock

Nursing Diagnoses

- *Alteration in tissue perfusion related to the response to the release of endotoxins*
- *Alteration in cardiac output (decreased) related to decreased cardiac function*

Interventions

- Monitor vital signs every 4 hours
- If hypotension is present, place patient flat in bed or in Trendelenburg position
- Assess skin color, temperature, and moisture every 4 hours
- Assess organ systems for malfunctions due to ischemia
- Monitor ECG for evidence of arrhythmias
- Monitor laboratory values closely
- Obtain specimens for culture and sensitivities
- Administer antibiotics
- Provide oxygen therapy
- Administer vasopressive drugs
- Administer pain medication

Nursing Diagnoses

- *Ineffective breathing patterns related to pulmonary edema and metabolic acidosis*
- *Impaired gas exchange related to circulatory collapse and pulmonary edema*

Interventions

- Observe ventilatory function for difficulties: shallow respirations, tachypnea, dyspnea, frothy secretions, and jugular vein distention
- Auscultate lungs for evidence of impairment
- Monitor intake and output
- Measure CVP
- Obtain or assist with measurement of arterial blood gases
- Administer humidified oxygen therapy by mask
- Administer diuretics and decrease fluid intake
- Suction nasopharynx and lungs

Spinal Cord Compression

Nursing Diagnosis

- *Impaired physical mobility related to spinal cord compression*

Interventions

- Assess patient's level of function/mobility: sensory, motor, bladder, and sexual function
- Check for evidence of venous thrombosis
- Implement pain management program
- Establish activity regimen according to patient's physical status and physician order
- Obtain consultations with physical and occupational therapy for evaluation and assistance
- Encourage and assist patient to perform self-care
- Discuss and teach the use of assistive and supportive devices
- Arrange consultation or referral to rehabilitative services

Nursing Diagnosis

- *Alteration in bowel elimination, constipation related to decreased activity or immobility*

Interventions

- Obtain history of bowel elimination
- Assess abdomen each day (distention, bowel sounds)
- Monitor bowel movements
- Encourage fluids
- Increase bulk and fiber in diet
- Administer stool softeners, laxatives, bulk products, and lubricants
- Initiate bowel training program as necessary

Nursing Diagnosis

- *Potential/actual alteration in pattern of urinary elimination related to neurogenic bladder/loss of voluntary control of micturation*

Interventions

- Obtain history of bladder elimination patterns
- Assess abdomen
- Monitor urinary output
- Check for residual after each voiding
- Monitor laboratory values
- Assess for signs and symptoms of a urinary tract infection
- Culture urine as ordered
- Observe for presence of hyperreflexia
- Initiate bladder training program as necessary

Nursing Diagnosis

- *Alteration in sexual dysfunction related to disease process and treatment*

Interventions

- Examine own attitudes, knowledge, and skills in the area of sexuality, sexual function, and sexual counseling
- Provide a therapeutic environment
- Elicit a sexual history as appropriate
- Be respectful of social, cultural, and religious factors that may influence patient perceptions of sexuality
- Discuss the potential impact of disease and/or treatment on sexuality and/or sexual function
- Identify available resources and make referrals

Superior Vena Cava Syndrome

Nursing Diagnoses

- *Potential for decreased cardiac output related to decreased venous return related to vena cava obstruction*
- *Potential for impaired gas exchange related to venous congestion related to vena cava obstruction*

Interventions

- Assess patient for changes in cardiac function
- Provide oxygen therapy as ordered

- Position patient for comfort and enhancement of venous drainage from upper torso
- Prevent activities that increase intrathoracic or intracerebral pressure
- Assist patient with physical activities as needed
- Provide measures to decrease anxiety

Nursing Diagnoses

- *Potential for alteration in cerebral tissue perfusion related to upper torso venous stasis and decreased cardiac output*
- *Potential for alteration in thought process related to decreased cerebral tissue perfusion and impaired gas exchange*

Interventions

- Assess organ systems for malfunction related to ischemia
- Note any changes in mental status
- Monitor laboratory values closely
- Administer vasoactive drugs
- Provide oxygen as prescribed
- Institute safety measures

Syndrome of Inappropriate Antidiuretic Hormone Secretion

Nursing Diagnoses

- *Alteration in fluid volume: excess related to fluid retention (due to SIADH) and possible hyponatremia*
- *Potential for fluid volume deficit related to fluid restriction as treatment for SIADH*

Interventions

- Assess for signs or symptoms of alteration in fluid volume: Excess or Deficit
- Auscultate lungs for breath sounds every 4 hours
- Monitor cardiac function and tissue perfusion

- Monitor intake and output closely
- Obtain a daily weight
- Monitor laboratory values
- Obtain urine osmolality and specific gravity
- Monitor skin integrity and provide skin care

Bibliography

1. Bailes BK: *Disseminated intravascular coagulation principles, treatment, nursing management,* AORN J 55(2):517, 1992.

2. Bajorunas DR, editor: *Advances in the hypercalcemia of malignancy,* Semin Oncol 17(Suppl 5):1, 1990.

3. Barbiere CC: *Cardiac tamponade: diagnosis and emergency intervention,* Crit Care Nurse 10(4):20, 1990.

4. Braunwald E: Pericardial disease. In Braunwald E and others, editors: *Harrison's principles of internal medicine,* ed 11, New York, 1991, McGraw-Hill.

5. Byrne TN: *Spinal cord compression from epidural metastases.* N Engl J Med 327:614, 1992.

6. Calafato A and Jessys AL: Body fluid composition, alteration in: hypercalcemia. In McNally JC and others, editors: *Guidelines for oncology nursing practice,* ed 2, Philadelphia, 1991, WB Saunders.

7. Cawley M: Alteration in cardiac output, decreased: related to superior vena cava syndrome. In McNally JC and others, editors: *Guidelines for oncology nursing practice,* ed 2, Philadelphia, 1991, WB Saunders.

8. Delaney TF and Oldfield EH: Spinal cord compression. In DeVita VT, Hellman S, and Rosenberg SA, editors: *Cancer: principle and practice in oncology,* ed 4, Philadelphia, 1993, JB Lippincott.

9. Dyck S: *Surgical instrumentation as a palliative treatment for spinal cord compression,* Oncol Nurs Forum 18(3):515, 1991.

10. Ellerhorst-Ryan JM: Septic shock: understanding and managing a crisis. In *Challenges in treatment and management, Proceedings of the Sixth National Conference on Cancer Nursing,* Atlanta, 1992, American Cancer Society.

11. Epstein C and Bakanauskas A: *Clinical management of DIC: Early nursing interventions,* Crit Care Nurs 11(10):42, 1991.
12. Gentzch P: Mobility, impaired physical, related to spinal cord compression. In McNally JC and others, editors: *Guidelines for oncology nursing practice,* ed 2, Philadelphia, 1991, WB Saunders.
13. Gilbert MR and Grossman SA: *Incidence and nature of neurologic problems in patients with solid tumors,* Amer J Med 81:951, 1986.
14. Gray BH and others: *Safety and efficacy of thrombolytic therapy for superior vena cava syndrome.* Chest 99:54, 1991.
15. Grossman SA and Lossignol D: *Diagnosis and treatment of epidural metastases,* Oncology 4(4):47, 1990.
16. Hilderley LJ: Spinal cord compression: the nurse's role in early detection and rehabilitation. In *Challenges in treatment and management, Proceedings of the Sixth National Conference on Cancer Nursing,* Atlanta, 1992, American Cancer Society.
17. Hogan CM: Sexual dysfunction related to disease process and treatment. In McNally JC et al, editors: *Guidelines for oncology nursing practice,* ed 2, Philadelphia, 1991, WB Saunders.
18. Kern L and Omery A: *Decreased cardiac output in the critical care setting,* Nurs Diagnosis 3(3):94, 1992.
19. Kratcha-Sveningson L: Body fluid composition, alteration in: syndrome of inappropriate antidiuretic hormone (SIADH). In McNally JC and others, editors: *Guidelines for oncology nursing practice,* ed 2, Philadelphia, 1991, WB Saunders.
20. Larkin M and Benson LM: Ineffective airway clearance. In Clark JC and McGee RF, editors: *Core curriculum for oncology nursing,* ed 2, Philadelphia, 1992, WB Saunders .
21. Lindaman C: *SIADH is your patient at risk?* Nursing 22(6):60, 1992.
22. Mangan CM: *Malignant pericardia effusions: pathophysiology and clinical correlates,* Oncol Nurs Forum 19(8):215, 1991.

23. McFadden ME and Sartorius SE: *Multiple systems organ failure in the patient with cancer. Part I: Pathophysiologic perspectives,* Oncol Nurs Forum 19(5):719, 1992.

24. McFadden ME and Sartorius SE: *Multiple system organ failure in the patient with cancer Part II: Nursing implications,* Oncol Nurs Forum 19(5):727, 1992.

25. McMorrow ME and Cooney-Daniello M: *When to suspect septic shock,* RN, 54(10):32, 1991.

26. Miaskowski C: Oncologic emergencies. In Baird SB, McCorkle R, Grant M, editors: *Cancer nursing a comprehensive textbook.* Philadelphia, 1991, WB Saunders.

27. Mundy G: *Options for correcting hypercalcemia of malignancy,* Hospital Therapy, Feb:52, 1988.

28. Olopade OI and Ultmann JE: *Malignant effusions,* CA 41(3):167, 1991.

29. Sahn SA: *Diagnosis pleural effusion,* Hosp Med, 28(9):66, 1992.

30. Schruber JA: Impaired gas exchange. In Clark JC and McGee RF, editors: *Core curriculum for oncology nursing,* ed 2, Philadelphia, 1992, WB Saunders.

31. Smith EL: *Dyspnea and quality of life, Quality of Life—A Nursing Challenge* 1(1):31, 1992.

32. Truett L: *The septic syndrome,* Cancer Nurs 14(4):175, 1991.

33. Warrell RP: Metabolic emergencies. In Devita VT, Hellman S and Rosenberg SA, editors: *Cancer: principles and practice in oncology,* ed 4, Philadelphia, 1993, JB Lippincott.

34. Yahalom J: Superior vena cava syndrome. In DeVita VT, Hellman S, and Rosenberg SA, editors: *Cancer: principles and practice in oncology,* ed 4, Philadelphia, 1993, JB Lippincott.

35. Zimberg M and Mahon SM: *Understanding delirium: an impediment of quality of life,* Quality of Life—A Nursing Challenge 1(1):3, 1992.

Section III

Cancer

Treatment

Modalities

Surgery

20

The four primary modalities for the treatment of cancers are surgery, chemotherapy, radiation therapy, and biotherapy. Surgery can be the initial and preferred treatment of choice for many cancers. Advances in surgical techniques, a better understanding of the metastatic patterns of individual tumors, and intensive postoperative care have now made it possible for tumors to be removed from almost any part of the body.

Applications for Surgical Oncology

Diagnosis of Disease

Surgical techniques that are used to obtain tissue samples for examination include: incisional biopsy, excisional biopsy, needle biopsy, or endoscopy. The type of biopsy technique depends on a tumor's location, size, and growth characteristics.

Staging of Disease

Surgical staging is reserved for tumors that are inaccessible, difficult to evaluate, and incorrectly staged by any other means. A staging laparotomy may be performed before radical surgery to obtain tissue samples and determine disease sites.

Treatment of Disease

Surgical treatment of the cancer process focuses on five primary areas: primary treatment, adjuvant treatment, salvage treatment, palliative treatment, and combination treatment.[3,5]

Primary treatment involves the removal of a malignant tumor and a margin of adjacent normal tissue. *Local excision* is the simple excision of a tumor and a small margin of normal tissue. *Wide excision* or en bloc dissection involves removal of the primary tumor, regional lymph nodes, intervening lymphatic channels, and involved neighboring structures. *Extended wide excision*, in which wide tumor infiltration in a particular region is removed. *Surgical treatment of cancer in situ* is accomplished by several special surgical techniques.

Adjuvant treatment involves the removal of tissues to decrease the risk of cancer incidence, progression, or recurrence and includes *cytoreductive therapy* or *debulking*.[17]

Salvage treatment involves the use of an extensive surgical approach to treat local recurrence after implementing a less extensive primary approach.[17]

Palliative treatment is used to decrease disease or treatment-related symptoms without trying to cure the cancer surgically. Examples of palliative procedures include:

- Bone stabilization
- Relief of life-threatening obstruction or bleeding
- Removal of solitary metastasis
- Treatment of oncologic emergencies
- Treatment of complications from chemotherapy and radiation therapy
- Ablative surgery, or removal of a hormone source
- Management of cancer pain.

Combination treatment involves the use of surgery with other treatment modalities with the goals of improving tumor resectability, decreasing the extent of tumor removed, limiting the change in physical appearance and functional ability, and improving treatment outcomes.

Insertion and Monitoring of Therapeutic and Supportive Hardware

Therapeutic and supportive hardware (ventricular reservoirs, central venous catheters, implantable vascular devices) can be surgically implanted to promote patient comfort and/or ease the delivery of treatment.

Second-look procedures involve follow-up surgery within a predetermined time frame after the original surgery and/or adjuvant treatment to check for the presence or absence of disease. Sites and volume of residual tumor are identified and resected when possible. Second-look procedures are usually done for those cancers that tend to recur locally.[9]

Reconstruction involves the reconstruction of anatomic defects caused by cancer surgery. Its purpose is to improve function and/or cosmetic appearance. Reconstructive surgery may be immediate and permanent, immediate and temporary, or postponed for safety reasons or until suitable graft tissue can be prepared and transferred.[13]

Prevention of Disease

Surgery is the preferred treatment for precancerous and in situ lesions of all epithelial surfaces.

Principles of Surgical Oncology

When considering surgery for the patient with cancer, the surgeon critically evaluates the following: tumor factors, tumor cell kinetics, and patient variables.[3,5,13]

Tumor factors
- Anatomic location
- Histologic type
- Tumor size

Tumor cell kinetics
- Growth rate or biologic aggressiveness
- Invasion
- Metastatic potential or pattern and extent of metastatic spread

Patient variables
- General state
- Host resistance or immune competence
- Desire for treatment
- Quality of life

Special Surgical Techniques

Several special surgical techniques are used in the treatment of cancer. These include electrosurgery, cryosurgery, chemosurgery, lasers, and photodynamic therapy.

Electrosurgery

Eliminates cancer cells by using the cutting and coagulating effects of high-frequency electrical current applied by needles, blades, or electrodes.

Cryosurgery

Involves application of liquid nitrogen probes to selectively destroy tumor tissue by deep-freezing them.

Chemosurgery

The combined use of layer-by-layer surgical resection of tissue and topical application of chemotherapeutic agents.[1]

Lasers

Light Amplification by Stimulated Emission of Radiation (Laser) therapy is used for local excision. Lasers destroy cancer cells by intensive thermal energy and can be used for cancers of the larynx, female reproductive tract, and skin.[8,16]

Photodynamic Therapy

Involves the intravenous injection of a light-sensitizing agent (hematoporphyrin derivative [HPD]) with uptake by cancer cells, followed by exposure to a laser light within 24 to 48 hours of injection. This results in fluorescence of cancer cells and cell death.[16]

Special Considerations in Surgical Oncology

Nutrition

Protein-calorie malnutrition generally results from: decreased oral intake, increased enternal losses as a result of malabsorp-

tion or intestinal fistulas, and/or increased nutritional requirements due to hypermetabolism or the presence of a tumor.

The results are: poor wound healing, anemia, infection, sepsis,
pneumonia, further malnutrition, and increased morbidity. Nutritional management is aimed first at reversing protein-calorie
malnutrition and preventing weight loss. Once this has been accomplished, the nutrition plan can be as aggressive as the cancer
treatment plan.[10,14]

Blood Disorders

Anemia is common among cancer patients and should be corrected preoperatively with packed red cell transfusions to a hematocrit equal to or greater than 35. It is generally accepted that
50,000 functionally active platelets per cubic millimeter are sufficient for surgery. An insufficient preoperative platelet count
can result in postoperative bleeding and fatal hemorrhage, especially if the patient receives large volumes of blood products.[11,14]

Complications of Multimodal Therapy

Radiation can cause fibrosis and obliteration of lymphatic and
vascular channels, causing long-term damages to underlying tissues. Postoperative wound healing is thus affected in the patient
who has been irradiated previously in the same area. Tissue that
has been irradiated is not biologically normal, and once surgery
disrupts tissue integrity, infection, wound dehiscence, and necrosis can occur. Chemotherapy drugs often decrease the cancer
patient's red blood cell, white blood cell, and platelet counts.
The nadir may not occur for ten to fourteen days after initial
drug administration. Monitoring of the patient's blood counts
and knowledge of the drug's schedule and effects can alert the
nurse to potential complications of wound infection and bleeding.[1]

Surgical Risks in Older Patients

All surgical procedures must be considered high-risk for the older
cancer patient. Careful preoperative assessment of physiologic
parameters and correction of nutritional deficits and fluid and
electrolyte imbalances should begin as early as possible.

The physiologic changes related to the aging process that
can affect surgical outcome include cardiovascular, respiratory,

urinary, musculoskeletal, gastrointestinal, metabolic and immune systems.[4,12]

Nursing Management

Preoperative Care

Preoperative nursing care of the cancer patient focuses on assessment and intervention. See Table 20-1 for information specific to preoperative assessment of physiologic parameters in the surgical oncology patient.

Nursing Diagnosis

- *Body image disturbance:*
  Related to surgical removal of body part
  Related to diagnosis of cancer

Interventions

- Encourage patient to discuss feelings and concerns with health care providers and significant others
- Help patient identify, label, and express feelings about the significance of the lost body part, treatment modalities, and anticipated prognosis

Nursing Diagnosis

- *Fluid volume deficit*
  Related to surgical procedure (loss of 15% to 20% of total blood volume during surgery)

Interventions

- Administer drugs as ordered to maintain BP, increase cardiac output
- Administer fluids and volume expanders as ordered
- Assess skin for color, temperature, and elasticity
- Maintain accurate intake and output
- Monitor arterial blood gases, respiratory rate and pattern, and urine output

Nursing Diagnosis

- *Infection: potential for*
    *Related to preoperative immunocompromised status,
    as a result of disease and/or previous therapy*

Interventions

- Monitor vital signs (increased pulse; low-grade, intermittent fever)
- Observe body secretions, excretions, and exudates for signs of infection; report abnormalities
- Monitor hydration and electrolyte balance
- Monitor changes in WBC count
- Turn patient frequently; instruct in deep breathing

Nursing Diagnosis

- *Injury: potential for*
    Related to peritonitis secondary to breakdown of anastomosis caused by decreased tissue healing resulting from chemotherapy, radiation therapy, poor nutritional status, and/or tumor

Interventions

- Assess for signs/symptoms:
    Moderate to sever abdominal pain
    Burning ache aggravated by any motion, even respiration
    Anorexia, Nausea, Vomiting
    Fever within 48 hours after surgery
    Chills, thirst, scanty urine
    Inability to pass feces or flatus
    Abdominal distention
    Tachycardia with weak, thready pulses
    Rapid, shallow respirations

Nursing Diagnosis

- *Injury: potential for*
    Related to hypercoagulability and postoperative inactivity

Table 20-1 Preoperative Assessment of Physiologic Parameters[6,11,15]

Physiologic Parameters	Factors That Increase Surgical Risk	Assessment Factors	Laboratory Tests/Others
Nutritional status	Debilitation and malnourishment as a result of disease and/or previous therapy	Anorexia Eating habits, Special diets Food restriction Supplementation Nausea, Vomiting, Stomatitis Smell or taste changes Recent weight loss	Decreased serum albumin
Cardiovascular system	Congestive heart failure as a result of previous and prolonged chemotherapy	Dyspnea, Fatigue Anorexia Abdominal distention Right upper quadrant pain Tachycardia Weak, thready pulse Hypotension Rapid, labored respiration Frothy, blood-tinged sputum Moist rales Weight gain Peripheral edema	Increased pulmonary capillary pressure Decreased cardiac output Increased right atrial pressure

Pulmonary system	Pulmonary edema and/or fibrosis as a result of previous and prolonged chemotherapy	Nasal flaring Labored, noisy breathing Diaphoresis Rales, Wheezing Persistent cough Restlessness Hypotension Tachycardia Sudden weight gain Swollen feet or ankles Chest pain	Decreased vital capacity Decreased minute volume Decreased cardiac output $PaCO_2$ PaO_2 pH K^+ Na^+ Pulmonary capillary wedge pressure Pulmonary artery pressure Sputum specimens for culture and sensitivity Serial chest x-ray reports
Genitourinary system	Renal insufficiency as a result of previous and prolonged chemotherapy	Frequency of voiding Dysuria, Anuria Infection Urine (color, clarity)	Decreased creatinine clearance Increased BUN and uric acid levels Increased serum creatinine levels

Continued.

Table 20-1 Cont'd.

Physiologic Parameters	Factors That Increase Surgical Risk	Assessment Factors	Laboratory Tests/Others
Fluid and electrolyte status	Dehydration and electrolyte imbalance as a result of disease and/or previous therapy Hypovolemia as a result of disease	Intake and output Vomiting, Diarrhea Bleeding	K^+, Mg^{++}, Ca^{++}, H^+
Liver function status	Metastatic liver disease	Jaundice, Ascites Vague upper abdominal pain Anorexia Weight loss Splenomegaly Dependent edema	Total bilirubin
Hematologic factors	Platelet dysfunction as a result of disease and/or previous therapy Hypercoagulability as a result of disease	Easy bruising Excessive bleeding Dyspnea Previous thrombophlebitis	PT, PTT Platelet count RBC and WBC count Hgb, HCT

Potential for postoperative complications	Preoperative infection as a result of immuno-competence and/or previous therapy Previous radiation therapy	Cough Sore throat Fever Rashes Radiation skin damage in relation to anticipated surgical incision	WBC count Throat and sputum culture

Interventions

- Assess calves daily
- Observe for signs/symptoms of thrombophlebitis:
    Calf pain, tenderness
    Homan's sign
    Dilated superficial veins
    Edema of involved extremity

Nursing Diagnosis

- *Nutrition, altered, less than body requirements*
    Related to surgical procedure for cancer that interferes with mechanical process of eating
    Related to surgical procedure for cancer that interferes with absorption of essential salts and nutrients

Interventions

- Assess for signs/symptoms of protein-calorie malnutrition:
    Edema
    Dyspigmentation and thinning of the hair
    Muscle wasting
- Perform nutrition assessment:
    Assess problem area, food preferences, patterns and behaviours related to food intake, intake and output, and calorie count
- Provide relaxed environment without pain
- Consult with dietician to provide diet and supplements that meet patient's needs
- Care for and monitor intravenous total parenteral nutrition and feeding tubes

Nursing Diagnosis

- *Pain*
    Related to surgical procedure
    Related to complications at therapeutic hardware's insertion sites

Interventions

- Incorporate the following in assessing patient's pain status:
    - Location, onset, frequency, intensity, quality
        - Effective and ineffective pain control measures
        - Pain expression style
        - Movement
        - Effect of pain on postoperative activities and sleep/wake patterns
- Identify strategies that eliminate or control pain
- Administer medication per physician's orders and protocols using appropriate delivery system:
    - Monitor effect at frequent intervals
    - Graphically record pain assessment data
    - Provide physician with evidence of need to change medication

Nursing Diagnosis

- *Skin integrity, impaired*
    - *Related to tissue damage and/or poor tissue healing as a result of chemotherapy, radiation therapy, and/or poor nutritional status*

Interventions

- Asses for signs/symptoms of dehiscence:
    - Monitor amount and color of drainage
    - Call physician immediately
    - Obtain vital signs
    - Prepare patient for surgery
- Assess for signs of evisceration:
    - Apply sterile moist towels over extruded intestine or omentum

Preoperative Patient Teaching Priorities:

Include information regarding:
- The surgery to be performed
- General preoperative activities and rationale
- General postoperative behaviours expected of the patient and rationale

- Techniques such as TCDB, incisional splinting, ROM exercises, incentive spirometry
- Types of apparatus to be used before and after surgery
- Plan of care and rationale for procedures
- Anticipated care settings, equipment and experiences related to surgery
- Self-care strategies to prevent and minimize complications of surgery

Outcomes of preoperative teaching:
The patient and/or significant other is able to:

- State that anxiety is decreased regarding surgery
- Demonstrate an understanding of preoperative and postoperative procedures and routines by return demonstration, verbal feedback, etc.

Postoperative Patient Teaching Priorities

Include information regarding:

- Changes in self-care activities and other activities resulting from surgery
- Progressive return to maximum activity level
- Anticipated discharge medications
- Wound management
- Proper use of assistive or prosthetic devices
- Symptoms to observe for: fever, pain, vomiting, diarrhea, bleeding, malnutrition
- Who and when the patient should call if problems arise
- Where to get additional information about cancer or treatment
- Where support groups are located and how to contact them: Reach to Recovery, Make Today Count
- Resources or agencies that might be helpful to the patient: physical therapy, occupational therapy, speech therapy, ostomy outpatient clinics, prosthetic fitting devices, home care agencies
- Where the patient can get medical supplies
- Follow-up care that may be needed
- When the patient can return to work
- Any job retraining that may be necessary
- When the patient can drive a car
- When the patient can resume sexual activity

Geriatric Considerations

- Physiologic changes: cardiovascular, respiratory, renal, gastrointestinal, immune, metabolic, and muscoloskeletal systems may be compromised
- Anesthesia risk for hypoxemia
- Postoperative risk for pulmonary edema myocardial infarction, decreased cardiac output, pulmonary thromboembolism, and aspiration pneumonia
- Discharge plan will require assessment for need of additional resources, such as homecare agency, American Cancer Society and/or social services

Bibliography

1. Alexander HR: Vascular access and other specialized techniques of drug In DeVita VT, Jr, Hellman S, and Rosenberg SA, editors: *Cancer: principles and practice of oncology,* Philadelphia, 1993, JB Lippincott.
2. Bender CM and Yasko JM: Nursing role in management: problems with abnormal cell growth. In Lewis SM and Collier IC, editors: *Medical-surgical nursing: assessment and management of clinical problems,* ed 3, St Louis, 1992, Mosby.
3. Cady B and Quinlan R: Overall principles of cancer management: surgery, In Ostean RT: *Cancer Manual* ed 8, 1990 American Cancer Society, Atlanta.
4. Derby SA: Cancer in the older patient. In Ashwander P, Belcher AE, Mattson EAH, Moskowitz R, and Riese NE, editors: *Oncology nursing: advances, treatments and trends into the 21st century,* Rockville, MD, 1990, Aspen Publishers.
5. Eberlein TJ and Wilson RE: Principle of surgical oncology, In Holleb AI and others (editors): *ACS Textbook of Clinical Oncology,* 1991 American Cancer Society, Atlanta.
6. Frogge MH and Goodman M: Surgical therapy. In Groenwald SL, Frogge MH, Goodman M, and Yarbo CH, editors: *Cancer nursing: principles and practice,* ed 2, Boston, 1990, Jones and Bartlett.

7. Howland WS: Preoperative evaluation of the cancer patient for emergency surgery. In Turnbull AD, editor: *Surgical emergencies in the cancer patient,* Chicago, 1987, Year Book Medical Publishers.

8. Lehr P: *Surgical lasers: how they work, current applications,* AORN J 50(5):972, 1989.

9. Liotta LA and Stetler Sterenson WG: Principles of molecular cell biology of cancer: cancer metastasis. In DeVita VT Jr, Hellman S, and Rosenberg SA, editors: *Cancer principles and practice of oncology,* Philadelphia 1993, JB Lippincott.

10. Luckmann J and Sorenson KC: *Medical-surgical nursing: a psychophysiologic approach,* ed 4, Philadelphia, 1991, WB Saunders.

11. Maxwell M: General principles of therapy. In Groenwald SL, Frogge MH, Goodman M, and Yarbo CH, editors: *Cancer nursing: principles and practice,* ed 2, Boston, 1990, Jones and Bartlett.

12. Patterson WB: *Surgical issues in geriatric oncology,* Semin Oncol 16:57, 1989.

13. Rosenberg SA: Principles of surgical oncology. In DeVita VT Jr, Hellman S, and Rosenberg SA, editors: *Cancer: principles and practice of oncology,* ed 4, Philadelphia, 1993, JB Lippincott.

14. Szopa TS: *I*mplications of surgical treatment for nursing. In Clark SC and McGee RF, editors: *Core curriculum for oncology nursing*, ed 2, Philadelphia, 1992, WB Saunders.

15. Thompson JM and others: *Clinical nursing*, ed 2, St Louis, 1989, Mosby.

16. Tootla J and Easterling A: *PDT: destroying malignant cells with laser beams...photodynamic therapy*, Nurs 19(11):48, 1989.

17. Wong RJ and DeCosse JJ: *Cytoreductive surgery*, Surg Gynecol Obstet 170(3):276, 1990.

Radiation Therapy

21

Radiation therapy is the use of high energy ionizing rays or particles to treat cancer. It is a localized treatment that is used alone or in conjunction with other treatments such as surgery, chemotherapy, or both. Approximately 60% of all persons with cancer will be treated with radiation therapy at some point in their illness.[5]

Principles of Radiation Therapy

High-energy ionizing radiation destroys the cancer cell's ability to grow and multiply. Some cells are directly damaged by the ionizing rays or particles. However, more cells are indirectly affected when the ionizing rays or particles penetrate the cell's nucleus and interact with the water content of the nucleus to form oxygen radicals.[1,11,12]

The radiosensitivity of cancer cells is dependent upon several factors:

- Type of cell (e.g. lymphoma, leukemia, seminoma, squamous cell)
- Phase of cell life—cells in the resting stage are less sensitive to radiation than those in active cellular division
- Division rate of the cell—rapidly dividing cells are more sensitive to radiation than slowly dividing cells because more cells will be in the active cellular division stage
- Degree of differentiation—poorly differentiated cells are more sensitive to radiation therapy than well-differentiated cells
- Oxygenation—well-oxygenated tissues are more sensitive to radiation therapy because oxygen is needed to form the chemically active substances. Body tissues have limits to the amount of radiation that can be tolerated. Exceeding those limits can result in serious complications

Administation of Radiation Therapy

External beam radiation (teletherapy) uses a treatment machine placed at some distance from the body. Radiation can also be delivered by implanting a sealed radioactive source in or near the cancerous area to provide a localized treatment (brachytherapy). Radioactive materials may be injected intravenously or taken orally for a systemic effect (nonsealed sources). The radioactive substance travels to areas of the body requiring treatment. Tumor-specific antibodies that have been coupled with radioactive isotopes combine the science of immunology with radiation therapy to maximize tumor treatment while minimizing normal tissue toxicity. These antibodies are designed to be attracted to specific antigens on certain tumor cells while sparing normal tissues.[11]

External Radiation Therapy

Treatment Planning

A plan is developed to determine the best way to deliver the radiation therapy treatments. A major part of the planning process is the localization procedure which uses a simulator. A *simulator* is a machine that simulates the treatment machine in its movement and positioning. A variety of radiographic studies such as CT scans, MRI studies, barium enemas, and intravenous pyelograms help define the exact area whithin the body that needs treatment. Marks or small tattoos placed on the body are used to position the patient for treatment. These marks assure that treatment delivery will be consistent. Special plastic or plaster forms or molds may be constructed to help support and assist the patient to maintain a precise position during each treatment. The area of treatment is shaped with special shielding devices called blocks. These blocks, made of lead or high-density alloys, help to minimize radiation exposure to normal tissues near the treatment area. A compensating filter may be used to differentially absorb the radiation beam to provide a uniform dose to the treatment volume. The treatment planning session usually lasts 1 to 2 hours.[1,5,11]

Treatment Delivery

External radiation treatments are usually administered daily, Monday through Friday, for 2 to 8 weeks. Palliative treatments, such as for pain from bone metastasis, may be delivered at higher daily doses for fewer numbers of treatment. The actual treatment takes 2 to 5 minutes.

A variety of machines are used in radiation therapy, depending on the type and extent of the tumor. These machines vary according to the energy produced as well as ionizing particles delivered. Linear accelerators are commonly used in cancer therapy. The higher the energy produced by the machine, the greater the depth of penetration of the radiation beam. With higher energies the maximum effect of the radiation occurs below the skin surface and the dose to the skin is minimized.

Because a single large dose of radiation is too toxic to normal tissues, the total radiation dose is divided into small daily doses or fractions to be given over time. This process is called *fractionation*. The dose is usually the same each day. With fractionation of the total dose, more radiation can be delivered to the tumor while minimizing the damage to normal tissues, because fractionation allows normal cells to repair the sublethal damage after each treatment. Some treatment schemes deliver treatments two to three times a day with at least 5 to 6 hours between each fraction. This is called *hyperfractionation*.[9,11,12]

Total Body Irradiation

In conjunction with bone marrow transplantation, supralethal radiation in the form of total body irradiation and chemotherapy is administered to reduce the tumor volume and provide immunosuppression to prevent the rejection of the marrow graft. A variety of techniques provide a homogenous dose of radiation to the entire body (Figure 21-1). Doses range from 8 to 14 Gy, depending on fractionation.[11]

Half-Body Irradiation

This procedure delivers a single treatment to the upper or lower half of the body and frequently results in dramatic pain relief.

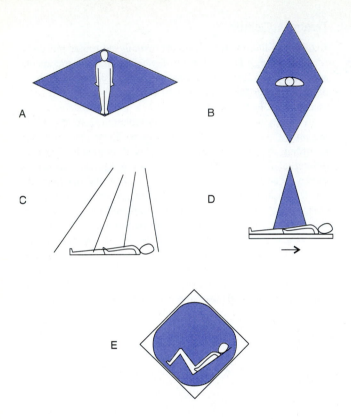

Figure 21-1. Methods of delivery of total body irradiation. **A,** Lateral opposed beams. **B,** Floor and ceiling parallel opposed beams. **C,** Supine and prone treatment using three matching fields. **D,** Supine and prone—patient moves horizontally through treatment beam field. **E,** Horizontal shrinking field technique—patient in sitting position. (From Quast U: *Total body irradiation,* Radiother Oncol 9:95, 1987, and Novack DH and Kiley JP: *Total body irradiation,* Front Radiat Ther Onc 21:69, 1987.)

Hyperthermia

Hyperthermia enhances the effects of radiation therapy on certain radioresistant and hypoxic tumor cells because heat affects more S-phase (synthesis) cells and poorly vascularized tumors are less able to dissipate heat. Hyperthermia is usually applied locally or regionally immediately after a radiation treatment. The number of treatments depends on the tumor site and its extent. Approximately 72 hours between treatments provides maximum benefit from hyperthermia. Local hyperthermia may be accomplished with microwaves, ultrasound, deep heating with electromagnetic wave applicators, and interstitial hyperthermia with probes implanted in or near the tumor. Regional hyperthermia involves perfusing heated solutions through a part of the body. The optimal therapeutic temperature is 41°C to 45°C for approximately 45 minutes. Interstitial temperature probes are usually inserted within the body part as well as placed superficially to monitor the heat.[17]

Intraoperative Radiation Therapy

Intraoperative radiation therapy provides direct visualization and treatment of tumors to control local recurrence of cancer (gastric, colorectal, bladder, pancreatic, cervical). After surgical exposure, a targeting cone is placed directly on the tumor site. The treatment machine is carefully aligned with the cone. All persons leave the treatment room for the 15 to 25 minutes it takes to deliver the fairly large dose of electron irradiation (approximately 2000 cGy). Anesthesia personnel monitor the patient through a closed-circuit television.[10]

Radiosensitizers

Chemical radiosensitizing compounds are used to increase the lethal effects of radiation therapy. Non-hypoxic sensitizers such as iododeoxyuridine (IUdR) incorporate into the DNA and increase the susceptibility of the cell to radiation damage. Hypoxic cell sensitizers such as metronidazole, misonidazole, SR2508, and Ro-03-8799 increase oxygen to hypoxic cells and promote damage of the DNA, preventing cell repair.[1]

Stereotactic External-Beam Irradiation

Stereotactic irradiation involves treatment of the relatively small intracranial volumes with a three dimensional distribution of the treatment beam (Arteriovenous malformations, astrocytomas and brain metastases). Various methods such as gamma units using cobalt ("gamma knife") and modified cobalt or linear accelerator units are used. To perform this treatment, a sterotactic frame is fixed to the patient's skull and used to target the treatment beam. Treatment is usually given in a single fraction. Steroid medications are used to minimize cerebral edema.[15]

Nursing Management

Nursing Care Related to External Radiation Therapy

Nursing Diagnoses

- *Impaired skin integrity related to radiation therapy*
- *Infection related to skin breakdown*
- *Activity intolerance related to radiation therapy*
- *Altered nutrition, less than body requirements related to anorexia*
- *Altered oral mucous membrane related to head and neck irradiation*
- *Sensory-perceptual alterations: gustatory, related to head and neck irradiation*
- *Impaired swallowing related to esophagitis*
- *Alteration in comfort related to cough*
- *Altered nutrition, less than body requirements, related to nausea and vomiting*
- *Diarrhea related to pelvic irradiation*
- *Altered patterns of urinary elimination related to pelvic irradiation*
- *Ineffective individual coping related to alopecia*
- *Disturbance in self-esteem related to alopecia*
- *Anxiety about radiation therapy*
- *Knowledge deficit about radiation therapy and self-care measures*

General Side Effects

Skin

The skin overlying the areas being treated may develop a reaction as soon as 2 weeks into the course of treatment. Skin erythema may range from mild, light pink to deep and dusky. Skin reactions vary but tend to be greater in those receiving large doses of radiation. Also, treatments with electron beams usually produce more intense skin reactions because of the superficial concentration of the radiation dose. Areas having skin folds such as the axilla, under the breasts, perineum, groin, and gluteal fold are also at increased risk for developing a skin reaction because of increased warmth and moisture and lack of aeration.[4,16]

Fatigue

Assess for the presence and pattern of fatigue. Evaluate factors that increase or decrease fatigue. Monitor blood counts for anemia, which can compound fatigue. Assure adequate pain management with pharmacologic and nonpharmacologic measures. Assure the person is maintaining an adequate nutritional intake. Evaluate the patient's and family's understanding of the causes of fatigue and their ability to modify activities to maintain or improve function.

Anorexia

Assess the loss of appetite in patients receiving radiation therapy. Assist the patient and family to plan ways to improve appetite to help the patient eat adequately and maintain body weight. Instruct the patient and family to have high-calorie, high-protein foods readily available at all times. Specially prepared nutritional supplements and carefully selected convenience foods can provide additional calories and protein.

Bone Marrow Suppression

Blood counts must be monitored from bi-weekly, weekly, to every 3 weeks depending on other concomitant therapies. Assess for infections, bleeding, and fatigue. Plan and implement education for the patient and family about precautions for neutropenia, thrombocytopenia, and anemia.

Hypopituitarism

The symptoms may develop slowly within the first year after radiation therapy or up to 24 years following treatment (alopecia, amenorrhea, short stature in children, lactation failure, decreased sexual libido). During times of stress such as surgery or acute illness, the consequences of hypoadrenalism can be life-threatening. Adrenal insufficiency is treated with adrenocortical replacement, and sex hormone deficits are replaced with appropriate hormone therapy.[11,12]

Chest

Common side effects of radiation therapy to the chest are esophagitis and cough. Late effects include pneumonitis and rarely, lung fibrosis.

Esophagitis

Approximately 2 to 3 weeks from the start of therapy, the patient may note difficulty or pain with swallowing and complain of a "lump in the throat." Assist the patient and family to plan a soft, bland, or liquid diet that provides a high calorie and protein intake. Use of anesthetic and coating mouth rinses before meals can decrease the discomfort associated with eating and allow the patient to continue with therapy.[7]

Cough

Assess the character, intensity, and frequency of cough and monitor changes in lung sounds. Humidification of the air and avoiding irritants such as smoke can reduce the cough. Use of cough preparations that contain codeine may be indicated for severe dry, hacking coughing that results in fatigue or disrupts sleep.[14]

Radiation Pneumonitis

Radiation pneumonitis can occur approximately 1 to 3 months after radiation therapy to the lung. Symptoms include fever and dyspnea. The effect is similar to the adult respiratory distress syndrome (ARDS).

Radiation Fibrosis

Radiation fibrosis may occur 6 to 12 months after treatment is completed. The primary symptom is shortness of breath.

Abdomen

Nausea and vomiting usually occur within the first 6 hours following treatments and may last for 3 to 6 hours. Assess patients for occurence and pattern of nausea and vomiting. Prophylactic use of antiemetics before treatment each day and as needed following treatment can minimize and relieve nausea and vomiting from radiation therapy.[4]

Pelvis

Diarrhea

Assess the patient's usual bowel pattern. If diarrhea occurs, help the patient and family plan measures to minimize diarrhea. Instruct the patient and family on the use of a low-residue diet. Decreasing the amount of fat in the diet can also be helpful because fats are difficult to digest. Evaluate the patient's and family's understanding and use of measures to minimize diarrhea and tenesmus in order to maintain the patient's usual pattern of elimination.[4]

Cystitis

Cystitis occurs if the bladder is within the treatment field. Symptoms include dysuria, small bladder capacity, urinary frequency and urgency, nocturia, and urinary hesitancy. Rarely, bleeding occurs. Hyperbaric oxygen therapy has shown therapeutic benefits in treating chronic radiation-induced cystitis that is refractory to conventional therapy. Assess and monitor symptoms of cystitis, including signs of hematuria. Instruct the patient to maintain an adequate fluid intake.

Erectile Dysfunction

Allow the patient and his partner to discuss concerns and feelings regarding changes in sexual functioning and body image.

Vaginal Stenosis

Vaginal stenosis can be minimized or prevented by use of a vaginal dilator. Vaginal dilation needs to be performed three times a week for at least 1 year. A well-lubricated dilator is inserted into the vagina for 5-10 minutes then withdrawn.

Ovarian Failure

Replacement hormonal therapy with midcyclic estrogens and progesterone reverses the clinical effects of early menopause.

Testicles

The testicles are usually shielded from radiation. However, if exposure is needed or unavoidable, spermatogenesis will stop, usually resulting in permanent sterility.

Brain

Cerebral Edema

Symptoms include headaches, nausea, vomiting, seizures, vision changes, motor function disabilities, slurred speech, and changes in mental status. Steroids are usually indicated during the course of treatment to minimize cerebral edema.

Alopecia

Alopecia, which occurs within the treatment area, depends upon the dose and extent of radiation to the scalp. Prepare the patient and family in advance for alopeica. Assess its significance. Provide information on what can be done to cover and care for the scalp.

Hair Texture and Color

Gentle brushing and combing of the hair is recommended. Permanent waves and hair coloring are contraindicated because they can irritate the scalp. Using a scarf, turban, hat, or cap to protect the scalp from the wind, cold, and sun is advisable. A wig may be worn. Assure that the wig lining is comfortable and does not further irritate the scalp. A mild shampoo may be used, but excessive shampooing should be avoided.

Internal Radiation Therapy

Brachytherapy

Radioactive implants deliver relatively large amounts of radiation to a specific site over a short time. Tumors may be treated with an implant alone, but more commonly, an implant is done following a course of radiation therapy to provide a boost of radiation to the tumor. Cancers of the brain, tongue, lips, esophagus, lung, breast, vagina, cervix, endometrium, rectum, prostate, and bladder may be treated with brachytherapy. Implants are usually placed temporarily within the body cavity or structure with specifically designed applicators. The radioactive material, in the form of ribbons, wires, seeds, capsules, needles, or tubes is encapsulated (sealed) so that there is no contamination of bodily fluids. Intracavitary placement of implants within the vagina or uterus is performed with general or spinal anesthesia.[1,3,8,13] Interstitial brain implants for recurrent brain tumors allow treatment of a highly localized area within the brain. Catheters are placed using a sterotactic frame with CT guidance.[55] Interstitial radioactive implants with needles, wires, seeds, or catheters are placed directly into the tissues. These implants may be temporary or permanent. Head and neck and breast cancers are commonly treated with temporary interstitial implants.

Nonsealed Radioactive Therapy

When radioactive isotopes are injected intravenously or taken orally (nonsealed sources), the patient and the body secretions may be radioactive, and nursing care must follow specific radiation safety precautions. Depending on the isotope used, the patient usually must be isolated because of radioactivity for approximately 3 to 4 days. The amount of radioactivity emitted is carefully monitored during the patient's hospitalization. Examples of radioactive isotopes include: Iodine131 and 125; Phosphorus 32, Iridium 192, Cesium 137, and Radium 226.

Minimizing Nurse's Exposure to Radiation

When the nurse works with patients with a radioactive implant or systemic radiation, he or she should anticipate the patient's needs and use the principles of time, distance, and shielding to minimize radiation exposure.[3,4]

- Time

    Minimize time spent in close proximity to the patient. Radiation exposure is directly related to the time spent within a specific distance of the source of radioactivity.

    Use time efficiently by organizing patient care activities and assembling necessary supplies before entering the patient's room. Before leaving the patient's room, place personal items within reach of the patient to avoid needing to reenter the room. Direct care is usually limited to one-half hour per person per shift. Encourage the patient to perform self-care activities.

- Distance

    Maximize the distance from the radioactive material. The amount of radiation decreases according to the inverse square law. Visit frequently with the patient at the door to the patient's room.

- Shielding

    When appropriate, use shielding to decrease exposure to radiation. With radium or cesium implants, a lead bed shield 1 inch thick is needed to attenuate the radiation. These shields are usually placed at the patient's bedside. Most nursing care is provided from behind the shields. The lead aprons used in diagnostic radiology are not sufficiently thick to stop gamma rays and therefore are not recommended.[15]

Patient Teaching Priorities:
External Beam Radiation Therapy[2,6]

Instruct patient and family about:
    Use of radiation therapy to treat cancer.

Events that occur before, during, and after a course of radiation therapy: consultation, simulation, daily treatment, routine evaluations during course of therapy, and follow-up.

Time factors: length of simulation, length of daily treatment, length of course of radiation therapy.

Environmental information: description of surroundings, treatment room, and machine

Effects and side effects of radiation therapy (general and site-specific):

That radiation therapy is a localized treatment and expected side effects are general as well as site specific.

What happens, why it occurs.

When these effects are experienced.

How long these effects last and when they resolve.

That patient is *not* radioactive; there is not need to isolate the patient from family and friends.

Measures that patients and families can use to minimize or prevent side effects:

General effects: skin care, nutrition, energy conservation.

Site-specific effects.

Delayed effects to monitor: skin care, fatigue, site-specific effects.

Follow-up care: routine follow-up with health care providers and adherence to recommendations for healthy living.

Patient Teaching Priorities: Internal Radiation Therapy—Sealed and Nonsealed Sources[2,6]

Instruct the patient and family about:

Use of internal radiation therapy to treat cancer.

Patient preparation before therapy.

Procedures involved in the therapy.

Visitation restrictions: no one under 18 years of age, no one who is or may be pregnant.

Isolation requirements: temporary isolation, patient remains in room, nursing care for essential activities only, time spent in close proximity will be limited. If the patient with nonsealed radioactive source has bathroom privileges, the patient is instructed to flush the toilet 2 to 3 times after each use.

Patient activity may be restricted depending on the procedure; diversional activities such as watching television or reading a book are recommended.

Discharge from the hospital: monitor for delayed effects such as fatigue; pelvic implants: diarrhea, urinary symptoms such as bladder infections, women are instructed to perform vaginal dilation 3 times a week for up to 1 year after the implant.

Geriatric Considerations[4]

Compromised body systems in the elderly place them at risk for developing side effects sooner and with greater severity:

Skin: monitor for excessive dryness and early skin reactions.

Energy stores may be depleted and increase fatigue.

Medications prescribed for symptom management may need dosage adjustments to minimize adverse reactions.

Head and neck irradiation: normally decreased oral secretions predispose the elderly to oral complications.

Check the fit and comfort of oral prostheses.

Taste acuity may be altered prior to start of irradiation.

Sexuality: assess changes experienced. Provide education about the effects of radiation therapy. Because of the importance of preventing vaginal stenosis so that vaginal intercourse and pelvic examinations are feasible, instruct women who have received radiation therapy involving the vaginal vault to perform vaginal dilation 3 times a week for up to 1 year. Radiation therapy further decreases vaginal secretions. Women are instructed to use water-based lubricants for comfort. Some men experience erectile dysfunction with aging as a result of vascular changes. Pelvic irradiation may further damage the pelvic vasculature and cause nerve damage. Provide counseling or referral to specialist.

Social concerns:

Radiation therapy is usually delivered Monday through Friday for up to 7 weeks. The elderly may need to rely on public transportation. In many situations, the patient is caring for a spouse or child and being away from home is difficult without a caretaker. Many elderly are on fixed incomes, and the added expense of therapy, transportation, out-of-town housing, and additional medications needed during therapy is a hardship.

Bibliography

1. Bentel GC, Nelson CE, and Noell KT: Elements of clinical radiation oncology. In Bentel GC, Nelson CE, and Noell KT, editors: *Treatment planning and dose calculation in radiation oncology,* ed 4, New York, 1989, Pergamon Press.

2. Brandt, B: *Informational needs and selected variables in patients receiving brachytherapy,* Oncol Nurs Forum 18:1221, 1991.

3. Bruner DW: *Report on the radiation oncology nursing subcommittee of the American College of Radiology task force on standards development,* Oncology 4:80, 1990.

4. Bruner DW, Iwamoto R, Keane K, and Strohl R, editors: *Manual for radiation oncology nursing practice and education,* Pittsburgh, 1992, Oncology Nursing Society.

5. Bucholtz J: Radiation therapy. In Ziegfeld CR, editor: *Core curriculum for oncology nursing,* ed 2, Philadelphia, 1992, WB Saunders.

6. Campbell-Forsyth L: *Patients' perceived knowledge and learning needs concerning radiation therapy,* Cancer Nurs 13:81, 1990.

7. Dunne CF: *Oral analgesics to relieve radiation-induced esophagitis,* Oncol Nurs Forum 18:785, 1991.

8. Greenburg S, Petersen J, Hansen-Peters I, and Baylinson W: *Interstitially implanted I-125 for prostate cancer using transrectal ultrasound,* Oncol Nurs Forum 17:849, 1990.

9. Hagopian GA: *The effects of a weekly radiation therapy newsletter on patients,* Oncol Nurs Forum 18:1199, 1991.

10. Haibeck SV: *Intraoperative radiation therapy,* Oncol Nurs Forum 15:143, 1988.

11. Hendrickson FR and Withers HR: Principles of radiation oncology. In Holleb AL, Fink DJ, and Murphy GP, editors: *American Cancer Society textbook of clinical oncology,* Atlanta, 1991, American Cancer Society.

12. Hilderley LJ: Radiotherapy. In Groenwald SL, editor: *Cancer nursing principles and practice,* ed 2, Boston/ Monterey, 1990, Jones and Bartlett.

13. Jordan LN and Mantravadi RVP: *Nursing care of the patient receiving high dose rate brachytherapy,* Oncol Nurs Forum 18:1167, 1991.

14. Ladd L: *The dry mouth dilemma,* Oncol Nurs Forum 18:785, 1991.

15. Larson DA, Wasserman TH, Drzymala RE, and Simpson JR: Stereotactic external-beam irradiation. In Perez CA and Brady LW, editors: *Principles and practice of radiation oncology,* ed 2, Philadelphia, 1992, JB Lippincott.

16. Margolin SG and others: *Management of radiation-induced moist skin desquamation using hydrocolloid dressing,* Cancer Nurs 13:71, 1990.

17. Perez CA and others: Hyperthermia. In Perez CA and Brady LW, editors: *Principles and practice of radiation oncology,* ed 2, Philadelphia, 1992, JB Lippincott.

Chemotherapy 22

Chemotherapy is the use of cytotoxic drugs in the treatment of cancer. It is one of the four modalities—surgery, radiation therapy, chemotherapy, and biotherapy—that provide cure, control, or palliation. Chemotherapy is systemic as opposed to localized therapy such as surgery and radiation therapy. There are four ways chemotherapy may be used:[10]

- *Adjuvant therapy*—a course of chemotherapy used in conjunction with another treatment modality (surgery, radiation therapy, and biotherapy) and aimed at treating micrometastases
- *Neoadjuvant chemotherapy*—administration of chemotherapy to shrink the tumor prior to surgical removal of the tumor
- *Primary therapy*—the treatment of patients with localized cancer for which there is an alternative but less than completely effective treatment
- *Induction chemotherapy*—the drug therapy given as the primary treatment for patients with cancer for which no alternative treatment exists
- *Combination chemotherapy*—administration of two or more chemotherapeutic agents in the treatment of cancer, allowing each medication to enhance the action of the other or to act synergistically

Principles of Chemotherapy

Cell Generation Cycle
The cell cycle is the sequence of events resulting in mitosis (the replication of DNA and equal distribution into daughter cells). Normal cells and cancer cells go through the same division cycle, characterized by the following phases: G_0—resting, or dormant

phase; G_1—phase in which protein synthesis takes place in preparation for the S phase DNA synthesis; and G_2— phase for further protein synthesis in preparation for the M phase—mitosis and cell division. The generation time, or length of time it takes for a cell to complete the phase or cycle, varies from hours to days. Chemotherapuetic drugs are most active against frequently dividing cells, or in all the phases of the cell cycle except G_0. Normal cells with rapid growth changes most commonly affected by chemotherapeutic agents include bone marrow (platelets, and red and white blood cells), hair follicles, mucosal lining of the gastrointestinal tract, skin and germinal cells (sperm and ova). Chemotherapy is given according to schedules that are most effective for tumor kill and are planned to allow recovery of the normal cells.[10]

Tumor Growth

The regulatory mechanism controlling the growth of cancer cells differs from that of normal cells. Unlike normal cells, cancer cells grow via a pyramid effect; however, they grow at the same rate as the tissue from which they originated (e.g., breast cancer develops at the same rate of growth as normal breast tissue development). The time required for a tumor mass to reach a certain size is called doubling time. Tumors probably have undergone approximately 30 doublings from a single cell before they are clinically detected. Between the seventh and tenth doubling time there is the possibility for the tumor to shed cells, a process called *micrometastasis*. During the early stages of tumor growth, doubling time is more rapid than at later stages. This pattern of growth is called Gompertzian function. Tumor cells are more sensitive than normal cells to chemotherapy agents that are toxic to rapidly dividing cells.[10,11]

Drug Classification

Chemotherapeutic agents are classified according to their pharmacologic action and their interference with cellular reproduction. The basic groups and their potential action are as follows:[10,18]

> Cell-cycle phase specific drugs are active on cells undergoing division in the cell cycle; examples include antimetabolites, vinca plant alkaloids, and miscellaneous

agents such as asparaginase and dacarbazine. These drugs are most effective against actively growing tumors that have a greater proportion of cells cycling through the phase in which the drug attacks the cancer cell. Cell-cycle phase specific drugs are given in minimal concentration, via continuous dosing methods.

■ Cell-cycle phase nonspecific drugs are active on cells in either a dividing or resting state; examples include alkylating agents, antitumor antibiotics, nitrosureas, hormone and steroid drugs, and miscellaneous agents such as procarbazine. These agents are active in all phases of the cell cycle and may be effective in large tumors with few active cells dividing at the time of administration. Drugs of this nature are often given as single bolus injections.

■ Alkylating agents are cell-cycle phase nonspecific. They act primarily to form a molecular bond with the nucleic acids, which interferes with nucleic acid duplication, preventing mitosis.

■ Antibiotics (antitumor agents) are cell-cycle phase nonspecific. These drugs disrupt DNA transcription and inhibit DNA and RNA synthesis.

■ Antimetabolites are cell-cycle phase specific. They exhibit their action by blocking essential enzymes necessary for DNA synthesis or become incorporated into the DNA and RNA so that a false message is transmitted.

■ Hormones are cell-cycle phase non-specific. These chemicals, secreted by the endocrine glands, alter the environment of the cell by affecting the cell membrane's permeability. By manipulating hormone levels, tumor growth can be suppressed.

■ Antihormonal agents derive their antineoplastic effect from their ability to neutralize the effect or inhibit the production of natural hormones used by hormone-dependent tumors.

■ Nitrosureas are cell-cycle phase nonspecific. They have the ability to cross the blood-brain barrier. Their action is similar to that of the alkylating agents; DNA and RNA synthesis are both inhibited.

- Corticosteroids provide an antiinflammatory effect on body tissues (e.g., they reduce intracranial or spinal cord compression and suppress lymphocytes).
- Vinca plant alkaloids are cell-cycle phase specific. They exert a cytotoxic effect by binding to microtubular proteins during metaphase, causing mitotic arrest. The cell loses its ability to divide and so dies.
- Miscellaneous agents may be cell-cycle phase specific or nonspecific or both. These drugs act by a variety of mechanisms. For example, enzyme products that act primarily by inhibiting protein synthesis.

Cell Kill Hypothesis

A single cancer cell is capable of multiplying and eventually killing the host. Every tumor cell must be killed to cure cancer. With each course of the drug therapy, a given dose of chemotherapeutic drug kills only a *fraction, not all* of the cancer cells present (Figure 22-1). Repeated courses of chemotherapy must be used to reduce the total number of cancer cells.[18,20,23]

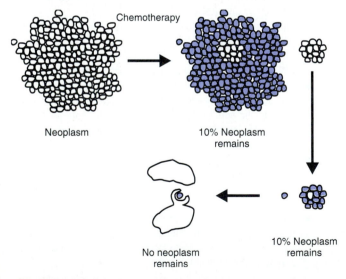

Figure 22-1. Cell kill hypothesis. (From Goodman MS: *Cancer: chemotherapy and care.* Bristol Laboratories, Division of Bristol-Myers Co, Evansville, Indiana.)

Factors Considered in Drug-Selection

- Patient's eligibility for chemotherapy (confirmed diagnosis; bone marrow, nutritional, hepatic, and renal status; expectation of longevity; history of chemotherapy and radiation therapy)
- Cancer cell type (e.g., squamous cell, adenocarcinoma)
- Rate of drug absorption (e.g., treatment interval and routes —oral, intravenous, intraperitoneal)
- Tumor location (many drugs do not cross the blood-brain barrier)
- Tumor load (larger tumors are generally less responsive to chemotherapy)
- Tumor resistance to chemotherapy (tumor cells can mutate and produce variant cells distinct form the tumor stem cell of origin)[6,7,13,29]

Combination Chemotherapy

Chemotherapeutic drugs are most frequently given in combination. This enhances the effect of the drugs on the tumor cell kill. Considerations for drugs used in combination include verified effectiveness as a single agent, results in increased tumor cell kill, increased patient survival, presence of a synergistic action, varied toxicities, different mechanisms of action, and administration in repeated courses to minimize the immunosuppressive effects that might otherwise occur. See Box 22-1 for examples of commonly used combination therapies.[13,14,15,19]

Chemotherapy Administration

Calculation of Drug Dosage

Drug dosage for cancer chemotherapy is based on body surface area (BSA) in both adults and children. Drug calculations should be verified by a second person to ensure the accuracy of the dose. The dosage range of a drug may vary with different drug regimens.[8,28]

The dosages of some drugs are calculated proportionally to the BSA of the patient. BSA is calculated in square meters (m^2). A nomogram is used to correlate height with weight to determine BSA. The drug dose is ordered in milligrams per square meter. For example[8,28]:

$$
\begin{aligned}
\text{Height} &= 68 \text{ inches} \\
\text{Weight} &= 150 \text{ pounds} \\
m^2 &= 1.80 \text{ BSA} \\
\text{Dose} &= 75 \text{ mg/m}^2 \\
1.80 \times 75 &= x \text{ dose} \\
x &= 135 \text{ mg dose}
\end{aligned}
$$

Drug Reconstitution

Pharmacy staff should reconstitute all drugs and preprime the intravenous tubings under a class II biologic safety cabinet.

When preparing and reconstituting the drugs, use aseptic technique in accordance with current manufacturer's recommendations. Immediately label all the syringes of reconstituted drugs with the name of the drug.

Box 22-1
___

Combination Chemotherapy Regimens
___

Breast
CMF—Cyclophosphamide, Methotrexate, 5-Fluorouracil
FUVAC—5-Fluorouracil, Vinblastine, Adriamycin, Cyclo-
    phosphamide
Lung
CAV—Cisplatin, Adriamycin, Vinblastine
CAMP—Cyclophosphamide, Adriamycin, Methotrexate,
    Procarbazine
Hodgkin's
ABVD—Adriamycin, Bleomycin, Vinblastine, Dacabazine
MOPP—Nitrogen Mustard, Oncovin, Prednisone,
    Procarbazine
Lymphoma
CHOP-BLEO—Cyclophosphamide, Adriamycin, Oncovin,
    Prednisone, Bleomycin
PROMACE-CytaBOM—Prednisone, Oncovin, Methotrexate,
    Adriamycin, Cyclophosphamide, Etoposide, Cytarabine,
    Bleomycin, Leucovorin, Dexamethasone, Trimethoprim
    Sulfa
Testicular
VBP—Vinblastine, Bleomycin, CisPlatin
VPV—VP-16 (etoposide), Cisplatin, Vinblastine

Guidelines for Administration[22,25]

Routes

Oral—emphasize importance of compliance by the patient with prescribed schedule. Plan and assess for drugs with emetic potential to be taken with meals; drugs requiring hydration (cytoxan) need to be taken early in the day.

Subcutaneous and intramuscular—demonstration with a return demonstration may be needed if the patient is giving self-injections. Be sure to rotate injection sites for each dose.

Topical—cover surface area with thin film of medication; instruct the patient to wear loose-fitting, cotton clothing. Wear gloves and be sure to wash hands thoroughly after procedure. Caution the patient not to touch area of topical ointment application.

Intraarterial—requires catheter placement in artery near tumor site. Because of arterial pressure, administer the drug in a heparinized solution by means of an infusion pump.

Throughout the infusion, monitor vital signs, color and temperature of extremity, and potential for bleeding at the site with temporary catheter placement. Instruct the patient and family on care components of catheter and infusion pumps if chemotherapy is given in home setting.

Intracavity—instill the drug into the bladder through a catheter and/or through a chest tube into the pleural cavity. Follow prescribed premedication dosage to minimize potential local irritation caused by drugs given through the intracavity route.

Intraperitoneal—warm the infusate solution (with dry heat) to body temperature of 38°C before administration. Deliver the drug into the abdominal cavity through the implantable port and/or external suprapubic catheter. Monitor the patient for abdominal pressure, pain, fever, and electrolyte status. Measure and record abdominal girth for 48 hours.

Intrathecal—reconstitute all intrathecal medications with preservative-free, sterile normal saline or sterile water. Infusion of medication may be given through an Ommaya reservoir, if available, and/or through lumbar puncture procedure. Usual volume of medication instilled is 15 mL or less. The medication should be injected *slowly*. If chemotherapy drugs Ara-C or methotrexate are given in high doses, monitor the patient closely for potential neurotoxicity. Only a physician may administer intrathecal drugs. *Intravenous route*—the medication may be given through central venous catheters or peripheral venous access. Methods of administration include the following:

- Push (bolus) – medication administered through a syringe directly into the vein
- Piggyback (secondary setup) – drug administered using a secondary bag (bottle) and tubing; primary infusion concurrently maintained throughout drug administration[25,26]
- Side arm – drug administered through a syringe and needle into the side port of a running (free-flowing) intravenous infusion
- Infusion – drug added to the prescribed volume of fluid IV bag or bottle

Check for blood return before, during, and after infusion of chemotherapeutic drugs. Follow the agency guidelines for frequency of monitoring continuous chemotherapeutic infusions. For continuous infusion of a vesicant drug, suggestions include validating blood return every 2 hours; for continuous infusion of a non-vesicant drug, validate blood return every 4 hours.

Vein Selection and Venipuncture

Selection of the appropriate site and equipment is determined by the patient's age, vein status, drugs to be infused, and expected period of infusion. The extremity should be observed and palpated. Use distal veins first, and choose a vein above areas of flexion. The distal veins of the hands and arms should be used first and subsequent venipuncture should be proximal to previous sites. Select the shortest catheter with the smallest gauge appropriate for the type and duration of the infusion. Veins commonly used include the basilic, cephalic, and metacarpal.

Procedure for Chemotherapeutic Drug Administration

- Verify the patient's identification, drug, dose, route, and time of administration with the physician's order
- Review drug allergy history with the patient
- Anticipate and plan for possible side effects or major system toxicity

- Review appropriate laboratory data and other tests
- Verify informed consent for treatment
- Select appropriate equipment and supplies
- Calculate the dose and reconstitute the drug using aseptic technique; follow safe handling guidelines
- Explain the procedure to the patient and the patient's family.
- Administer antiemetics or other prescribed medications.
- Initiate peripheral IV site and/or prepare central venous access site
- Administer chemotherapeutic agents
- Monitor the patient at scheduled intervals throughout the course of drug administration
- Dispose of all used supplies and unused drugs in approved puncture-proof, leakproof containers outside of patient area
- Document procedure according to agency policy and procedure

Drug Preparation

To ensure safe handling, all chemotherapeutic drugs should be prepared according to the package insert in a class II biologic safety cabinet (BSC). Venting to the outside is desirable where feasible. Personal protective equipment includes disposable surgical latex gloves and a gown made of lint-free low-permeability fabric with a closed front, long sleeves, and elastic or knit cuffs. Wear eye-protective splash goggles or a face shield when preparing drugs if not using a biologic safety cabinet.

Change gloves between preparation and administration of the drug, and at least every 30 minutes during preparation and administration.[1,25,27,30]

Suggestions to minimize exposure include the following:
- Wash hands before and after drug handling
- Limit access to drug preparation area
- Keep labeled drug spill kit near preparation area
- Apply gloves before drug handling
- Prepare drugs using aseptic technique
- Avoid eating, drinking, smoking, chewing gum, applying

cosmetics, and storing food in or near drug preparation area

- Place absorbent pad on work surface
- Use Luer-Lok equipment
- Open drug vials and ampules away from body
- Vent vials with a hydrophobic filter needle or pin to prevent spray of drug
- Wrap alcohol wipe around neck of ampule before opening
- Prime lines containing drugs inside BSC using original drug vial or a zip-close plastic bag
- Cover tip of needle with sterile gauze or alcohol wipe when expelling air from syringe
- Label all chemotherapeutic drugs
- Clean up any spills immediately
- Transport drugs to delivery area in a leakproof container

Drug Administration

- Wear protective equipment (gloves, gown, and eyewear)
- Inform the patient that chemotherapeutic drugs are harmful to normal cells and that protective measures used by personnel minimize their exposure to these drugs
- Administer drugs in a safe and unhurried environment
- Place a plastic-backed absorbent pad under the tubing during administration to catch any leakage
- Do not dispose of any supplies or unused drugs in patient care areas.

Disposal of Supplies and Unused Drugs

- Do not clip or recap needles or break syringes
- Place all supplies used *intact* in a leakproof, puncture-proof, appropriately labeled container
- Place all unused drugs in containers in a leakproof, puncture-proof, appropriately labeled container; keep these containers in every area where drugs are prepared or administered so that waste materials need not be moved from one area to another
- Dispose of containers filled with chemotherapeutic supplies and unused drugs in accordance with regualtions of hazardous wastes, for example, licensed sanitary landfill or incineration at 1000°C

Management of Chemotherapy Spills

Chemotherapy spills should be cleaned up immediately by properly protected personnel trained in the appropriate procedures. A spill should be identified with a warning sign so that other persons will not be contaminated. The following are recommended supplies and procedures to manage a chemotherapy spill on hard surfaces, linens, personnel, and patients.[27]

Supplies

- Chemotherapy spill kit:
  Respirator mask for airborne powder spills
  Plastic safety glasses or goggles
  Heavy-duty rubber gloves
  Absorbent pads to contain liquid spills
  Absorbent towels for cleanup after spill
  Small scoop to collect glass fragments
  Two large waste disposal bags
- Protective disposable gown
- Containers of detergent solution and clear tap water for postspill cleanup
- Puncture-proof and leak-proof container approved for chemotherapy waste disposal
- Approved, specially labeled, impervious laundry bag
- Eyewash faucet adapters or fountain in or near work area[27]

Caring for Patients Receiving Chemotherapeutic Drugs

Personnel handling blood, vomitus, or excreta from patients who have received chemotherapy within the previous 48 hours should wear disposable surgical latex gloves and gowns to be appropriately discarded after use. Linen contaminated with chemotherapeutic drugs, blood, vomitus, or excreta from a patient who has received these drugs within 48 hours before should be placed in a specially marked impervious laundry bag according to procedures for drug spills or linen.[27]

Employment Practices Regarding Reproductive Issues

The handling of chemotherapeutic agents by women who are either pregnant or actively trying to conceive, and by those who are breast-feeding, remains a sensitive and unsettled issue. Some suggest offering these personnel the opportunity to transfer to areas that do not involve chemotherapeutic agents. All safe handling guidelines should be practiced with utmost care by all pregnant personnel.[3,30]

Extravasation Management

Extravasation is the accidental infiltration of vesicant or irritant chemotherapeutic drugs from the vein into the surrounding tissues at the IV site. A vesicant is an agent that can produce a blister and/or tissue destruction. An irritant is an agent that is capable of producing venous pain at the site of and along the vein with or without an inflammatory reaction. Injuries that may occur as the result of extravasation include sloughing of tissue, infection, pain, and loss of mobility of an extremity. The degree of tissue damage is related to several factors such as drug vesicant potential, drug concentration, the quantity of drug extravasated, duration of tissue exposure,[1,6,31,44] vein-puncture site/device, needle insertion technique, and individual tissue responses.[5,11,16,21,26]

Box 22-2 Chemotherapeutic Drugs

Generic Name	Trade Name
Nonvesicant Chemotherapeutic Drugs	
Asparaginase	Elspar
Bleomycin	Blenoxane
Carboplatin	CBDCA
Cisplatinum	Cisplatin
Cyclophosphamide	Cytoxan
Cytarabine	Ara-C, Cytosar
Floxuridine	FUDR
Fludarabine	Fludara
Fluorouracil	5-FU

Continued.

Box 22-2 Cont'd.

Generic Name	Trade Name
Ifosfamide	Naxamide
Methotrexate	Mexate
Taxol	
Thiophosphoramide	Thiotepa
Topotecan	

Chemotherapeutic Drugs with Vesicant Potential

Amasacrine	AMSA
Bisantrene	ADAH
Dacarbazine	DTIC-Dome
Dactinomycin	Actinomycin D, Cosmegen
Daunorubicin	Cerubidine, Daunomycin
Doxorubicin	Adriamycin
Epirubicin	Epi-Epidoxrudicin
Esorubicin	Eso-Deoxydoxorubicin
Idarubicin	Ida-Idamycin
Mechlorethamine	Nitrogen Mustard, Mustargen
Mitomycin	Mutamycin
Vinblastine	Velban
Vincristine	Oncovin

Chemotherapeutic Drugs with Irritant Potential

Carmustine	BCNU
Etoposide	VP-16, VePesid
Mitoguazone	Methyl-GAG, MGBG
Mitoxantrone	Novantrone
Plicamycin	Mithracin
Streptozocin	Zanosar
Teniposide	VM-26
Vindesine	Eldisine

Prevention of Extravasation

Nursing staff responsibilities for the prevention of extravasation include the following:

- Knowledge of drugs with vesicant potential (Box 22-2)
- Skill in drug administration
- Identification of risk factors, for example, multiple veni-punctures, previous treatment

- Anticipation of extravasation and knowledge of approved management protocol
- Obtaining a new venipuncture site daily, if peripheral access used
- Consideration of central venous access for difficult peripheral access
- Most sources recommend 24 hour vesicant infusion via central venous access *only*
- Administration of drug in a quiet, unhurried environment
- Testing vein patency without using chemotherapeutic agents
- Providing adequate drug dilution, for example, side port infusion via free-flowing intravenous infusion
- Careful observation of access site and extremity throughout the procedure
- Validation of blood return from intravenous site before, during, and after vesicant drug infusion
- Educating patients regarding symptoms of drug infiltration, for example, pain, burning, and stinging sensations at intravenous site

Protocol for Extravasation Management at a Peripheral Site

Agency policy and procedure for management of extravasation with the responsible physician's prescription should be easily accessible to the staff. The approved antidotes should be readily available, and the following procedure should be initiated with a physician's prescription as soon as extravasation of a vesicant or irritant agent is suspected or occurs[26,27]

- Stop the chemotherapeutic drug
- Leave the needle or catheter in place
- Aspirate any residual drug and blood in the IV tubing, needle or catheter, and suspected infiltration site
- Instill the IV antidote
- Remove the needle
- If unable to aspirate the residual drug from the IV tubing, remove needle or catheter
- Inject the antidote subcutaneously clockwise into the infiltrated site using 25-gauge needle; change the needle with each new injection (see pp 655)

- Avoid applying pressure to the suspected infiltration site
- Photograph the suspected area of extravasation according to agency's policy and procedure for documentation and follow-up
- Apply topical ointment if ordered
- Cover lightly with an occlusive sterile dressing
- Apply cold or warm compresses as indicated
- Elevate the extremity
- Observe regularly for pain, erythema, induration, and necrosis
- Documentation of extravasation management:
  Date, time, insertion site/device, drug sequence, amount extravasated, patient comments, physician notification and nursing management of the extravasation.

Anaphylaxis

The nurse must be informed and prepared for the specific drugs known to be at risk for anaphylaxis. Test dosing prior to infusion of the drug and following the infusion precautions will decrease the anaphylaxis occurence. Emergency medications and supplies for management of anaphylaxis include the following:[4,6,14,17]

- Injectable aminophylline, diphenhydramine hydrochloride (Benadryl), dopamine, epinephrine, heparin, hydrocortisone
- Oxygen setup, tubing cannula, or mask and airway device
- Suction equipment
- IV fluids (isotonic solutions)
- IV tubings and supplies for venous access
- Immediately stop the drug infusion
- Maintain an intravenous line with isotonic saline
- Position the patient for comfort and to promote perfusion of the vital organs
- Notify the physician, nursing agency and/or emergency medical services
- Maintain the airway and anticipate the need for cardiopulmonary resuscitation
- Monitor the vital signs according to agency policy
- Administer the appropriate medications with an approved physician's order (see pp 652)

- Follow the nursing agency's protocol for follow-up care
- Document the incident in the patient's medical record

Alternative Care Settings

Improved drug delivery, cost containment, and considerations of the quality of life have affected trends in chemotherapy administration. Management of symptoms, such as control of nausea and vomiting and innovative pain management have reduced the need for hospitalization. Options to give chemotherapy in outpatient settings include ambulatory care centers, physicians' offices, extended care facilities, and home health agencies. Certain principles of chemotherapy administration and standards of care for patients must be maintained by the staff regardless of the setting.[9,14,24]

The oncology patient is now and will continue to be a major segment of home health care. Criteria specific to home administration of chemotherapy include: care giver(s) able and willing to assist; patient's physical condition stable and within range of home care capabilities; stable and suitable living conditions, including cleanliness, plumbing, refrigeration, telephone; and access to emergency assistance.

Nursing Management

Nursing Assessment and Intervention

Chemotherapeutic drugs may cause adverse side effects and major system toxicity and dysfunction. Side effects and toxicity vary in severity according to the patient's individual response to the drug therapy. The most frequent side effects are myelosuppression, nausea, and vomiting. Myelosuppression can be a dose-limiting toxicity. The chemotherapeutic drugs work by destruction and/or suppression of new leukocytes, platelets, and erythrocytes. Monitor these effects through an evaluation of the blood count at scheduled periodic intervals. The time or level at which a blood count reaches its lowest point is the nadir. The nadir varies with individual drugs but usually occurs between 7 and 21 days after the administration of chemotherapeutic drugs.

Nausea and vomiting are often the most distressing side effects of chemotherapy.[17,24] Nausea and vomiting may be acute, anticipatory, delayed, or persistent. Assessing and reporting their frequency, severity, patterns, and duration aid in prevention and management of symptoms. Prevention is best for nausea and vomiting. Behavioral interventions such as relaxation, distraction, and guided imagery may help with anticipatory nausea and vomiting. Administration of antiemetics 30 to 60 minutes before chemotherapy may alleviate the symptoms. Antiemetics should be continued at scheduled intervals throughout the expected duration of nausea and vomiting. Chemotherapy drugs with mild, moderate, and severe emetic potential are listed in Table 22-1. A parenteral antiemetic protocol is listed in Table 22-2.

Nursing Diagnosis

- *Knowledge deficit related to chemotherapeutic side effects*

Interventions

- Assess educational level, ability, desire to learn, and barriers to learning
- Evaluate understanding relative to the specific diagnosis, disease process, and potential treatment planned
- Determine availability of caregiver to participate in patient's care and treatment process
- Assess patient/family needs for consultation with varied resources (e.g., I Can Cope Support Group, Reach to Recovery, Look Good-Feel Better, Ostomy, and Laryngectomy Support Groups)

Nursing Diagnosis

- *Injury, potential for, related to alteration in immune system; clotting factors.*

Interventions

- Monitor CBC, hemoglobin, PT, PTT, and platelet count
- Assess type of therapy (chemotherapy, radiation therapy) and current drugs (aspirin, anticoagulants), which may alter bleeding and clotting time

- Assess factors (fever, sepsis, altered hepatic function, and bone marrow function) that may alter clotting process
- Observe and report symptoms: bruising, bleeding from venous access sites, nose, gums, vagina, rectum; hemoptysis, hematemesis; black, tarry, and/or gross blood in stools; increase in usual menstrual flow, change in vital signs, and spontaneous petechiae or hematomas

Nursing Diagnosis

- *Nutrition, alteration in: less than body requirement related to nausea and vomiting.*

Interventions

- Assess the amount, color, consistency and frequency of emesis, and nauseous episodes
- Determine what factors facilitate and/or prevent nausea and vomiting
- Assess baseline weight prior to illness, onset of illness, changes since onset of treatment, weight 1 month ago, and note weight gains/losses
- Monitor laboratory values: serum albumin, serum transferrin level, CBC, and electrolytes
- Assess dietary history: food habits, food likes/dislikes, and amount and type of food eaten at breakfast, lunch, supper, and snacks

Nursing Diagnosis

- *Disturbance in self-concept related to alopecia.*

Interventions

- Inform patient that hair loss is temporary and hair will regrow when the treatment is stopped; usual hair growth returns 2-6 months
- Provide resources for purchase/loan of wigs, scarves, and caps
- Inform patient about health care measures for scalp protection: use of gentle shampoos, avoidance of hair dryers and curling irons, permanents, and hair drying; protect scalp in winter and summer (cold/heat loss) and wear protective covering when outdoors

Nursing Diagnosis

- *Infection, potential for, immunosuppression, break in skin, or contamination of supplies.*

Interventions

- Monitor CBC and acute granulocyte count
- Monitor expectation of nadir related to chemotherapy
- Instruct and monitor prudent handwashing technique; prior to any nursing intervention, before/after meals, after bathroom use, and prior to any treatment-related activity for self-care
- Restrict visitors with potential infections, or recently immunized with attenuated live vaccines (DPT, MMR)

Patient Teaching Priorities for Chemotherapy

- Assess willingness, readiness to learn, and barriers to learning (acuity of illness, sensory deficits, pain, and/or fear and anxiety regarding diagnosis/treatment).
- Inform patient/family about schedule of activities for chemotherapy administration, and monitoring of laboratory and diagnostic tests.
- Encourage practice and repetition of newly learned skill to enhance the learner's performance for at risk procedures.
- Validate aseptic technique and skills of the patient or the caregiver, for prescribed self-administration and discontinuation of chemotherapy drugs.
- Provide written materials such as those from the National Cancer Institute "Chemotherapy and You," "What Are Clinical Trials All About?" 1-800-4-CANCER telephone number, and other materials as needed.
- Teach and review specific drugs and related side effects the patient may experience, and when, where, how, and who to call if problems arise.
- Provide information and list of resources for obtaining, storing, and disposing drugs and supplies.[9,24]

Geriatric Considerations

Potential for cardiac, renal, respiratory, and hepatic systems compromise: medication dosage and/or schedule of administration may be altered.

High-dose drug regimens have been associated with increased toxicity (e.g., neurotoxicity with high-dose cytarabine— patients over 50 years old are particularly susceptible to this toxicity).

Consider neuromuscular and sensory deficits that may be present, such as visual and hearing losses and arthritic joints; plan individualized teaching sessions; use printed materials with large print for reading ease; return demonstration techniques may require more simplistic steps to facilitate patient/family ease in learning the required technique.

Consider age-related changes in body function accommodations; bowel and bladder tonicity (unable to hold large volume hydration, unable to retain large volume bowel cleansing preparations); provide prompt and frequent elimination needs.

Premedications may cause drowsiness; encourage patient/family to utilize transportation resources (family, public, American Cancer Society) if receiving chemotherapy, and/or requires laboratory tests monitoring.

Query the patient/caregiver regarding over-the-counter and/or previous physician-prescribed medications; some of these medications may alter bleeding and clotting times and/or interfere with prescribed chemotherapy medications.

Assess ability of patient and caregiver and determine if additional resources, such as home-care agency, Meals on Wheels, and social services for financial assistance are needed.[6,7,9,14,24]

Bibliography

1. American Society of Hospital Pharmacists: *ASHP technical assistance bulletin on handling cytotoxic and hazardous drugs,* Am J Hosp Pharm 47(5):1033, 1990.

2. Baird and others: *Cancer Nursing: a comprehensive textbook,* Philadelphia, 1991, WB Saunders.
3. Barnicle MM: *Chemotherapy and pregnancy,* Semin Oncol Nurs 8(2):124, 1992.
4. Barton-Burke MS and others: *Potential toxicities and nursing management.* In *Cancer chemotherapy: a nursing process approach,* Boston, 1991, Jones and Bartlett.
5. Beason R: *Antineoplastic vesicant extravasation,* INS 13(2):111, 1990.
6. Bender C: Implications of antineoplastic therapy for nursing, In Clark JC and McGee RF editors, *Core curriculum for oncology nursing,* ed 2, 1992, Philadelphia, WB Saunders.
7. Brown JK and Hogan CM: Chemotherapy, In Groenwald SL, Frogge MH, Goodman M, and Yarbro CH: *Cancer nursing principels and practice,* Boston, 1992, Jones and Bartlett.
8. Brown M and Mulholland JL: *Drug calculations: process and problems for clinical practice,* ed 4, St Louis, 1992, Mosby.
9. Carey PJ and others: *Appraisal and caregiving burdens in family members caring for patients receiving chemotherapy,* Oncol Nurs Forum 18(8):1341, 1991.
10. DeVita VT Jr.: Principles of chemotherapy, In DeVita VT Jr., Hellman S, and Rosenberg SA, editors: *Cancer: Principles and practice of oncology,* ed 4, Philadelphia, 1993, JB Lippincott.
11. Dorr RT: *Antidote vesicant chemotherapy extravasation,* Blood Review 4:41, 1990.
12. Dudjak LA: *Cancer metastasis.* Semin Oncol Nurs 8(1):40, 1992.
13. Fields SM and Von Hoff DD: *New anticancer agents,* Highlights on Antineoplastic Drugs, 10(2):16, 1992
14. Finley RS: *Drug interactions in the oncology patient,* Semin Oncol Nurs 8(2):95, 1992.
15. Galassi A: *The next generation: new chemotherapy agents for the 1990s,* Semin Oncol Nurs 8(2):83, 1992.
16. Hessen JA: *Protocol for treatment of vesicant antineoplastic extravasation,* Hosp Pharm 24(9):705, 1989.

17. Kane B and Kuhn JG: *Therapeutic drug monitoring in antineoplastic drug development.* Highlights on Antineoplastic Drugs 10(2):21, 1992.

18. Lind J: *Tumor cell growth and cell kinetics,* Semin Oncol Nurs 8(1):3, 1992.

19. Lobert S and Correia JJ: *Antimiotics in cancer chemotherapy,* Cancer Nursing 15(1):22, 1992.

20. Madeya ML and Pfab-Tokarsky JM: *Flow cytometry: an overview,* Oncol Nurs Forum 19(3):459, 1992.

21. McCaffrey D and Engelking C: *Ten fallacies associated with the nature and management of chemotherapy extravasation,* Progressions 2(4):3, 1990.

22. McGovern K: *10 Golden rules for administering drugs safely,* Nursing 22(3):49, 1992.

23. McMillan SC: *Carcinogenesis,* Semin Oncol Nurs 8(1):10, 1992.

24. McNally JC and others: *Guidelines for oncology nursing practice,* ed 2, Philadelphia 1991, WB Saunders.

25. Oncology Nursing Society Cancer Chemotherapy: *Guidelines and recommendations for nursing education and practice,* 1992, Pittsburgh, Pa.

26. *Oncology Nursing Society Clinical Practice Committee Module V of the Cancer Chemotherapy guidelines revised,* Oncol Nurs Forum 16(2):275, 1989.

27. US Department of Labor, Office of Occupational Medicine, Occupational Safety and Health Administration: *Work practice guidelines for personnel dealing with cytotoxic (antineoplastic) drugs,* No 8-1.1, Washington, DC, 1986, US Government Printing Office.

28. Weinstein SM: *Math calculations for intravenous nurses,* INS 13(4):231, 1990.

29. Wujcik D: *Current research in side effects of high-dose chemotherapy,* Semin Oncol Nurs 8(2):102, 1992.

30. Xistris D and Schulmeister L: *Complying with the new OSHA regulations.* Problem solving in Office Oncology Nursing, 6(4):1, 1992.

31. Yarbro JW: *Oncogenes and cancer suppressor genes,* Semin Oncol Nurs 8(1):30, 1992.

Biotherapy

23

The rapid introduction of novel agents and approaches has opened an exciting era in cancer therapy. Traditionally, surgery, radiation therapy, and chemotherapy, either singly or in combination, have been the mainstays of cancer therapy. Recently, however, biotherapy, or biologic therapy, has emerged as an important fourth modality for treating cancer.[9,26,31]

Definition

Biotherapy may be defined as treatment with agents derived from biologic sources and/or affecting biologic responses. The subcommittee on biologic response modifiers (BRMs) to the National Cancer Institute Division of Cancer Treatment defines BRMs as "agents or approaches that modify the relationship between tumor and host by modifying the host's biologic response to tumor cells with a resultant therapeutic effect.

Although nonspecific immunomodulating agents such as BCG and *C. parvum* are still used, a variety of newer agents such as interferons, interleukins, monoclonal antibodies, and hematopoietic growth factors are now undergoing clinical investigation. Many of these are naturally occurring body substances that act as messengers between cells. A generic term for these messengers is *cytokine*, which refers to protein products from cells that serve as cell regulators. More specifically, lymphokines are products of lymphocytes, and monokines are products of monocytes. The name *interleukin* refers to proteins that act as messengers between cells.[5]

In general, BRMs can be classified into three major divisions: agents that augment, modulate, or restore the host's immunologic mechanisms; agents that have direct antitumor activity (cytotoxic or antiproliferative mechanisms); and agents that possess other biologic effects (those that affect differentiation or maturation of cells, that interfere with the ability of a tumor cell to metastasize, or that affect initiation or maintenance of neoplastic transformation).[10,19]

Major Agents in Use

Interferons

There are three major classes, according to antigenic type: alpha, beta, and gamma. While alpha- and beta-IFNs are primarily produced by leukocytes and fibroblasts respectively, gamma-IFN is made primarily by T-lymphocytes. The interferons may be termed a family of glycoprotein hormones possessing pleiotropic biologic effects. All IFNs mediate their cellular effect after binding to a specific receptor. Alpha- and beta-IFN share a receptor, while gamma-IFN uses a different one. The interferons possess a wide range of biologic effects: antiviral, antiproliferative, and immunomodulatory. The Food and Drug Administration has approved two recombinant alpha-IFN products for the treatment of hairy-cell leukemia, AIDS-related Kaposi's sarcoma, condyloma acuminata, chronic hepatitis non-A, non-B/C, and chronic hepatitis B, chronic myelogenous leukemia, low-grade lymphomas, multiple myeloma, melanoma, renal cell cancer, ovarian carcinoma, and superficial bladder carcinoma. Routes of administration are intramuscular and subcutaneous, intravenously, intralesionally, intraperitoneally, intravesically, intraarterially and intrathecally.[15,21,28,33,37]

Side Effects

In general, side effects are similar for all classes of interferon, with slight variations according to dosage, schedule, and type:

- Flulike symptoms
- Fever spikes up to 40°
- Myalagias
- Malaise
- Anorexia
- Lethargy
- Mild thrombocytopenia
- Proteinuria
- Asymptomatic hypotension
- Chills
- Headaches
- Arthralgias
- Fatigue
- Weight loss
- Neutropenia
- Elevated transaminase levels

Gastrointestinal effects such as:
- Nausea
- Diarrhea
- Vomiting
- Altered taste

Central nervous system or neurologic changes such as:
- Depression
- Decreased libido
- Mood alterations
- Memory problems

Inflammation at the injection site, reactivation of herpes simplex, rash, exacerbation of psoriasis, and mild alopecia have all been reported.

Interleukins

Interleukin-2

Interleukin-2 is a glycoprotein mainly produced by activated T-helper cells. IL-2 supports the growth and maturation of sub-populations of T-cells both in vitro and in vivo, stimulates cytotoxic T cells, stimulated the proliferation and activity of NK cells, and develops the capacity in lymphoid cells incubated with IL-2 to lyse fresh tumor cells.[8,11] IL-2 has been approved by the FDA for the treatment of renal cell cancer and melanoma. The most common route of administration is intravenous, using either bolus or continuous infusion. In patients receiving adoptive immunotherapy with either LAK or TILs, the majority of side effects are attributable to IL-2. Chills and fever are the major side effects noted with cell infusions. These are readily treatable with meperidine. A further risk is that of infection, because lymphocytes incubated in culture medium for 3 to 4 days may be contaminated with viruses or bacteria. Major side effects alter the cardiovascular, pulmonary, renal, gastrointestinal, endocrine, integumentary and central nervous systems and hematologic and hepatic functions.[12,28]

Interleukin-4

Interleukin-4 stimulates the growth of resting B cells in vitro; increases production of immunoglobulin in vitro; may stimulate certain T-cell lines in vitro; produces CSF-like activity in vitro; and may stimulate growth and maturation of mast cells in vitro.

Hematopoietic Growth Factors

Colony-stimulating factors (CSFs) are a family of glycoprotein hormones responsible for the proliferation differentiation, and maturation of hematopoietic cells in vitro. The four classic CSFs are granulocyte-macrophage colony-stimulating factor (GM-CSF), granulocyte colony stimulating factor (G-CSF), macrophage colony-stimulating factor (M-CSF), and IL-3 (multi-CSF).

In vitro studies suggest that the CSFs may have clinical value in a variety of settings; decrease myelosuppression, speed marrow recovery after bone marrow transplant; restore bone marrow function in aplastic anemia, myelodysplastic syndrome, myelomas, leukemias, and acquired and congenital neutropenias; enhance effector cell functions further; and treat burns, overwhelming sepsis-related infections, and parasitic infections.[4,13,19,23,24]

GM-CSF

The most common route of administration is a 2 hour IV infusion beginning 2-4 hours after the autologous bone marrow infusion. Side effects are affected by the dosage, route of administration, patient population, and setting used (postchemotherapy, post-bone marrow transplantation). Common side effects are constitutional symptoms (chills and fever), bone pain, fatigue, anorexia, rashes, flushing, phlebitis, gastrointestinal disturbances, erythema at the injection site, hypotension, fluid retention, pericarditis, pleural and pericardial effusions, thrombocytopenia, and thrombus formation at the catheter tip. These effects are generally reversible with cessation of therapy.

G-CSF

G-CSF is administered subcutaneously or intravenously. Side effects include medullary bone pain, and erythema at the subcutaneous injection site.

M-CSF

Subcutaneous administration doses up to 12,800 μg/m^2 have been administered. In general, toxicity has been mild consisting of local reaction, arthralgia, and fatigue.[22]

Interleukin-3

Both subcutaneous and intravenous routes are used, with doses up to 1000μg/m^2/day being fairly well tolerated. The most common toxicities experienced are low-grade fever and headaches with occasional flushing, erythema at injection sites, bone pain, lethargy, and nausea and vomiting.[24]

Erythropoietin

Patients are generally started at a dosage of 50 to 100 U/kg three times a week intravenously or subcutaneously. Maintenance doses are generally titrated in 25-unit increments to keep the hematocrit in a chosen target range, for example 36% to 38%.[2,27]

Tumor Necrosis Factor

Current efforts are focused on phase II investigations and on evaluating combination therapy of TNF with other cytokines, and chemotherapy (actinomycin).

TNF

TNF is administered by intramuscular, subcutaneous, intravenous (via both bolus and continuous infusion), and intraperitoneal routes.

Side effects are similar to those seen with other biologic agents, are dose dependent, and in general, resolve upon discontinuation of therapy. Dose-limiting toxicities with IV administration have been constitutional symptoms and shocklike manifestations, including fever and hypotension. Occasional side effects include hematologic changes (leukopenia, thrombocytopenia), cardiovascular changes (hypotension, dizziness), hepatic changes (elevated transaminases, hyperbilirubinemia), elevated triglycerides, and decreased serum cholesterol. These changes are usually reversible with cessation of therapy.[18,23,28]

Other Immunomodulating Agents

Bacillus Calmette-Guerin

Developed in the early 1900s, it is an attenuated form of the living bovine tubercle bacillus. It is believed to have a non-specific immunostimulating effect. BCG is approved for the treatment of bladder cancer by intravesical instillation. BCG can be administered intralesionally; intradermally by scarification, the tine technique, or the Heafgun; or intracavitarily (to the pleura, peritoneum, or bladder). Side effects can include local inflammatory reactions, flulike symptoms, hypersensitivity, and the serious complication of disseminate BCG infection.[14,26,34]

Levamisole

Levamisole is an orally active synthetic agent that is an isomer of tetramisole, a broad-spectrum antihelminthic agent. Ergamisol (levamisole) is now approved by the FDA for use with 5-FU as an adjuvant treatment for colon cancer (Duke's stage C). Toxicity has been minimal with levamisole alone, and no more severe than expected for fluorouracil alone, when the two drugs were combined.[26,31]

Tumor Antigens

Tumor vaccines employ tumor cells or purified components of tumor cell membrane. To increase the immunogenicity of the cells, the surface is often treated with viruses, irradiation, or neuramidase. Tumor vaccines are also given in combination with other immunostimulants such as BCG or *C. parvum*. Vaccines are usually administered by multiple intradermal injections, with patients receiving vaccines prepared from their own tumor cells.[16]

Handling Issues

Handling the issues are a concern to all oncology nurses. To date there has been no formal research on the safest way to handle IFNs or other BRMs. Many institutions place BRMs in the same classification as chemotherapy, instructing staff to follow institutional policy on the handling and disposal of cytotoxic drugs.

Nursing Management

Nursing Diagnoses for Patients Receiving Biotherapy

Neurologic function
- Sensory/perceptual alterations (specify)
- Sleep pattern disturbance
- Social interaction, impaired
- Thought processes, altered

Renal function
- Urinary elimination, altered patterns

Hematologic function
- Potential for injury re: weakness or bleeding
- Potential for infection re: decreased WBC
- Activity intolerance re: anemia

Skin
- Skin integrity, impaired

Gastrointestinal system
- Nutrition altered less than body requirements
- Diarrhea
- Oral mucous membranes, altered
- Skin integrity, impaired, potential re: diarrhea

Cardiovascular system
- Tissue perfusion, altered re: hypotension
- Fluid volume deficit

Pulmonary system
- Impaired gas exchange, potential
- Anxiety re: respiratory distress

Miscellaneous
- Fatigue
- Activity intolerance
- Body temperature, altered, potential
- Pain
- Self-care deficit
- Knowledge deficit (specify)

Psychosocial adjustment
- Coping, ineffective, individual or family
- Decisional conflict (specify)
- Hopelessness
- Sexuality patterns, altered

Assessment and Planning[25,29,32]

- Perform a baseline assessment using a body systems approach, including psychosocial concerns, before the patient starts therapy. Include current symptoms related to disease or previous treatment, level of functional status, and hopes, fears, and expectations related to therapy.
- Obtain medication profile.
- Evaluate symptoms for duration, frequency, and severity in order to plan appropriate care. Information and care plans should be documented in the patient's medical record.
- Assess treatment plan to develop a plan of care and intervene appropriately. Such questions include the following:
- Will the therapy be given in the hospital, in an ambulatory care setting, or both? In the ambulatory care setting, assessment of the patient's compliance with the therapeutic plan is especially important.
- What types of laboratory tests (routine lab work, special lab work, and pharmacology) and diagnostic procedures will be required?
- What agent or agents will the patients receive, and what are the associated side effects?
- Is the agent under investigation or FDA approved?
- If under investigation, has informed consent been secured?
- What is the nature of the agent? Are there special handling precautions or storage requirements?
- Are any special equipment or emergency supplies needed?
- What type of teaching will the patient need (self-administration techniques, side effects and management, and so on)?
- What type of monitoring will be required? Are special vital signs necessary, such as orthostatic blood pressures?

Management of Side Effects

Neurologic Side Effects

Assess patient before therapy for baseline data and regularly during therapy for changes in level of consciousness, orientation, and mental status. Evaluate patient's medication profile for other drugs that can contribute to CNS toxicity. Observe for problems such as confusion, disorientation, and somnolence. Protect patient from injury, when appropriate, implement fall precautions or bed sensors. Patient should be reoriented as needed.[6]

Renal Side Effects

Evaluate for renal toxicity: obtain BUN, creatinine levels; obtain strict intake and output measures; weigh regularly; administer diuretics, fluids and vasopressors as ordered.

Hematologic Side Effects

Monitor changes in CBC, (differential and platelet counts). Observe for symptoms of thrombocytopenia and infection.

Hepatic Side Effects

Assess patient for changes in serum transaminases and bilirubin, and for jaundice or hepatomegaly.

Skin Changes

Observe skin daily for infection and breakdown. Therapeutic measures for dry skin include gently cleansing (avoid scrubbing the skin), tepid versus hot baths, frequent use of water-based lotions and creams, soft cotton clothing, and bath oils. Teach patient to avoid perfumed lotion, as it can further irritate already sensitive skin. Implement measures to diminish pruritus—soft clothing, use of colloidal oatmeal baths, and administer antipruritic medications.[19,21]

Gastrointestinal Side Effects

Assess baseline nutritional status and dietary intake. Offer small, frequent meals and calorie supplements; administer antiemetics, antidiarrheals as ordered. Assess oral cavity for mucositis.

Cardiovascular/Pulmonary Side Effects

Evaluate cardiovascular status by monitoring heart rate, blood pressure (including orthostatic checks), central venous pressure as indicated, and other cardiac indices. Obtain accurate daily weight and strict intake and output measures. Assess for presence of edema and abdominal ascites. Assess pulmonary status by monitoring respiratory rate, ausculation of breath sounds, monitoring lab values or oxygenation, and heeding complaints of shortness of breath or altered breathing patterns.[12,28]

Constitutional Symptoms

Chills followed by fever are seen with almost all biologic agents. Premedicate patient with acetaminophen or other NSAID's. Keep patient warm with blankets during chills. Observe and monitor chills/fever patterns. Administer fluids, observe for signs and symptoms of infection.[23]

Fatigue

Teach patient about the side effect and its management. Stress that fatigue is chronic, not acute, and that more sleep often exacerbates the problem.[18,35]

Geriatric Considerations

Factors affecting medication dosage and administration
- Alteration in hepatic and renal function may necessitate adjustment of dosage and or schedule.
- Decreases in cardiovascular function may require lower doses of biologic response modifiers (BRMs) such as interferon and interleukin-2, whose side effects may stress cardiovascular system.

- Alterations in neurosensory/perceptual protective mechanisms may place elderly patient at higher risk for problems with CNS-associated side effects of BRMs such as confusion, depression, memory loss, or slowed thinking.
- Decreased functional status may place patient at a higher risk for intolerance of fatigue associated with many BRMs.
- Altered nutritional intake (less than body requirements) may be increased due to anorexia associated with some BRMs.
- Decreased tissue, skin and mucous membrane integrity may place patient at higher risk for IL-2-related skin toxicity.
- Evaluation of patient's current medication profile should occur to determine drugs that may be contraindicated with BRMs and/or cause addictive toxicity.

Factors affecting patient teaching
- Assess for neuromuscular and sensory deficits (e.g., vision problems, hearing losses, arthritic joints) that may inhibit teaching/learning. Utilize appropriate teaching tools for deficits present (e.g., large print, minimal illustrations for patient with vision problems).
- Asses for reading level and comprehension, as many people 65 and older have completed eight or fewer years of formal schooling. Utilize reading materials targeted for appropriate reading level and/or audiovisual aids. Reinforce information presented often.[25,29]

Factors affecting social support systems
- Approximately 30% of patients 65 or older live alone, the majority being women. The difficulties of living alone are often intensified by poverty, having few relatives or other social supports, and decreased functional status.
- Many BRMs are given on an outpatient basis; hence patients are required to learn self-care. Evaluation of formal and informal support networks, functional capacity and economic status should be incorporated into nursing assessment, and referrals made to community resources as needed.
- Spouses should be evaluated for early indicators of caregiver role strain, and appropriate interventions initiated.

Bibliography

1. Amgen: *Neupogen (Filgrastim), package insert*, Thousand Oaks, CA, 1991, Amgen.

2. Amgen, Inc., *Epogen (Epoetin alfa), package insert*, Thousand Oaks, CA, 1989, Amgen.

3. Baird SB (Ed): *New perspectives on the management of myelosuppression,* Oncol Nurs Forum 18(2) Suppl, 2, 1991.

4. Bajorin DF, Cheung NV, and Houghton AN: *Macrophage colony-stimulating factor: biological effects and potential applications for cancer therapy,* Semin Hematol 28(2) Suppl 2:42, 1991.

5. Brophy LR and Rieger PT: Biotherapy. In Clark JC and McGee RF, editors: *Core curriculum for oncology nursing,* ed 2, Philadelphia, 1992, WB Saunders.

6. Brophy LR and Sharp EJ: *Physical symptoms of combination biotherapy: a quality-of- life issue,* Oncol Nurs Forum 18(1) suppl: 25, 1991.

7. Cetus Oncology Corp: *Proleukin® (Aldesleukin) for injection, package insert,* Emeryville, CA, 1992, Cetus Oncology.

8. Dawson MM: *Lymphokines and interleukins,* Boca Raton, 1991, CRC Press.

9. DeVita VJ, Hellman S, and Rosenberg SA, editors: *Biologic therapy of cancer,* Philadelphia, 1991, JB Lippincott.

10. Dillman RO: Antibody therapy. In RK Oldham, editor: *Principles of cancer biotherapy,* New York, 1991, Marcel Dekker.

11. Dinarello CA: *Interleukin-1 and interleukin-1 and interleukin-antagonism,* Blood 77(8):1627, 1991.

12. Farrell MM: *The challenge of adult respiratory distress syndrome during interleukin-2 therapy,* Oncol Nurs Forum 19(3):475, 1992.

13. Gabrilove JL: Colony-stimulating factors: clinical status. In DeVita VT Jr, Hellman S, and Rosenberg SA, editors: *Important advances in oncology,* Philadelphia, 1991, JB Lippincott.

14. Galazka AR and others: Lymphokines and cytokines. In RK Oldham, editor: *Principles of cancer biotherapy,* New York, 1991, Marcel Dekker.

15. Genentech: *Actimmune (Interferon gamma 1b), package insert*, San Francisco, CA, 1991, Genentech.

16. Grossbard ML and Nadler LM: Immunotoxin therapy of malignancy. In DeVita VT Jr, Hellman S, and Rosenberg SA, editors: *Important advances in oncology,* Philadelphia, 1991, JB Lippincott.

17. Hoechst-Roussel Pharmaceuticals, Inc.: *Prokine, package insert,* Sommerville, NJ, Hoechst-Roussel, 1991.

18. Hogan CM: *Coping with biotherapy: physiological and psychosocial concerns,* Oncol Nurs Forum 18(1) Suppl 1:19, 1991.

19. Hood LE and Abernathy E: Biological response modifiers. In Baird SB, McCorkle R, and Grant M, editors: *Cancer nursing: comprehensive textbook*, Philadelphia, 1991, WB Saunders.

20. Immunex Corporation: *Leukine (Sargramostim), package insert,* Seattle, WA, 1991, Immunex.

21. Jassak PF: Biotherapy. In Groenwald SL, Hansen Frogge M, Goodman M, and Yarbro CH, editors: *Cancer nursing: principles and practice,* ed 3, Boston, 1993, Jones and Bartlett.

22. Lyman AD and Williams DE: *Biological activities and potential therapeutic uses of steel factor,* Am J Ped Hem/Oncol 14(1):1, 1992.

23. Mayer DK: *Biotherapy: recent advances and nursing implications,* Nurs Clin N Am 25(2):291, 1990.

24. Mendelsohn J: Antibodies to growth factors and receptors. In DeVita VT Jr, Hellman S, and Rosenberg SA, editors: *Biologic therapy of cancer,* Philadelphia, 1991, JB Lippincott.

25. Morra ME and Grant M (Eds.): *Cancer patient education,* Semin Oncol Nurs 7(2):79, 1991.

26. Oettgen HF and Old LJ: The history of cancer immunotherapy. In DeVita VT Jr, Hellman S, and Rosenberg SA, editors: *Biologic therapy of cancer,* Philadelphia, 1991, JB Lippincott.

27. Ortho Biotech: *Procrit (epoetin alfa), package insert, Raritan,* NJ, 1993, Ortho Pharmaceutical.

28. Rieger PT: *The pathophysiology of selected symptoms associated with BRM therapy.* Monograph, 1992, Cetus.

29. Rieger PT and Rumsey KA: Responding to the educational needs of patients receiving biotherapy. In Carroll-Johnson RM, editor: *The biotherapy of cancer V—Monograph,* Pittsburgh, 1992, Oncology Nursing Press, p. 10.

30. Roche Laboratories: *Roferon-A package insert,* Nutley, NJ, 1990, Hoffman-LaRoche.

31. Rosenberg SA: *The immunotherapy and gene therapy of cancer,* J Clin Oncol 10(2):180, 1992.

32. Rumsey KA and Rieger PT, editors: *Biological response modifiers: a self-instructional manual for health professional,* Chicago, IL, 1992, Precept Press.

33. Schering Corp: *Intron A: Interferon alpha-2b recombinant for injection, Kenilworth,* NJ, 1992, Schering.

34. Siegel JP and Puri RK: *Interleukin-2 toxicity,* J Clin Oncol 9(4):694, 1991.

35. Vitetta ES and Thorpe PE: Immunotoxins. In DeVita VT Jr, Hellman S, and Rosenberg, SA, editors: *Biologic therapy of cancer,* Philadelphia, 1991, JB Lippincott.

36. Winningham ML: How exercise mitigates fatigue: Implications for patients receiving cancer therapy. In Carroll-Johnson RM, editor: *The biotherapy of cancer V—Monograph.* Pittsburgh, 1992, Oncology Nursing Press.

37. Yarbo JW, Bornstein RS, and Mastrangelo MJ: *Management of anemia in oncology,* Semin Oncol 19(3) Suppl 8:1, 1992.

38. Yarbo JW, Bornstein RS, and Mastrangelo MJ: *Interferon: advances in biotherapy,* Semin Oncol 18(5) Suppl 7:1, 1991.

Bone Marrow Transplantation

24

Bone marrow is a spongy tissue found in the inner cavities of bone. Normal functioning marrow is rich in progenitor or stem cells, which eventually proliferate into mature erythrocytes, leukocytes, and platelets. Bone marrow transplantation (BMT) is the process of replacing diseased or damaged bone marrow with normal functioning bone marrow.

Types of Bone Marrow Transplantation

There are two major types of BMT: autologous and allogeneic. The type of transplant is identified by the relationship of the recipient to the donor. An autologous BMT is a transplant in which the patient's own bone marrow is collected (harvested), placed in frozen storage (cryopreserved), and reinfused to the patient following the conditioning regimen. An allogeneic BMT is a transplant in which the patient receives someone else's bone marrow. There are several types of allogeneic BMT, each type named according to the donor. They are: *syngeneic*—occurs when the donor is the patient's identical twin; *related*—the donor is related to the recipient and is usually a sibling; *unrelated*—the donor is no relation to the recipient. Autologous BMT is primarily used for the treatment of diseases in which the patient's own bone marrow contains adequate stem cells that can eventually generate functioning erythrocytes, leukocytes, and platelets. The major criterion for an allogeneic BMT is finding a suitable donor. Tissue typing of the patient and potential donors is the first step in identifying whether a patient has a compatible donor. To determine a person's tissue type, a small amount of peripheral blood is drawn and antigens on the surface of the leukocytes are analyzed. These antigens make up the human leukocyte antigen (HLA) system, which plays a role in immune surveillance by constantly identifying "self" from "non-self."[25] The best match is one in which the antigens of the patient and potential donor match. The best chance of finding a matched donor occurs among full siblings. The chances of matching someone in the general population are approximately one in 20,000. When possible donors are identified from HLA typing, a mixed lymphocyte culture (MLC) is performed. The MLC is done to further ensure compatibility between donor and patient.

The last option for donor availability is the attainment of an unrelated donor. The National Bone Marrow Donor Registry Program (NBMDR) was established in 1987 for this purpose. The registry contains over 600,000 available bone marrow donors, all of whom have had tissue typing completed and have expressed a desire to donate bone marrow.

Peripheral Blood Stem Cell

PBSCs are collected through the process of aspheresis, which extracts the various blood cells, separates them, retains the peripheral stem cells, and returns the remaining cells back to the patient. This is accomplished by an apheresis machine to which the patient is connected via IV lines, usually for 2 to 6 hours. Typically, 6 to 8 apheresis sessions are required to collect a sufficient number of peripheral stem cells for transplantation. The concentration of stem cells in bone marrow can be 100 times greater than in the peripheral system. After collection, the peripheral stem cells are cryopreserved to be transplanted at a later time. Diseases treated with PBSC transplantation: acute leukemia, brain tumors, breast cancer, Hodgkin's disease, multiple myeloma, neuroblastoma, non-Hodgkin's lymphoma, ovarian cancer, small cell lung cancer, and testicular cancer.

Bone marrow transplantation is a treatment modality for a variety of malignant and nonmalignant diseases. The type and stage of the disease, the patient's age and performance status, and donor availability determine the type of transplant that can be done and the chances of survival. Allogeneic transplants are more frequently done for leukemia and nonmalignant diseases. Autologous transplants are more common in the treatment of malignant lymphoma and solid tumors.

Hematologic Malignancies

Leukemia
- Acute lymphocytic leukemia
- Acute myelogenous leukemia
- Chronic myelogenous leukemia

Lymphoma
- Hodgkin's
- Non-Hodgkin's lymphoma

Other Hematologic Malignancies
- Myelodysplastic syndrome
- Multiple myeloma

Solid Tumors

- Breast cancer
- Testicular cancer
- Neuroblastoma
- Ewing's sarcoma
- Rhabdomyosarcoma
- Wilm's tumor
- Malignant melanoma

Non-Malignant Diseases

- Aplastic anemia
- Severe combined immunodeficiency syndrome
- Myelofibrosis

Bone Marrow Transplantation Procedure

Pretreatment Work Up

An extensive evaluation is performed on the bone marrow transplant recipient prior to transplant. This is done to establish the recipient's physical and psychosocial status. For allogeneic transplants, the donor is also thoroughly assessed. The assessment is done on an outpatient basis and includes a variety of tests, procedures, and consultations (Box 24-1).

Marrow Harvest

Box 24-1

Pretransplantation Evaluation

Bone marrow recipient
History and physical examination
Bone marrow biopsy and aspiration with cytogenetics
Chemistry profile
Complete blood count, platelets, reticulocyte count
ABO and Rh typing
Coagulation profile
Serum immunoelectrophoresis
Quantitative immunoglobulins
Hepatitis screen
Cytomegalovirus, HIV, and herpes simplex virus titers
Urinalysis, creatinine clearance, and protein quantification
Chest x-ray
Electrocardiogram, echocardiogram, or radionucleotide
    ventriculogram
Pulmonary function testing
Sinus x-ray
Allergy testing
Audiology consultation
Physical therapy consultation
Dental consultation
Dietary consultation
Social work consultation
Psychology/psychiatry consultation
Opthamology consultation
Surgery consult—insertion of multiple lumen catheter

Bone marrow donor
History and physical examination
Chemistry profile
Complete blood count, platelet count
ABO and Rh typing
Hepatitis screen
Cytomegalovirus, HIV, and herpes simplex virus titers
Chest x-ray
Electrocardiogram
Urinalysis

Harvesting is the process of obtaining bone marrow for transplantation. This procedure occurs in the operating room, typically under general anesthesia. Bone marrow is obtained by performing multiple punctures with a large bore needle into the patient's posterior and occasionally anterior iliac crests. Multiple punctures are necessary since each aspiration obtains only 2 to 5 mL of bone marrow. The amount of bone marrow collected depends on the size of the recipient and donor as well as the type of bone marrow transplant (autologous vs. allogeneic). Usually 10 cc per kilogram of body weight will yield the amount of needed stem cells. Once collected, the marrow is mixed with a heparinized solution, filtered to remove bone fragments and fat, and placed in a blood bag to be treated or purged. For an autologous transplant, the collected marrow is mixed with the preservative dimethylsulfoxide (DMSO), placed in a blood bag, and cryopreserved. It will be thawed and transplanted at a later date.

Conditioning Regimens

The conditioning regimen is the process of preparing the patient to receive bone marrow. It accomplishes three vital functions: obliterate the malignant disease; destroy the patient's preexisting immunologic state; and create space in the marrow cavity for the proliferation of the transplanted stem cells. The conditioning regimen consists of high-dose chemotherapy with or without total body irradiation. There are several regimens using various combinations of chemotherapy and/or radiation that last 4 to 10 days. The side effects in response to the chemotherapy and/or radiation can continue for several weeks following BMT. Management of these side effects focuses on control of the symptoms, prevention of further complications, and maintenance of patient comfort (Table 24-1).

Transplantation of Marrow

Following completion of the conditioning regimen, the bone marrow must be infused. If the regimen was one in which chemotherapy was the last treatment given, there is a rest period of 24 to 72 hours prior to transplant. This rest period is necessary because of the drug's half-life.

Table 24-1 Side Effects of Conditioning Regimens

	Major Side Effects	Management
Busulfan	Nausea, vomiting, diarrhea, seizures (possible during administration and up to 48 hours after last dose)	Administer antiemetic at scheduled intervals Check emesis for busulfan tablets and replace 1 for 1 Establish seizure precautions and monitor for seizure activity Administer anticonvulsant at scheduled intervals as ordered
Carmustine (BCNU)	Nausea, vomiting, diarrhea Hypotension Alcohol intoxication (drug is reconstituted in an alcohol base) Stomatitis Veno-occlusive disease (hepatic failure occurs in first 4 weeks)	Administer antiemetic at scheduled intervals Monitor BP throughout administration Maintain adequate hydration Monitor for possible intoxication, maintain safe environment, and keep patient in bed during administration and several hours afterward Monitor for ascites, edema, and elevated liver function Administer diuretics, lactulose, albumin, and fluid restriction as ordered
Cyclophosphamide (Cytoxan)	Nausea, vomiting, diarrhea Hemorrhagic cycstitis Alopecia	Administer antiemetic at scheduled intervals Maintain adequate hydration Monitor for blood in urine

Cardiac toxicity		Maintain continuous bladder irrigation as ordered and provide foley catheter care Administer MESNA and pain medications as ordered Ensure that EKG is done and checked prior to administration of each dose
Cytarabine (Ara-C)	Nausea, vomiting, diarrhea Erythema Neurotoxicity Hemorrhagic conjunctivitis Alopecia	Administer antiemetics at scheduled intervals Monitor palms and soles for erythema, provide creams and assistance with ADLs as needed Monitor for cerebellar toxicity—ataxia Administer steroid eye drops at scheduled intervals up to 48 hours after last dose
Etoposide (VP-16)	Nausea, vomiting, diarrhea Hypotension Atopecia	Administer antiemetics at scheduled intervals Monitor BP throughout administration Maintain adequate hydration

Continued.

Table 24-1 Cont'd.

	Major Side Effects	Management
Total body irradiation (TBI)	Nausea, vomiting, diarrhea Stomatitis Alopecia Veno-occlusive disease Fever Parotitis Erythema	Administer antiemetics 30 minutes before treatment and immediately following Monitor for ascites, edema, and elevated liver function Administer diuretics, lactulose, albumin, and fluid restriction as ordered Monitor temperature every 2 to 4 hours and observe fever pattern Assess for signs and symptoms of infection Administer antipyretics as ordered Apply hot/cold packs to affected areas Administer pain medications as ordered Monitor skin integrity and keep skin clean and dry Avoid harsh soaps and irritants. If desquamation occurs, use dressings, ointments, only as ordered

For autologous transplants, the frozen marrow is brought to the recipient's room for transplantation. The bag of marrow is thawed in a normal saline bath, drawn up in large syringes, and given rapid IV push via central venous catheter. The entire process takes approximately 20 to 30 minutes depending on the volume of bone marrow being transplanted.

For allogeneic transplants, the marrow is infused on the same day as it is collected. This procedure resembles a red blood cell transfusion in that the bag of marrow is hung and transfused via the patient's central venous catheter. Unfiltered tubing must be used in order to prevent precious stem cells from becoming trapped and not getting infused. The total time of infusion depends on the amount of marrow, but usually lasts between 1 and 5 hours.

Engraftment Period

The engraftment period is the time immediately post transplant when the transfused stem cells migrate, by some unknown phenomenon, to the patient's bone marrow space and begin to regenerate. This usually takes 2 to 3 weeks and is evidenced by increasing blood counts. During this period the patient experiences severe pancytopenia and immunosuppression.

Complications of Marrow Transplantation

BMT recipients experience toxic complications associated with the immunosuppressive therapy necessary to allow the graft to occur. The major complications characteristic of BMT are: graft

Table 24–2 Major Complications Following BMT

Complication	Appearance	Signs/Symptoms	Management
GRAFT REJECTION	1–4 weeks	Absent/prolonged neutropenia Partial marrow recovery Hypoplasia Hemolysis	Blood component therapy Retransplantation
INFECTION Bacterial Fungal Viral Herpes Cytomegalovirus Varicella zoster	1–5 weeks 1–5 weeks 1–3 months 3 months 1st year	Fever Dry, nonproductive cough Change in breath sounds Erythema—oropharynx/catheter site Diarrhea Lesions—skin or mucous membranes Hypotension	Maintain protective environment Provide good hygiene Monitor vital signs frequently Frequent head-to-toe systems assessments Administer colony stimulating factors CMV negative blood products Adminsiter broad spectrum antibiotics Administer acyclovir and/or ganciclovir Intravenous immunoglobulins

PNEUMONITIS			
Interstitial	1-4 months	Fever	CMV negative blood products
Toxic	1-6 months	Dry nonproductive cough	Leukocyte poor blood products
		Shortness of breath	Colony stimulating factors
		Tachypnea	Ganciclovir
		Interstitial changes on x-ray	Intravenous immunoglobulins
ACUTE GVHD	3-14 weeks	Maculopapular skin rash	Immunosuppression with cyclosporine-A, steroids, and/or methotrexate
		Nausea, vomiting, uncontrollable diarrhea	Symptomatic treatment of skin, GI tract, and/or liver
		Jaundice	
		Elevated liver function tests	
		Hepatomegaly	
CHRONIC GVHD			
Skin	months-years	Hyper- or hypopigmentation; patch erythematous scaling; thickening, hardening resembling scleroderma; hair loss in involved areas	Immunosuppresion with cyclosporine-A, steroids, azathioprine (Imuran), and/or thalidomide (investigational)

Continued.

Table 24-2 Cont'd.

Complication	Appearance	Signs/Symptoms	Management
Mouth		White striae and erythema on mucosa; decreased salivary flow with dryness of mouth	Symptom management of affected organ or system
Eyes		Dryness, redness, itching/burning; corneal thickening	
Sinuses		Chronic sinusitis; predisposition to gram positive infections	
GI tract		Difficulty swallowing; retrosternal pain; abdominal discomfort; diarrhea	
Pulmonary		Productive cough; progressive dyspnea, wheezing, pneumothorax	
Vagina		Inflammation; dryness; stenosis	
Muscle		Occasional polymyositis; proximal weakness	
GU tract		Cystitis; mild nephrotic syndrome	
Hematopoietic		Eosinophilia; thrombocytopenia; hypoplastic marrow; marrow fibrosis	

Lymphoid		Hypocellularity and atrophy of lymph tissues; functional asplenia	
Endocrine		Decreased growth rates; delayed pubertal development; autoimmune hyperthyroidism	
Nervous system		Entrapment neuropathy; peripheral neutropathy; myasthenia gravis	
LATE EFFECTS			
Cateracts	1-6 years	Loss of vision	Surgical intervention
Gonad dysfunction	variable	Dryness	Replacement sex hormones
		Infertility	Psychosexual counseling
		Menopause	
Growth failure	variable	Impaired growth of facial skeleton and dentition (< 6 y/o)	Supplemental growth hormone
		Absent growth spurts	Replacement sex hormones
		No height changes	

Continued.

Table 24-2 Cont'd.

Complication	Appearance	Signs/Symptoms	Management
Hypothyroidism	1-15 years	Dry skin Hoarse speech Lethargy/apathy Weight gain with appetite loss Increased susceptibility to cold	Replacement hormones
Secondary malignancy	months-years	Specific to disease	Determined by type and extent of disease as well as by patient's physical and psychological status
RECURRENCE	months-years	Signs/symptoms of original disease	Determined by extent of disease and patient's physical and psychological status

rejection, infections, pneumonitis, graft-versus-host disease
(GVHD), and recurrence of original disease (Table 24-2).

Nursing Management

Nursing Diagnosis

- *Body image disturbance, potential*
    Related to treatment process

Interventions

- Encourage patient to verbalize feelings about appearance
  and perceptions of life-style changes
- Validate perceptions and assure that responses are appropriate
- Promote acceptance of positive, realistic body image
- Suggest ways that the patient can cope with body image
  changes

Nursing Diagnosis

- *Comfort, alteration, potential*
    Related to side effects of treatment regimens

Interventions

- Assess patient's pain:
    Location, onset, frequency, intensity, quality
- Identify effective pain control measures
- Administer medications as ordered and needed
- Assess for effectiveness of pain control measures
- Intervene at onset of pain
- Instruct patient in relaxation techniques (see Chapter 28)

Nursing Diagnosis

- *Coping, ineffective, individual*
    Related to transplant process
    Related to potential life style changes

Interventions

- Assess patient's level of distress and anxiety related to:

Uncertainty of future
Bothersome symptoms
Changes in self-concept
- Assess for signs of maladaptive or risky behaviors that interfere with responsible health practices
- Identify patient's support system, resources, and communication patterns
- Encourage verbalization of fears
- Assist patient with problem solving as needed
- Provide reassurance that anxiety or distress are common feelings among transplant patients
- Initiate referrals to social work, psychology, or community resources as appropriate (see Chapter 30)

Nursing Diagnosis

- *Injury, potential for*
  Related to thrombocytopenia

Interventions

- Monitor platelet count and anticipate nadir.
- Assess for signs and symptoms of bleeding:
  Petechiae, ecchymosis, epistaxis
  Vaginal or rectal bleeding
- Administer platelet transfusions as ordered.
- Observe patient for signs of transfusion reaction and response to transfusions.
- Teach patient to avoid:
  Shaving with razor
  Flossing teeth
  Picking nose or scabs
  Forceful nose-blowing

Nursing Diagnosis

- *Knowledge deficit*
  Related to transplant process

Interventions

- Evaluate patient and family readiness to learn
- Identify barriers to learning such as language, physical deficiencies, psychological deficiencies, intellectual de-

velopment
- Determine patient and family knowledge of the transplant process
- Provide written or audiovisual education materials and review with patient and family
- Allow adequate time for verbalization of questions, concerns and fears

Nursing Diagnosis

- *Sexuality patterns, altered*
    Related to treatment process
    Related to late effects

Interventions

- Assess for physical symptoms that may affect libido
- Assess for fear, anxiety, depression, and diminished self-concept
- Promote open communication about sexual issues by bringing up the subject
- Instruct patient on appropriate hygiene and contraceptive measures (see Chapter 31)

Refer to Tables 24-1 and 24-2 for nursing management of fluid and electrolyte imbalance, growth and development altered infection, nutrition altered, and skin integrity impaired.

Bibliography

1. Atkinson K: *Chronic graft-versus-host disease following marrow transplantation,* Marrow Transplantation Reviews 2:1, 1992.
2. Ayash LJ and others: *Hepatic venoocclusive disease in autologous bone marrow transplantation of solid tumors and lymphomas,* J Clin Oncol, 8:1699, 1990.
3. Barlogie B and Gahrton G: *Bone marrow transplantation in multiple myeloma,* Bone Marrow Transplant 7:71, 1991.
4. Belec RH: *Quality of life: Perceptions of long-term survivors of bone marrow transplantation,* Oncol Nurs Forum 19:31, 1992.

5.   Benisinger WI and Berenson RJ: *Peripheral blood and positive selection of marrow as a source of stem cells for transplantation,* Prog Clin Biol Res 337:93, 1990.
6.   *BMT Newsletter, Peripheral stem cell transplants,* BMT Newsletter, 11:1, 1992.
7.   Chielens D and Herrick E: *Recipients of bone marrow transplants: Making a smooth transition to an ambulatory care setting,* Oncol Nurs Forum 17:857, 1990.
8.   Deeg HJ: *Delayed complications of marrow transplantation,* Marrow Transplant Rev 2:10, 1992.
9.   Ersek M: *The process of maintaining hope in adults undergoing bone marrow transplantation for leukemia,* Oncol Nurs Forum 19:883, 1992.
10.   Gale RP, Armitage JO, and Dicke KA: *Autotransplants: Now and in the future,* Bone Marrow Transplant 7:153, 1991.
11.   Gaston-Johansson F, Franco T, and Zimmerman L: *Pain and psychological distress in patients undergoing autologous bone marrow transplantation,* Oncol Nurs Forum, 19:41, 1992.
12.   Gorin NC: *Autologous bone marrow transplantation in hematological malignancies,* Am J Clin Oncol 14(Suppl 1):S5, 1991.
13.   Kessinger A: *Autologous peripheral stem cell transplantation,* Marrow Transplant Rev 25, 1992.
14.   Klob HJ and Bender-Gotze CH: *Late complications after allogeneic bone marrow transplantation for leukemia,* Bone Marrow Transplant 6:61, 1990.
15.   Marks DI and Goldman JM: *Bone marrow transplantation in chronic myelogenous leukemia,* Marrow Transplant Rev 2:17, 1992.
16.   McGlave P: *Bone marrow transplants in chronic myelogenous leukemia: An overview of determinants of survival,* Semin Hematol 27:23, 1990.
17.   McMillan A and Goldstone A: *What is the value of autologous bone marrow transplantation in the treatment of relapsed or resistant Hodgkin's disease?* Leuk Res 15:237, 1991.
18.   Moss TJ: *Bone marrow transplantation for solid tumors in pediatrics,* Cancer Treat Res 50:279, 1990.
19.   Rabinowe SN and others: *The impact of myeloid growth*

factors on engraftment following autologous bone mar-row transplantation for malignant lymphoma, Semin Hematol 28(Suppl 2):6, 1991.

20. Seeger RC and Reynolds CP: *Treatment of high-risk solid tumors of childhood with intensive therapy and autologous bone marrow transplantation,* Ped Clin North Am 38:393, 1991.

21. Sullivan KM: *Prevention and treatment of chronic graft-versus-host disease,* Marrow Transplant Rev 2:8, 1992.

22. Ulich TR and others: *Acute and subacute hematologic effects of multi-colony stimulating factor in combination with granulocyte colony stimulating factor in vivo,* Blood 75:48, 1990.

23. Vitale V, Barra S and Frazone P: *Total body irradiation in the conditioning regimen for hematological malignancies,* Bone Marrow Transplant 8(Suppl 1):28, 1991.

24. Volker DL: *Clinical characteristics of cytomegalovirus infection,* Nursing Acumen 3:1, 1992.

25. Whedon MB, editor: *Bone marrow transplantation principles, practice and nursing insights,* Boston 1991, Jones and Bartlett.

Cancer
Clinical
Trials

25

Historical Perspective of Clinical Trials

Oncology as a medical and nursing specialty has grown rapidly over the past 20 years. The efforts of a nation-wide network of physicians and nurses performing clinical trials resulted in improved surgical outcomes, new chemotherapy agents, less toxic radiation therapy, and the testing of numerous biologic agents and growth hormones. The United States federal government founded the National Institutes of Health (NIH) in 1887. The purpose of the NIH is to support research in the cause, diagnosis, prevention, and cure of human disease. As one of the largest biomedical research facilities in the world, the NIH is part of the U.S. Department of Health and Human Services.

In 1937, Congress unanimously passed the National Cancer Institute Act, which appropriated $700,000 to establish the National Cancer Institute (NCI), now the largest of the 12 NIH institutes. The NCI underwent numerous reorganization and expansions over the next decades. The motivated efforts of a public and private campaign ultimately resulted in the signing of the National Cancer Act in 1971. This created a national cancer program administered by the NCI with its director appointed by and reporting to the president of the United States. Increased power and funding created new opportunities for physicians, improving the quality and increasing the accessibility of cancer care for patients across the country.[5,20] The following programs, initiated by the NCI since 1971, increased the number of cancer specialists and organized a structure to coordinate national research and to translate research advances into clinical practice.

Oncology Training Programs

The NCI funded fellowship programs in medical oncology and radiotherapy. There were 100 medical oncologists in the 1960s; now there are more than 4,000.

Comprehensive Cancer Centers

Designation as a comprehensive cancer center requires meeting eight criteria established by the NCI. These include basic research, mechanisms for technology transfer, clinical research, program of high priority clinical trials, cancer prevention and control research, research training and continuing education programs, cancer information services, and community service and outreach activities.

Cooperative Research Groups

Cooperative research groups consist of researchers who jointly develop and conduct cancer treatment clinical trials in a multi-institutional setting.[5] These groups are funded by the National Cancer Institute through cooperative agreements (Box 25-1).

The goals of cooperative group research are:

- To improve survival and quality of life for cancer patients
- To conduct basic scientific research on cancer biology, pathology, epidemiology, and supportive care
- To serve as a research base for the conduct of cancer control research
- To conduct oncology nursing research[11,19,20]

Community-Based Research Programs

Cooperative Group Outreach Program

The program consists of individual community oncologists, surgeons, or radiation therapists contracting with a member institution of a cooperative group to register patients on research protocols.

Community Clinical Oncology Program

The community clinical oncology program institutions are groups of community-based physicians linked to cooperative groups and cancer centers that serve as their research bases.[5]

Box 25-1

NCI-Funded Cooperative Research Groups

Brain Tumor Cooperative Group (BTCG)
Cancer and Leukemia Group B (CALGB)
Children's Cancer Study Group (CCSG)
Eastern Cooperative Oncology Group (ECOG)
European Organization for Research and Treatment of Cancer
(EORTC)
Gynecological Oncology Group (GOG)
Intergroup Rhabdomyosarcoma Study (IRS)
National Surgical Adjuvant Project for Breast and Bowel
Cancers (NSABP)
National Wilms' Tumor Study (NWTS)
North Central Cancer Treatment Group (NCCTG)
Pediatric Oncology Group (POG)
Radiation Therapy Oncology Group (RTOG)
Southwest Oncology Group (SWOG)

Cancer Control

Cancer control research is implemented through the cooperative group mechanism. Each cooperative group has a standing cancer control committee composed of interested oncology nurses, physicians, epidemiologists, and statisticians.[15,27]

Minority-Based CCOPS

Minority-based CCOPs accrue patients on both treatment and cancer control studies. These are located in areas that serve ethnic minorities and poor populations.

Drug Development

The NCI is the largest, single sponsor of studies using antineoplastic agents. More than 100 such agents are currently in clinical testing and even larger numbers are in preclinical testing. New drugs are also being developed by pharmaceutical companies. The drug development process encompasses drug identification, screening, formulation and production, toxicity testing, new drug application and approval by the FDA.[5,13,14,18,24]

Cancer Protocols

A protocol is a formal document written to clearly describe the proposed experiment. It provides the rationale for the proposed study, the study objectives or questions to be answered, and a concise description of the treatment involved. The protocol is written by the principal investigator and must be approved by the study sponsor prior to distribution to participating investigators. It is then followed by everyone involved in the study—physicians, nurses, data managers, pharmacists, study sponsor, and statisticians.

Ethical Issues/Regulations

Institutional Review Boards

To protect human subjects from research abuses, the Department of Health and Human Services (DHHS) requires all federally-funded institutions to have institutional review boards. The Office for Protection from Research Risks (OPRR) is the administrative subdivision of DHHS that negotiates assurances of compliance with individual institutions.

The institutional review board is composed of at least five members with professional competence, experience, and qualification. The board should include both men and women and should represent a variety of backgrounds, races, and cultural considerations. At least one member should be a nonmedical professional and one person must have no direct affiliation with the institution performing the research.[2,6,8]

Informed Consent

Informed consent is defined as "the knowing consent of an individual or his legally authorized representative so situated as to be able to exercise free power of choice without inducement or any element of force, fraud, deceit, or any other form of constraint or coercion." The patient must be allowed to ask questions, and the physician must verify that the patient has understood what has been said.[6,21,26]

Required Elements

- Statement of research, its purpose, expected duration of participation, description of procedures including identification of any experimental procedures.
- Description of risks and benefits of the study treatment.
- Disclosure of alternative procedures or treatments that may be advantageous to the subject.
- Description of confidentiality; disclosure of possibility of FDA inspection.
- Explanation as to whether compensation and medical treatments are available if injury occurs.
- Whom to contact about research, patient's rights, and research-related injury.
- Instruction that participation is voluntary and results in no penalty or loss of benefits to which the subject is otherwise entitled.

The following factors assist in the process of informing the patient:

- Allow the patient to take the consent form home to read before making a decision.
- Write down treatment information.
- Draw a diagram of randomization and treatment schedule.
- Provide "What Are Clinical Trials All About" pamphlet from the NCI.
- Encourage the patient to call the NCI hotline (1-800-4-CANCER) for information regarding disease and treatment.
- Show audiovisual information about chemotherapy and side effects.
- Assess the patient's anxiety level and integration of new information.
- Question the patient to determine whether he or she understands the treatment.
- Continue to review and reinforce information throughout treatment.

Phases of Clinical Research

Phase I

The purpose of a phase I trial is to determine the maximum tolerated dose (MTD) in humans, to determine the most effective schedule of administration, and to identify and quantify toxic effects in normal organ systems. Phase I trials are usually performed in single institutions so the data can be monitored very closely by the study sponsor. Data is submitted biweekly and study summaries are required every 6 months to comply with FDA regulations. The first occurrence of any toxic reaction is reported by telephone to the Cancer Therapy and Evaluation Program for NCI-sponsored drugs, for rapid information dissemination to other investigators using the agent.[7]

Phase II

Phase II evaluation of a new anticancer drug is designed to determine whether or not the compound has objective antitumor activity in a variety of cancers. Attention is focused on the types of tumors that respond and the dose-response relationship. Depending on the drug and disease under study, previous treatment with chemotherapy and/or other treatment modalities may or may not be allowed. Adequate hematologic, hepatic, renal, and cardiac parameters are specified by the protocol. Life expectancy of at least 8 weeks is required and patients must be capable of partial self-care to be eligible for most phase II trials. The phase II study is a plan to ensure that adequate numbers of patients with the greatest probability of benefit are treated with the optimal dose and schedule of the drug. The recommended dose and schedule from phase I are tested in a variety of tumor types.[3,24]

Phase III

A phase III trial establishes the value of the new treatment relative to standard treatments by a randomized or comparative study. Eligibility for a phase III trial is similar to phase II in that patients must have a histologically confirmed disease that is bidimensionally measurable, have adequate major organ function, and be capable of performing at least partial self-care. Patients in phase III trials have received little or no previous therapy.

Phase III trials are large studies that involve hundreds of patients and multiple institutions. These trials are often randomized, meaning that the patient is arbitrarily assigned to one of two or more possible treatments. Neither the physician nor patient knows which treatment will be assigned until after informed consent is given and the registration is completed. The purpose of randomization is to remove potential biases in allocating patients to each treatment so that similar numbers of "like" patients receive each treatment.[24,25]

Ineffective Cancer Therapies

The American Cancer Society defines unproven cancer therapies as "those diagnostic tests or therapeutic modalities which are promoted for cancer prevention, diagnosis, or treatment and which are, on the basis of careful review by scientists and/or clinicians, not deemed proven or recommended for current use."[1] Furthermore, The American Society of Clinical Oncology's Subcommittee on Unorthodox Therapies states that the term *quackery* implies a knowing intent to misrepresent, whereas belief based on inadequate knowledge may be the underlying promotional incentive rather than the deliberate intent to defraud.[13,17,22]

Recognizing Ineffective Cancer Therapy

The American Society of Clinical Oncologists' Subcommittee on Unorthodox Therapies published its paper "Ineffective Cancer Therapy: A Guide for the Layperson" in 1983. The committee identified 10 ways to recognize ineffective therapy:

- Is the treatment based on an unproven theory?
- Is there a need for special nutritional support when the remedy is used?
- Is there a claim made for harmless, painless, nontoxic treatment?
- Are claims published frequently in the mass media?
- Are claims of benefit the result of the power of suggestion?
- Are the major promoters recognized experts in cancer treatment?
- Do the promoters back up their claims with controlled studies?
- Is there a claim that only specially trained physicians can produce results with their drug, or is the formula a secret?
- Do the promoters attack the medical and scientific establishments?
- Is there a demand for "freedom of choice" regarding drugs?

Types of Ineffective Therapy

More than 100 types of ineffective therapy have been or are available. Examples include Koch antitoxin therapy, Hoxsey method, Krebiozen, Laetrile, DMSO (Dimethylsulfoxide), biologic products, metabolic therapies (macrobiotic diet), psychologic/spiritual/mystical techniques and immunologic therapy. Patient motivations for the use of ineffective therapy are fear, family pressure, disease recurrence, progression and mistrust of the medical system. The American Cancer Society and Food and Drug Administration have files on unproven treatments accessible to both professionals and lay persons.

Nursing Management

Nursing Diagnoses

- *Knowledge deficit related to disease pathology and new diagnosis*
- *Knowledge deficit related to clinical trials process, randomization process, informed consent process*
- *Knowledge deficit related to experimental chemotherapy and side effects*
- *Anxiety related to new diagnosis or disease progression*
- *Anxiety related to treatment with experimental agent or procedure*
- *Coping, ineffective; potential for related to new diagnosis or change in prognosis and new treatment*

Nursing Interventions in Phase I, II, and III Clinical Trials

Phase I

- Assess the adequacy of informed consent and notify the physician if the patient doesn't fully understand the risk-benefit relationship
- Know the mechanism of drug action, route of administration, absorption, metabolism, and excretion of drug
- Know results of animal toxicology studies to anticipate human toxicities

- Assess for, evaluate, and document unexpected adverse drug reactions
- Provide nursing care to minimize disease and treatment-related morbidity
- Understand disease process to distinguish between disease-related and treatment-related effects
- Carefully document objective and subjective response to treatment
- Document acute, chronic, delayed, and cumulative side effects[8,10,12]
- Perform and document results of pharmacokinetic studies
- Participate in decisions concerning dose escalation, schedule manipulation, and determination of optimal dose[16,19]

Phase II

- Know results of phase I drug studies:
  Side effects
  Dose-limiting toxicities
  Method of administration
  Drug metabolism and escretion
- Provide patient education and support:
  Treatment plan
  Expected side effects
  Symptom management
  Disease process

Phase III

- Ensure drug doses are calculated correctly
- Document toxicities and grade correctly
- Modify doses correctly and consistently
- Evaluate tumor measurements appropriately for response determination
- Ensure the patient's understanding of randomization process
- Assess for new and unexpected side effects of the drug
- Assess performance status
- Administer "Quality of Life" assessment tools
- Follow-up after treatment completion:
  Teach the patient the importance of follow-up visits even years after treatment is completed

Report data on survival and late effects until the patient dies

Develop systems to maintain contact with patients who have moved or changed physicians

Encourage patients to return to a healthful lifestyle in light of knowing cancer may recur

Teach recommendations for screening and early detection appropriate to age

Counsel other family members of patients at high risk for developing cancer[21,23]

Geriatric Considerations

■ Cancer Clinical Trials and Cancer Control Research have established eligibility criteria for patient accrual; refer to age-related guidelines.

■ Consider sensory and neuromuscular deficits (e.g., visual, hearing, mobility) in selection of educational materials.

■ Review current prescription and over-the-counter medication guidelines that may interact with scheduled drugs/treatments.

■ Additional limitations such as fixed-income transportation, caregiver resources, and age-related functional status will require assessment and intervention strategies.[10,16]

Bibliography

1. AMA Council on Scientific Affairs: *Viability of cancer clinical research: patient accrual, coverage, and reimbursement*, J Natl Cancer Inst 83(4):254, 1991.

2. Belmont Report: *Ethical principles and guidelines for the protections of human subjects of research*, DHEW Publication No. (05)-78-0012, Washington DC, 1978, US Government Printing Office.

3. *The Cancer Letter,* 17(40):6, October 18, 1991.

4. Cassidy J and Macfarlane DK: *The role of the research nurse in clinical cancer research*, Cancer Nurs 14(3):124, 1991.

5. Cheson BD: *Clinical trials programs*, Semin Oncol Nurs 7(4):235, 1991.

6. Department of Health and Human Services: *Protection of human subjects: informed consent.* Washington DC, Federal Register, January 27, 1981, Part IX.

7. DeVita VT: Principles of chemotherapy. In DeVita VT, Hellman S, and Roseberg SA, editors: *Cancer principles and practice of oncology*, ed 4, Philadelphia, 1993, JB Lippincott.

8. Donocan CT: Ethics in cancer nursing practice. In Groenwald S and others, editors: *Cancer nursing: practice and principles*, ed 2, Boston, 1991, Jones and Bartlett.

9. Durant J: *Current status of clinical trials*, Cancer 65(suppl):2371, 1990.

10. Engelking C: *Clinical trials: impact evaluation and implementation considerations.* Semin Oncol Nurs 8(2):148, 1992.

11. Friedman MA: *Patient accrual to clinical trials*, Cancer Treat Rep 71:557, 1987.

12. Galassi A: New antineoplastic agents. In Hubbard SM, Greene PE, and Knobf MT, editors: *Current issues in cancer nursing practice*. Philadelphia, 1991, JB Lippincott.

13. General Accounting Office: *Off label drugs: initial results of a national survey.* Washington, DC, US General Accounting Office, (GAO/PEDM-91-12BR), 1991.

14. *Grant guidelines for cancer control: areas of programmatic interest*, US Department of Health and Human Services.

15. Greenwald P, Cullen JW, and Weed D: *Cancer prevention and control,* Semin Oncol 17(4):383-390, 1990.

16. Guy JL: New challenges for nurses in clinical trials, Semin Oncol Nurs 7(4):297-303, 1991.

17. Henney JE: Unproven methods of cancer treatment. In DeVita VT, Hellman S, and Rosenberg SA, editors: *Cancer principles and practice of oncology*, ed 4, Philadelphia, 1993, JB Lippincott.

18. Investigators' Handbook, *Cancer Therapy Evaluation Program, Division of Cancer Treatment*, National Cancer Institute, Bethesda, MD, 1986.

19. Jenkins J and Curt G: Implementation of clinical trials, In Baird SB, McCorkle R, and Grant M: *Cancer nursing: a comprehensive textbook*, Philadelphia, 1991, WB Saunders.

20. Jenkins J and Hubbard S: *History of clinical trials*, Semin Oncol Nurs 7(4):228, 1991.

21. Kelly ME: Informed consent. In Northrup CE and Kelly ME, editors: *Legal issues in nursing*, St Louis, 1987, Mosby.

22. Kessler DA: *The regulation of investigational agents*, N Engl J Med 320(5):281, 1989.

23. McEvoy MD, Cannon L, and MacDermot ML: *The professional role for nurses in clinical trials*, Semin Oncol Nurs 7(4):268, 1991.

24. Melink TJ and Whitacre MY: *Planning and implementing clinical trials*, Semin Concol Nurse 7(4):243, 1991.

25. *Update*, National Cancer Institute, October 1993, Bethesda, MD.

26. Varricchio CG and Jassak PF: *Informed consent: an overview*, Semin Oncol Nurs 5(2):95, 1989.

27. Winn R: *From opera to chemoprevention*. Oncol Issues 7(2):13, 1992.

Section IV

Cancer Care
Supportive
Therapies

Home Care and Alternative Care Settings

26

The advent of rising health care costs and efforts to contain these costs have resulted in the increased emphasis upon home care and alternative care settings. It is essential that the health care professional accurately assess and identify the specific needs of the client and, if available, the family's ability to take on the caregiving role. Identification of the presence or absence of adequate caregiving supports is central to determining if home care or alternative care settings are appropriate. The discharge planning process is an organized systematic approach commonly utilized in the acute care setting to facilitate the transition from the hospital and/or clinic to home.[4,14]

The Discharge Planning Process

The Assessment

The nurse can effectively assess, identify, and respond to new patient posthospitalization/postclinic visit needs as these needs surface, if the nurse is continuously cognizant of the importance of discharge planning. This process necessitates not only thorough assessment and evaluation, but also extensive planning and coordination.

The screening process should be followed by (1) the client interview, (2) identification of the specific posthospitalization or postclinic problems or needs, and (3) development of a plan for solving client problems or needs.[3,4,13]

The Client Interview

1.   Introduction (if necessary).
2.   Establish the relationship of the client to: (a) spouse, (b) family, including children, (c) neighbors, (d) church, and (e) senior citizen support activities.
3.   Establish how the client's illness has affected his or her role and function in the family with special attention to: (a) financial support, (b) shopping, (c) meal preparation, (d) transportation, and (e) living arrangements.
4.   Determine the client's prehospital daily routine.
5.   Assess the client's learning and comprehension ability.
6.   Assess the client's interest in discharge planning services.[13]

Identification of Post-Hospital Problems and Needs

1.   Inadequate or no support system.
2.   Inadequate financial resources.
3.   Poor environmental conditions.
4.   Inability to carry out treatment and medication regimen.
5.   Inability to carry out activities of daily living.
6.   Poor socialization.
7.   Potential problems (i.e., related to disease progression or treatment).

Planning

Development of a Plan for Solving Client Problem Needs

Identify the client's problems or needs using a collaborative process, involve the client, family or significant others, and health care professional. Address the following items to assist the client and family in the decision making process:[3,7,12]

1.   Assist client or family to identify the specific problem(s).
2.   Assist client or family to set priorities among the problems.
3.   Assist the client or family to identify the services or resources needed.
4.   Interpret services of the available resources of the client or family (extended care facility, skilled care nursing setting, home care agency).

5. Establish financial status.
6. Work out details of selected plan with client or family.

Settings For Care

In addition to the hospital, other settings for care include the home and extended care facilities.

Extended Care

There are four basic types of extended care facilities, which vary according to the amount and type of care needed by the client. These facilities include:

1. Skilled care facilities provide around-the-clock skilled nursing care and observation.
2. Intermediate care facilities provide around-the-clock basic nursing care for clients that are medically stable but unable to care for themselves.
3. Adult foster or sheltered care facilities are for individuals that require a protective living arrangement that provides general supervision and assistance with bathing, dressing, meals, and other personal needs.
4. Residential care facilities are for individuals that no longer wish to live alone or have no place to live and provide similar services as a sheltered care facility.[4,5,13]

Home Care

There are two types of home care services available to health care consumers: traditional home care and high-technology home care. Traditional home care services generally provide skilled nursing care including patient assessment and intervention, patient and family education; rehabilitative services such as physical, occupational, and speech and language therapies; social work intervention and home health aide support.[7,9,14]

High-technology home care for patients with cancer generally refers to the home management of infusional therapies such as: antifungal, antibiotic, and hydration therapy, hemotherapy, venous access and pain management, and TPN.

Patients and their families must be properly screened prior to initiating such therapies in the home setting to ensure that the treatment is both safe and efficacious.

Geriatric Considerations

Ill elderly people generally want to be home among family and familiar surroundings. Family members feel inadequate in their abilities to properly care for their parent/spouse and may be reluctant to bring them home. It is important that the nurse provide an opportunity for family members to discuss their fears, feelings, and concerns. Consideration should be also given to how this illness is affecting the family's ability to meet their continuing needs.[5,6,10,11]

The following set of questions enable the nurse to gain a more thorough awareness of the family's needs and coping abilities:

Criteria for patient screening, home infusion therapy

1. The patient must want to receive therapy at home.
2. The patient must be medically stable for home treatment.
3. The patient should have a venous access device in place or adequate venous access via the peripheral route (or a plan must exist should peripheral access become exhausted).
4. The patient or caregiver must be able to care for the central line and demonstrate proficiency and competency in maintaining the access device.
5. The patient or caregiver must be knowledgeable of the therapy: this knowledge includes:
   a. Name of drug(s)—both infusional and adjunct medications
   b. Dosage(s)
   c. Potential side effects
   d. Actions to take to prevent or minimize side effects
   e. Potential adverse reactions to medication
   f. Storage of drug(s)
6. The patient or caregiver must be knowledgeable and proficient in the functioning of the infusion pump as follows:
   a. Operation of the pump
   b. Using the alarm system
   c. How to check if the pump is working
   d. Troubleshooting the pump
7. The patient's home environment must be conducive to home care (e.g., physical layout, telephone access, support person[s], running water, electricity).
8. The patient must have the financial means to pay for home treatment (e.g., insurance, private pay).
9. The patient or caregiver must have an emergency 24-hour number to call for problems (e.g., clinic RN, doctor's office, home-care agency).

Figure 26-1. *Criteria for patient screening, home infusion therapy.* (From Maloney CH and Preston F: Oncol Nurs Forum 19(1):77, 1992)

Needs
1. What difficulties is the family experiencing with the medical treatment?
2. What are the sources of financial strain from direct and indirect costs related to the illness?
3. What changes are required in day-to-day living activities for the family?
4. What impact has the illness or its management had on the ability to meet their continuing needs?

Coping Strategies
1. What strategies does the family employ to help maintain a sense of normalcy in family life?
2. Who are identified supportive people or groups and what do they provide for the family?
3. What activities do the family members use to enhance positive coping strategies?

Hospice

Hospice is a philosphy of care that provides high quality, comprehensive care to persons with a terminal disease and their families. The setting for this care is usually in the home, however, hospitalization is available during acute medical crisis (uncontrolled pain, nausea, and vomiting), impending death, or to give the family a short (2 to 5 days) respite. The goal of hospice is to enhance the quality of life for the patient who is dying and for the surviving family members.[11]

Private Duty

There are many home care organizations that provide supplemental home care services on a fee for service basis (nursing housekeepers, nursing aides, companions).

Agencies that provide these services are required by law to be licensed and can be found in your local yellow pages.

Reimbursement Issues

Most health care insurances cover home care services. All require that the service is ordered by a physician and a medical plan of care is signed by the physician. Patients must also be *homebound,* unable to leave home without assistance of others and assistive devices. In addition, patients must also need skilled nursing care and have a medical condition that warrants ongoing assessment and evaluation.[3,14]

Patient and Family Teaching

The education process includes the steps of assessing, planning, implementing, and evaluating. The primary learner(s) in the family must be identified and his or her learning needs assessed. Following this assessment, a mutually acceptable plan to meet the identified educational needs is developed by nurse/teacher and client/learner. Appropriate teaching strategies are used to implement the plan, and it is mutually evaluated with the evaluation serving as a basis for further decision. Addressing the educational wants and needs of the family caregiver is of top priority if the patient is to receive proper care and be able to remain in the comforts of his home. Tools for assessment and planning may include Figures 26-2.[1,2,8,10,13]

Discharge Instructions

To help facilitate the transition to the home setting and ensure continuity of care and medical follow-up, it is very important to clearly convey specific discharge instructions to the patient and/or family members at the time of discharge. It is advisable to have specific written instructions to review and give the patient and family at the time of discharge.[4,13]

Identifying the needs of home givers of patients with cancer

Specifics related to illness	Emotional concerns
Specifics related to treatment and effects	Support groups/resources
Exercise/activity and rest	Family concerns
Safety	Rehabilitation
Financial issues	Adaptive techniques
Insurance issues	Returning to work
Social interactions	Long-term planning
Others: _____	

Figure 26-2. Sample topics for patients and families. (From Hileman JW: *Identifying the needs of home care givers of patients with cancer*, Oncol Nurs Forum 19(5):771, 1992)

Follow-up Appointments

There are several things that the nurse can do to help facilitate keeping follow-up appointments.

It is important to ask the patient or family member if transportation is a problem. The American Cancer Society and the American Red Cross are national organizations that have local offices that provide transportation to and from medical facilities at no charge or minimal cost. Many private companies provide transportation services for the disabled for a fee. Patients need to know what assistance is available when they arrive for their follow-up appointment. If a wheelchair is needed, how do they arrange to have one available? Advise patients and their families to bring with them the medications that they may need to take while still at the clinic. In particular, be sure to tell patients to bring any prn medications, especially pain medications. Tell patients and their families what to expect at the follow-up appointment, especially if the patient is going to receive a treatment or particular diagnostic test for the first time.

Follow-up Phone Call

A follow-up phone call to patients and/or their families should be made within 24 to 48 hours after discharge.

Ask family the following questions:
1. How are things going since you came home?
2. Have any problems occurred?
3. Do you have any questions that I can answer for you?

Ask specific questions related to the patient's illness and treatment plan to ensure accurate assessment of home situation. If you determine other resources are needed, refer the patient/family to see the physician and/or request from the physician a home care referral.

Durable Medical and Adaptive Equipment

Durable medical equipment (DME) includes hospital beds, wheelchairs, and assisting devices. Essential equipment such as hospital beds, wheelchairs, and bedside commodes should be in the home at the time of discharge. Most insurances provide coverage for some DME; however, a physician's order is usually required. DME companies in your community can be found in your local yellow pages.

Community Resources

There are many national and local community resources available to cancer patients and their families. The types of resources available range from personal services, informational services, social services, and support services. A phone call to the Cancer Information Service (1-800-4-CANCER) and the local American Cancer Society chapter is a good starting point when first attempting to identify resources available in your community.

Local community services often include agencies that provide and/or assist with: chore or housekeeping services, adult day care, companion, nutrition, and transportation services, and financial issues.

Nursing Management

Nursing Diagnosis

Impaired Home Maintenance Management related to: (specify)
- *Inability to perform household activities secondary to side effects of chemotherapy*
- *Inability to perform household activities secondary to disease progression*

Interventions

Assess for causative or contributing factors
    Lack of knowledge
    Insufficient funds
    Lack of necessary equipment or aids
    Inability to perform household activities
    Impaired cognitive and emotional functioning
    Impaired emotional functioning
Reduce or eliminate causative or contributing factors if possible
Lack of knowledge for home care
    Determine with the patient and family the information needed to be taught and learned:
    Monitoring skills needed
    Medication administration
    Treatment procedures
    Equipment use/maintenance

      Safety issues (e.g., environmental)

      Community resources

      Follow-up care

   Initiate the teaching and give detailed written instructions

   Refer to a community nursing (home care) agency for follow-up

Lack of necessary equipment or aids

   Determine the type of equipment needed, considering availability, cost, and durability

   Seek assistance from agencies that rent or loan supplies:

      Teach the care and maintenance of supplies that increase length of use

      Consider adapting equipment to reduce cost

Insufficient funds

   Consult with social service department for assistance

   Consult with service organizations for assistance

Inability to perform household activities

   Determine the type of assistance needed and assist the individual with resources

Impaired mental processes

   Assess the ability of the individual to safely maintain a household

   Initiate appropriate referrals

Impaired emotional functioning

   Assess the severity of the dysfunction

   Initiate appropriate referrals

Provide anticipatory guidance

Discuss the implications of caring for a chronically ill family member

      Amount of time involved

      Effects on other role responsibilities (spouse, children, job)

      Physical requirements (lifting)

Share alternatives to reduce strain and fatigue of caretaking responsibilities

      Acquire relief from responsibilites at least twice a week for at least 3 hours (sitter, neighbors, relatives)

      Enlist the aid of others to meet some of the needs of the ill person (hairdresser, transporting to physician's office)

Plan to utilize at least 1 hour a day as leisure time (after ill person is asleep)

Maintain contacts with friends and relatives even if only by phone; let friends know that you do use sitters so they can include you in some social activities

Allow the caretaker opportunities to share problems and feelings

Bibliography

1. Hileman JW, Lackey NR, and Hassanein RS: *Identifying the needs of home caregivers of patients with cancer*, Oncol Nurs Forum 19(5):771, 1992.

2. Hiromoto BM and Dungan J: *Contract learning for self-care activities,* Cancer Nurs 14(3):148, 1991.

3. Johnston and Clark B: *Orientation to home care: Maximizing Medicare reimbursement*, Home Health Care Nurse 8:45, 1990.

4. Kelly K and McClelland E: Discharge planning: home care considerations. In Martinson IM and Widmer A, editors: *Home health care nursing*, Philadelphia, 1989, WB Saunders.

5. Leiby SA and Supe DR: *Does home care lessen hospital readmissions for the elderly?* Home Health Care Nurse 10(1):37, 1992.

6. Magilvy JK and Lakomy JM: *Transitions of older adults to home care,* Home Health Care Serv Quart 12(4):59, 1991.

7. Maloney CH and Preston F: *An overview of home care for patients with cancer,* Oncol Nurs Forum 19(1):75, 1992.

8. Mathis EJ: *Family caregivers want education for their caregiving roles*, Home Health Care Nurse, 10(4):19, 1992.

9. McAbee RR, Grupp K, and Horn B: *Home intravenous therapy: part I—issues.* Home Health Care Serv Quart 12(3):59, 1991.

10. Perry G and Rhoades de Meneses M: *Cancer patients at home: needs and coping styles of primary caregivers*, Home Health Care Nurse 7(6):27, 1989.

11. Sankar A: *Dying at Home: a family guide for caregiving.* Baltimore: The Johns Hopkins University Press, 1992.

12. Sherry D: *Cost effectiveness and home care: myth or reality?* Home Health Care Nurse 10(1):27, 1992.
13. Slevin AP and Roberts AS: *Discharge planning: a tool for decision making,* Nurs Manage 18(12):47, 1987.
14. Smith JB: *Competition and continuity of care in home health nursing,* Home Health Care Nurse 9(1):9, 1992.

Nutrition

27

Cancer and its treatment may affect the nutritional status of the patient in a variety of ways. Besides being subject to metabolic effects, patients are emotionally stressed when nutritional intake is impaired. Because eating is a basic bodily function and often a social activity, inability to eat or difficulty in eating may have a profound physical and psychologic impact on the individual with cancer.[3,16]

Effects of Cancer on Nutritional Status

Systemic Effects

- Anorexia-cachexia
- Vitamin deficiencies: Vitamin A, B, C
- Fluid and electrolyte imbalance
- Hypercalcemia
- Syndrome of inappropriate secretion of antidiuretic hormone
- Immunocompetence

Local Effects

- Impaired ingestion (chewing, swallowing, obstruction, distention, and peristalsis)
- Pain
- Bowel fistula
- Malabsorption

Nutritional Consequences of Cancer Treatment

Effects of Various Modes of Treatment

Surgical alterations in any area of the alimentary tract from the mouth to the anus may cause temporary or occasionally permanent alterations in nutritional intake or absorptive capabilities.

- Partial or total gastrectomy
- Gastrojejunostomy
- Malabsorption of fat

Radiation therapy may affect the normal tissues surrounding the treatment areas. Patients with cancer of the head and neck have both acute and chronic symptoms. The normal tissues of the salivary gland, oral mucosa, muscle, and occasionally bone may be affected.

- Taste changes
- Xerostomia
- Pain
- Difficulty swallowing

Irradiation of the small intestine produces vomiting, anorexia, diarrhea, and gastric distention.

Chemotherapy may produce side effects that impair the patient's nutritional status. Chemotherapy causes nutritional deficiencies by promoting anorexia, stomatitis, alimentary tract disturbances, taste alterations, nausea, vomiting, aversions to specific foods, anorexia, and diarrhea.[7,8,10,12,24]

Nutritional Assessment

A nutritional assessment can screen for potential or existing problems in nutritional status, provide a data base for individuals at high risk, and determine response to treatment or dietary interventions; particular attention should be given to the elderly patient.[18] See box 27-1.

Box 27-1

Components of Nutritional Assessment

Nursing history
Date diagnosed
Type of cancer
Type and duration of therapy
Concurrent medications
Concomitant medical conditions
Surgical procedures
Side effects of therapy
Allergies

Biochemical measurements
Evaluation of nutrient
    composition
Hemoglobin, hematocrit
Serum transferrin
Total lymphocyte count
Creatinine
Urine urea nitrogen
Creatinine-height index
Skin testing

Anthropometric data
Height
Weight
Weight change over time
Triceps skin fold thickness
Midarm muscle circumference
Subscapular skin fold thickness

Psychosocial assessment
Home environment
Family support
Coping abilities
Self-image
Perceptions of
    role of nutrition
Cultural, religious
    considerations

Dietary evaluation
24-hour recall of intake
Food preferences
Food allergies
Use of vitamin
    supplements
Changes in diet or eating
    on life-style patterns
Observation of intake
Serum albumin

Physical assessment
General overall appearance
Hair texture
Skin turgor and integrity
Condition of mouth and
    gums
Performance status
Alterations in elimination,
    comfort

Nutritional Support

Oral Nutrition

Supplemental oral nutrition may range from simple measures such as adding gravies and sauces to more complex interventions. The degree of intervention is based on the severity of nutritional deficiency.

- Supplemental oral nutrition (Isocal, polycose, vivonex)
- Foods high in protein: cheese, fish, poultry, gravies, peanut butter, milk-shakes, pre-packaged puddings
- Alternative flavorings (vanilla)
- Cold foods
- Small frequent feedings

Enteral Nutrition

Assessment of nutritional status is essential for determining which patients are candidates for tube feedings. Generally, patients with functioning GI tracts who are unable to ingest adequate nutrients to meet their metabolic demands are candidates for tube feedings. Indications include numerous cancer diagnoses and related disorders.

Tube feedings can be administered by the nasogastric, nasoduodenal, nasojejunal, esophagostomy, gastrostomy, and jejunostomy routes. Obtain daily weights and serum proteins every 7 to 10 days while the patient is receiving enteral nutrition.[2,4,19]

ADMINISTRATION OF TUBE FEEDING.
The size of the tube selected for enteral feedings should be the smallest through which the food will flow. The volume and concentration of nutriment delivered by tube feeding should meet the individual's specific needs. Isotonic formulas are more easily tolerated than hypertonic formulas and do not require the same degree of dilution. The duodenum and jejunum are more sensitive than the stomach to both volume and osmolality. Therefore, duodenal or jejunal feeding should be low in osmolality and delivered by continuous drip or pump.

Bolus feedings of enteral formulas are administered usually at 250 to 400 mL over a few minutes, five to eight times daily. Patients who are intolerant of bolus feedings may have nausea, diarrhea, aspiration, abdominal distention, and cramps.[30] Gravity feedings may be intermittent or continuous. Feedings to the distal duodenum or jejunum should be given by continuous pump infusion to prevent dumping syndrome. Continuous feedings may be given during the night over 10 to 12 hours or around the clock. They should be started at 50 mL or less and advanced only if the patient shows no diarrhea, cramping, or other signs of intolerance. When the desired rate has been reached, the strength can be increased as tolerated.

Selection of equipment and supplies is based on the formula to be given, rate and frequency of feedings, tube site, and other considerations, including the care giver's preference. To prevent bacterial contamination when a large container is used, the amount of formula in the bag should approximate that which can be given over 8 hours.

New formula should not be added to formula that has already been hanging for 8 hours at room temperature. The container and tubing should be rinsed well before adding formula. With very careful cleaning, a feeding bag may be used for two days; however, discarding the bag after 24 hours is recommended.[13] An enteral pump is usually indicated if the patient is being fed by the small intestine, if the feedings are given continually around the clock, or if the desired rate is less than 200 mL per hour.[11,13,19,22,23]

Complications of Tube Feeding

Complications may be mechanical and metabolic and may affect the gastrointestinal and respiratory systems (Table 27-1).

Home Enteral Therapy

Once it is determined that a patient needs enteral therapy and discharge is anticipated, the patient is assessed. A caregiver is selected if the patient is unable to perform self-care. The capabilities of the caregiver are assessed, the home environment is discussed, and the caregiver is trained until he or she can independently care for the tube-fed patient. Home supervised visits may also be conducted, and occasionally tube feedings are initiated in the home. General care of the tube-fed patient at home includes tube care, feeding, and assessment of complications, and goal achievement.[1,17,22,23,32]

Table 27-1 Common Complications of Enteral Nutrition

Complication	Etiology
MECHANICAL	
Nasal irritation and erosion	Use of rigid, large-bore tubes
Esophagitis, pharyngitis	
Tube dislocation	Coughing or pulling on tube, tube migration
Tube occlusion	Kinked tube, inadequate irrigation, formula incompletely crushed, or incompatible medications
GASTROINTESTINAL	
Abdominal distention	Rapid infusion rate, delayed gastric emptying, formula intolerance
Nausea, vomiting	Rapid infusion rate, delayed emptying, formula intolerance, malabsorption, electrolyte imbalance, contaminated formula
Diarrhea	Rapid infusion rate, formula intolerance, malabsorption, contaminated formula
Constipation	Long-term use of low-residue solutions, inadequate fluid intake
RESPIRATORY	
Aspiration pneumonia	Gastric reflux of aspiration (especially with large-bore tubes), improper tube placement, large gastric residuals, patient positioned lower than 30° head elevation.
METABOLIC	
Hyperglycemia	Underlying diabetes, sepsis, stress, intolerance to infusion rate

Continued.

Table 27-1 Cont'd.

Hypokalemia	Concurrent diuretic, insulin, or antibiotic therapy
Hyperkalemia	Metabolic acidosis, renal insufficiency, excessive potassium in formula
Hypernatremia, dehydration	Insufficient water (especially if hyperosmolar, high-protein formulas are used)

Parenteral Nutrition

Total parenteral nutrition (TPN) supplies all of the daily requirements for protein and calories directly into the bloodstream. Parenteral nutrition is indicated for patients who have totally nonfunctioning gastrointestinal tracts, require bowel rest, or are intolerant of enteral therapy. Cancers of the GI tract and related obstructions, radiation enteritis and intractable diarrhea, are also indications for TPN.[1,6,14,15,20,28]

Peripheral Parenteral Nutrition
- Peripheral administration provides limited calories, generally fewer than 2,500 kcal/day, as well as a limited amount of protein, less than 100 grams per day
- Solutions administered peripherally can be very irritating to the vein, especially if dextrose is more than 10%
- Solutions may be stopped quickly; tapering and weaning are not needed
- Peripheral administration is useful for short-term nutritional support

Central Parenteral Nutrition
- Requires central venous access
- Central administration can provide a large amount of calories and protein
- Final dextrose concentration can be as high as 35% and final amino acid concentrations can be more than 5%
- These solutions cannot be discontinued suddenly. Abrupt cessation may induce profound hypoglycemia. Tapering

down the rate and concentration is the most effective method for discontinuation

Components of Parenteral Nutrition

The three main components of total parenteral nutrition (TPN) are glucose, amino acids, and fats. The glucose content of TPN, usually in the form of dextrose 50%, provides both immediate and long-term energy. Amino acids or proteins are provided with or without electrolytes and are usually ordered in concentrations of 5.5% or 8.5%. The lower concentration is indicated for patients with hepatic or renal dysfuntion or failure.

Administration of fats with TPN is required because the TPN solution stimulates the production of insulin, which in turn prevents fat from being metabolized. A fatty acid deficiency may result. Fat is provided through intralipids, usually in a concentration of 10% to 20%, and may be piggybacked or added to the TPN solution. Exact formulations are specific to the patient; they depend on individual requirements, tolerances, body chemistry, and disease processes.

A TPN formula that combines the dextrose, amino acids, and fat emulsion in one container is often called a three-in-one or total nutrient admixture. Eliminating the need for piggybacking lipids allows for a closed system that reduces the risk of infection, minimizes manipulations, and cuts waste. Often three-in-one solutions are ordered for patients receiving TPN at home because they are convenient and easy to administer. If lipids are piggybacked, TPN is generally given two to three times per week.[6]

Administration of Parenteral Nutrition

Total parenteral solutions may be given continuously or by cycling. Cycling is most often used for patients receiving TPN at home during the night because it allows them to be mobile during the day. The disadvantage of cycling TPN is that patients must be able to tolerate a high-volume load. Cyclic TPN may be increased slowly at the start and then tapered at the end of the cycle. Programmable pumps are widely used to prevent or minimize hyperglycemia and hypoglycemia as blood sugars rise and fall. Compact, portable TPN pumps are also available with programmable functions. The portable pump, worn in a backpack-type carrying bag, is best suited for the ambulatory patient.

An assessment of the patient's life-stype, home environment, family and support systems, body image, and perceptions about TPN should be conducted when it is started. During hospitalization frequent assessments are needed to assist in identifying patients who are candidates for TPN at home.

Monitoring the Patient and Complications of Therapy

Daily monitoring of vital signs, weight, and lab values may indicate metabolic changes requiring the adjustment of TPN formula or its rate of administration. The metabolic and technical problems sometimes associated with TPN are numerous. Some are related to the insertion of the central venous access device. Other problems include electrolyte imbalance, infection, and volume overload (Table 27-2).

Home Parenteral Nutrition

Screening patients for home TPN includes assessment of the home environment, availability of a care-giver, learning abilities or disabilities, physical limitations, and motivation to learn procedures. Teaching sessions over several days are best for teaching the complex procedures of administration of home TPN. Provision of a take-home booklet is recommended and return demonstrations performed by the caregiver are often beneficial. Teaching topics include: catheter care, preparation of medication, operation of equipment, assessments of complications, and goal achievement.

Follow-up visits in the home are essential. Although many patients may appear quite competent in the hospital, a home visit assures that procedures are followed appropriately. A home assessment also provides the opportunity to determine whether TPN formulas and supplies are stored correctly and whether infection control measures are observed.[1,5,9,21,30]

Ethical Considerations

Nutritional support of the terminally ill patient with cancer remains controversial. Frequently, family members insist on feeding their loved one. Nurses should advocate for the patient by teaching that loss of appetite often occurs. Nursing interventions should be directed at structural or functional deficits, such as stomatitis, nausea and vomiting, and then managing concurrent but exacerbating symptoms like fatigue and dyspnea. The use of intravenous hydration may be helpful in loosening pulmonary secretion, decreasing gastric secretions, and correcting fluid and electrolyte imbalances in select patients.[2,26,27,29,31]

Nursing Management

The additional nursing interventions listed below can be made depending on the specific alteration in intake or digestive abilities.

Nursing Diagnoses and Suggestions for Dietary Modifications for Common Problems that may Affect Intake

Nutrition, alterations in: less than body requirements related to:

Taste/olfactory changes
Use tart food to stimulate taste buds
Use extra seasoning
Try sauces and flavor additives
Substitute fish and chicken for red meat

Dysphagia
Eat soft or liquid foods
Use sauces and gravies
Eat small meals frequently
If eating is painful, eat bland foods

Dyspepsia
Avoid fatty and spicy foods
Avoid gas-producing foods
Use antacids
Avoid lying down after meals

Anorexia
Vary surroundings
Eat with family and friends
Try new foods and recipes
Use smaller plates

Table 27-2 Common Complications of Parenteral Nutrition

Complication	Etiology
NONMETABOLIC	
Allergy or sensitivity	Sensitivity to either the amino acid solution or the lipid emulsion
Infection	Catheter-related sepsis
Volume overload	Improper pump rate
Catheter placement	Puncture of or injury to nearby organs or vessels
Pneumothorax	
Arterial puncture	
Hematoma	
Thoracic duct puncture	
Brachial plexus injury	
Pulmonary embolism	
METABOLIC	
Hyperglycemia/Hyperosmolarity	Inability to metabolize high glucose concentration of formula
Hypoglycemia	When TPN is abruptly discontinued, high insulin levels cause rebound drop in blood sugar
Vitamin or mineral deficiencies	Administration of formulas lacking sufficient vitamins or micronutrients
Fatty acid deficiencies or overload	Insufficient or excessive administration of lipids
Hyponatremia	Formulas without sufficient sodium content
Hypokalemia, hyperkalemia	Insufficient or excessive potassium content
Hypocalcemia, hypercalcemia	Insufficient or excessive calcium content
Hypomagnesemia	Insufficient magnesium or increased metabolism of magnesium

Eat high-calorie snacks
Drink high-protein shakes
Try hard candy
Use distraction: radio, TV, etc.

Gastrointestinal mucositis
Avoid acidic fruits and juices
Eat cool foods
Use a topical analgesic before eating

Nausea and vomiting
Drink clear liquids and advance diet as tolerated
Drink flat beverages
Avoid sweet, rich, and fatty foods
Try dry foods (toast, crackers)
Try easily digested foods (rice)
Avoid food odors
Eat cool foods
Eat small, frequent meals
Use antiemetics 30 minutes before meals

Elimination, alterations in: related to:

Dumping syndrome
Avoid fatty foods
Avoid concentrated foods
Eat small, frequent meals
Drink liquids 30 minutes before and after meals

Constipation
Drink adequate fluids
Eat high-fiber foods
Exercise regularly
Avoid cheese and concentrated foods

Diarrhea
Drink adequate amounts of fluid
Drink fluids providing electrolytes
Avoid milk products
Avoid fatty, gas-producing foods
Avoid high-fiber foods
Eat high-potassium foods

Bibliography

1. American Society for Parenteral and Enteral Nutrition: *Standards for home nutrition support,* Nutr Clin Pract 7(2):65, 1992.

2. Benya R and Mobarhan S: *Enteral alimentation: administration and complications,* J Am Coll Nutr 10:209, 1991.

3. Brennan MF: Nutritional support. In DeVita VT, Hellman S, and Rosenberg SA, editors: *Cancer: principles and practice of oncology,* ed 4, Philadelphia, 1993, JB Lippencott.

4. Campos AC, Butters M, and Meguid MM: *Home enteral nutrition via gastrostomy in advanced head and neck cancer patients,* Head Neck 12(2):137, 1990.

5. Capka MB and others: *Nursing observations of central venous catheters. The effect on patient outcome,* J Intrav Nurs 14:243, 1991.

6. Chandra RK: *Protein-energy malnutrition and immunological responses,* J Nutr 122(3 suppl):597, 1992.

7. Chen MK, Souba WW, and Copeland EM: *Nutritional support of the surgical oncology patient,* Hematol Oncol Clin North Am 5:125, 1991.

8. Chlebowski RT: *Nutritional support of the medical oncology patient,* Hematol Oncol Clin North Am 5:147, 1991.

9. Clarke DE and Raffin TA: *Infectious complications of indwelling long-term central venous catheters,* Chest 97:966, 1990.

10. Daly JM and others: *Nutritional support of patients with cancer of the gastrointestinal tract,* Surg Clin North Am 71:523, 1991.

11. Davies L and Knutson KC: *Warning signals for malnutrition of the elderly,* J Am Diet Assoc 91:1413, 1991.

12. Dreizen S and others: *Nutritional deficiencies in patients receiving cancer chemotherapy,* Postgrad Med 87:163, 1990.

13. Eisenberg PG: *Pulmonary complications from enteral nutrition,* Crit Care Nurse Clin North Am 3:641, 1991.

14. Fry ST: *Ethical issues in total parenteral nutrition,* Nutrition 6:329, 1990.

15. Grant JP: *Proper use and recognized role of TPN in the cancer patient,* Nutrition 6(4 suppl):6, 1990.

16. Groenwald S: Nutritional disorders. In Groenwald S, editor: *Cancer nursing: principles and practice,* Boston, ed 3, 1993, Jones & Bartlett.

17. Horwarth CC: *Nutrition goals for older adults: a review,* Gerontologist 31:811, 1991.

18. Jeejeebhoy KN, Detsky AS, and Baker JP: *Assessment of nutritional status,* J Parenter Enteral Nutr 14(5 suppl):193, 1990.

19. Kohn CL and Keithley JK: *Enteral nutrition. Potential complications and patient monitoring,* Nurs Clin North Am 24:339, 1989.

20. Lehmann S: *Immune function and nutrition. The clinical role of the intravenous nurse,* J Intraven Nurs 14:406, 1991.

21. Mahmood T and Rubin AD: *Home-based intravenous therapy for oncology patients,* N J Med 89(1):43, 1992.

22. Mullan H, Roubenoff RA, and Roubenoff R: *Risk of pulmonary aspiration among patients receiving enteral nutrition support,* J Parenter Enteral Nutr 16:160, 1992.

23. Murphy JI: *Tube feeding problems and solutions,* Adv Clin Care 5(2):7, 1990.

24. Padilla GV: *Gastrointestinal side effects and quality of life in patients receiving radiation therapy,* Nutrition 6:367, 1990.

25. Pisters KM and Kris MG: *Management of nausea and vomiting caused by anticancer drugs: state of the art,* Oncology 6(2 suppl):99, 1992.

26. Robuck JT and Fleetwood JB: *Nutritional support of the patient with cancer,* Focus on Crit Care 19(2):129, 1992.

27. Roe DA: *Geriatric nutrition,* Clin Geriatr Med 6:319, 1990.

28. Segura M and Sitges-Serra A: *Clinical predictors of infection of central venous catheters used for parenteral nutrition,* Infect Control Hosp Epidemiol 12:407, 1991.

29. Stephany TM: *Nutrition for the terminally ill,* Home Health Nurse 9(3):48, 1991.

30. Viall CD: *Daily access of implanted venous ports. Implications for patient education,* J Intrav Nurs 13:294, 1990.

31. Wilmore DW: *Catabolic illness. Strategies for enhancing recovery,* N Engl J Med 325:695, 1991.

32. Young CK and White S: *Preparing patients for tube feeding at home,* Am J Nurs 92(4):46, 1992.

Pain Management

28

Nurses play a major role in the successful management of the person who is experiencing cancer pain by preventing the situation of pain.

Pain affects a person's sleeping pattern, family, work, and social relationships. Ultimately, it affects a patient's quality of life and possibly the will to live.[24,25,26]

Definitions

- *Pain*—"Whatever the experiencing person says it is, existing whenever the experiencing person says it does:" an unpleasant sensory and emotional experience associated with actual or potential tissue damage, or described in terms of such damage.
- *Suffering*—an experience, either physical or mental, that the person dislikes.
- *Drug tolerance*—the involuntary need for increasing doses of analgesic to achieve the same level of pain relief. Tolerance will develop more rapidly following IV or intraspinal administration than after oral or rectal administration, first there is a decreased duration of relief, then decreased level of pain relief.
- *Addiction*—the use of narcotics for the psychological euphoric effect and *not* for the analgesic effect; there is overwhelming involvement with obtaining and using drugs for other than approved medical reasons.
- *Physical dependence*—the body's adaptation to the use of opioids without withdrawal symptoms will occur based on physiologic changes. The person who is on opioids for longer than 3 to 4 weeks may become physically dependent.[8,14,16,21]

Theories of Pain

- *Specificity*—The intensity of nociceptive stimulus and perception of pain are directly correlated and travel along specific pathways from the pain receptors to the spinal cord.
- *Gate control theory*—Nociceptive impulses are transmitted via the spinothalamic tract but can be modulated in the spinal cord, brainstem, or cerebral cortex. Two types of afferent fibers have been identified: thinly myelinated A-delta fibers and unmyelinated C fibers. The substantia gelatinosa in the dorsal horn of the spinal cord is the proposed site of the "gating" mechanism.[9,16,21]

Types of Pain

- *Acute pain*—pain is brief in duration, the cause is usually known, the intensity may range from mild to severe, and the treatment is aimed at elimination of the cause.
- *Chronic pain*—extends beyond 3 to 6 months, the cause may or may not be known, it has not responded to treatment and/or does not subside after the injury heals, intensity may range from mild to severe and treatment varies.
- *Chronic cancer pain*—may be both *acute and chronic*. There is the time element of chronic pain, the intensity may be severe, the pain can be described as "intractable", and may be due to several etiologies.[9,14,21]

Etiologies of Cancer Pain

Direct Tumor Involvement[7,9,12]

- *Somatic pain* (nociceptive)—results from stimulation of afferent nerves in the skin, connective tissue, muscles, joints, or bones.
- *Visceral pain*—involves organs in the thoracic or abdominal area.
- *Neuropathic pain* (deafferentation)—results from peripheral or central nerve injury and is usually described as *"burning, shooting, or tingling."* Response to analgesics is usually poor.
- *Cancer Pain Syndromes*—different types of pain, different

etiologies of pain, and different methods of treatment.

- *Bone involvement*—multiple bony metastases are by far the most common cause of generalized bone pain.
- *Periperhal nerves*—sites where this may occur include the chest wall and retroperitoneal space, which may produce pain in the back, abdomen, or legs.
- *Brachial plexus*—usually a result of a primary lung tumor (Pancoat's syndrome).
- *Epidural spinal cord compression*—"Over 95% of patients with epidural spinal cord compression report pain, which may be focal or referred."

Cancer Treatment[9,11,16,21]

- *Postthoracotomy pain sydrome*—the intercoastal nerve may be damaged at the time of surgery.
- *Postmastectomy pain syndrome*—the intercostobrachial nerve may be damaged at the time of surgery.
- *Postamputation syndrome*—due to the formation of a neuroma which has both lancinating (shooting) and "burning" components, phantom sensation that exhibits both continuous dysesthesias, and "shooting" pain.
- *Multiple neural involvement*—may be several neural areas affected by chemotherapy.
- *Mucositis*—inflammation of the oral mucosa as a side effect of some of the chemotherapeutic agents.
- *Postradiation pain*—inadvertent damage to the spinal cord, mucosa, or bone.

Factors Affecting One's Response to Pain

Anxiety

Anxiety is considered to be the most important factor affecting an individual's response to pain because it affects a person's ability to tolerate and cope with pain.

Past Experience of Pain

The more experience of pain one has in childhood, the greater the perceptions of pain in adulthood; determine what measures have helped/not helped relieve pain in the past.

Culture and Religion

Acceptable responses to pain are learned at a very early age. Cultural and religious practices in one's family play an important role in the pain experience. Some cultures may view the expression of pain or suffering as a weakness, so they tend to minimize pain. Other cultures expect expression of pain so they may have greater overt manifestations of pain. It is important to realize that not all people manifest pain in the same way and that there is no right or wrong way. The nurse should accept all patients' expressions of pain, regardless of their cultural or religious backgrounds.[5,7,8,20]

Pharmacologic Interventions

Non-Opioid Analgesics

The non-opioids work primarily at the peripheral nervous system level and are used for mild to moderate pain especially of bone metastases, soft-tissue infiltration, or arthritis. The categories of non-opioids include aspirin, acetaminophen, and the nonsteroidal anti-inflammatory drugs (NSAID).

Non-opioids are often given together with opioids and therefore a lower dose of opioid may be effective (Table 28-1).[1,9,13]

Opioid Analgesics[1,24,25]

The opiates work primarily at the central nervous system (CNS) level and do not have a ceiling case effect.

Table 28-2 contains opioid analgesia guidelines for opioid-naive adults ≥ 50 kg; Table 28-3 opioid-naive adults < 50 kg and Table 28-4 drugs and routes of administration not recommended for treatment of cancer.

Special Issues of Opioids[18,23,27]

Titration/Escalating Doses

When it is determined that more medication is needed to manage an individual's pain, the safe plan of increasing the dose is: *increase 25-50% of the previous dose.*

Rescue Doses

"Rescue" medication should be the same drug as the scheduled analgesic; a liquid immediate-release formula will act more rapidly than a tablet form. This dose should equal 33% to 50% of the regularly scheduled every 4 hour dose, or calculate 10% of the total 24 hour requirement.

Decreasing Doses

If a person's pain decreases, the opioid requirements may indeed decrease dramatically.

Symptoms

Withdrawal during 1st 24 hours:
- Restlessness
- Lacrimation
- Rhinorrhea
- Yawning
- Perspiration
- Gooseflesh
- Restless sleep
- Mydriasis

Withdrawal during 24-72 hours:
- Twitching/muscular spasms
- Kicking movements
- Severe aches in back, abdomen, and legs
- Nausea, vomiting, diarrhea
- Coryza and severe sneezing
- Increase in all vital signs (T, P, BP, and R)

To safely "wean" the person from the opioids and prevent abstinence syndrome from occurring, the following formula is used:

Give 50% of the previous order for 48 hours and then reduce by 25% q48h until <10 to 15 mg (parenteral morphine equivalent) per 24 hours.[6,7,17]

Table 28-1 Nonopioid Analgesics

Drug	Recommended Dose and Interval	Comments
PARA-AMINOPHENOL DERIVATIVE		
Acetaminophen (Tylenol, Panadol, Anacin-3, Excedrin, Midol, Sine-Aid)	500-1000 mg q4-6 hr	Similar to aspirin in analgesic and antipyretic effects, but only slight anti-inflammatory effects. May not have effect on platelet aggregation. May cause liver toxicity
ACETYLSALICYLICS		
Acetylsalicylic acid (aspirin)	50-1000 mg q4-6 hr	First choice analgesic if able to tolerate; standard anti-inflammatory; increased bleeding time due to inhibition of platelet aggregation
NONACETYLATED SALICYLATES		
Choline magnesium trisalicylates (Trilisate)	1000-1500 mg q8-12 hr	Minimal effect on platelet aggregation (platelet-sparing); available in liquid
Diflunisal (Dolobid)	500-1000 mg q8-12 hr	Longer action; minimal antipyretic effect; minimal GI side effects
Salsalate (Disalcid; Salsitab)	750-1000 mg q8-12 hr	May have minimal effect on platelet aggregation; minimal GI side effects
NSAIDs (NONSTEROIDAL ANTI-INFLAMMATORY DRUGS)		
Propionic acid derivatives:		
Ibuprofen (Motrin, Nuprin, Advil, Medipren)	200-400 mg q4-8 hr	
Fenoprofen (Nalfon)	200 mg q4-6 hr	Available as oral suspension

Drug	Dose	Comments
Naproxen (Naprosyn)	250-500 mg q6-8 hr	Available as oral liquid
Naproxen sodium (Anaprox)	275-550 mg q6-8 hr	Faster onset than naproxen
Ketoprofen (Orudis)	25-50 mg q6-8 hr	
Indole acetic acid derivatives:		
Indomethacin (Indocin)	25-50 mg q8-12 hr	Available as oral suspension and rectal suppository; high incidence of side effects: GI symptoms
Sulindac (Clinoril)	150-200 mg q8-12 hr	Lower incidence of renal toxicity; GI side effects common
Tolmetin (Tolectin)	200 mg q6-8 hr	Weak analgesic effect
Anthranilics:		
Mefenamic acid (Ponstel)	250 mg q6 hr	Not recommended for use longer than 7 days
Meclofenamate (Meclomen)	50-100 mg q6-8 hr	Diarrhea may occur as well as other GI side effects
Oxicam:		
Piroxicam (Feldene)	10-30 mg q6 hr or 20 mg qd	Not recommended for patients with renal or liver dysfunction; effect may not be seen for 7-12 days
Pyrrololacetic acid:		
ketorolac (Toradol)	30 mg q6 hr	Only injectable NSAID; not recommended for use longer than 7 days; equivalent to 10 mg parenteral morphine; oral form also available

Note: It is important to remember that all of the NSAIDs have similar side effects, especially GI irritation. All of these drugs should be administered on a full stomach and with milk. In addition to GI irritation, GI bleeding can be a serious problem related to the inhibition of platelet aggregation and NSAIDs should be used with caution in thrombocytopenic patients. See note on choline magnesium trisalicyte.

Table 28-2. Dose equivalents for opioid analgesics in opioid-naive adults ≥ 50 kg[1]

Drug	Approximate equianalgesic dose Oral	Parenteral	Usual starting dose for moderate to severe pain Oral	Parenteral
Opioid agonist[2]				
Morphine	30 mg q3-4h (repeat around-the-clock dosing) 60 mg q3-4h (single dose or intermittent dosing)	10 mg q3-4h	30 mg q3-4h	10 mg q3-4h
Morphine, controlled-release[3,4] (MS Contin, Oramorph)	90-120 mg q12h	N/A	90-120 mg q12h	N/A
Hydromorphone[3] (Dilaudid)	7.5 mg q3-4h	1.5 mg q3-4h	6 mg q3-4h	1.5 mg q3-4h
Levorphanol (Levo-Dromoran)	4 mg q6-8h	2 mg q6-8h	4 mg q6-8h	2 mg q6-8h
Meperidine[5] (Demerol)	300 mg q2-3h	100 mg q3h	N/R	100 mg q3h

Methadone (Dolphine, other)	20 mg q6-8h	10 mg q6-8h	20 mg q6-8H	10 mg q6-8h
Oxymorphone[3] (Numorphan)	N/A	1 mg q3-4h	N/A	1 mg q3-4h
Combination opioid/NSAID preparations[6]				
Codeine (with aspirin or acetaminophen)[7]	180-200 mg q3-4h	130 mg q3-4h	60 mg q3-4h	60 mg q2h IM/SC)
Hydrocodone (in Lorcet, Lortab, Vicodin, others)	30 mg q3-4h	N/A	10 mg q3-4h	N/A
Oxycodone (Roxicodone, also in Percocet, Percodan, Tylox, others)	30 mg q3-4h	N/A	10 mg q3-4h	N/A

[1]Caution: Recommended doses do not apply for adult patients with body weight less than 50 kg. For recommended starting doses for adults < 50 kg body weight, see Table 28-5.

[2]Caution: Recommended doses do not apply to patients with renal or hepatic insufficiency or other conditions affecting drug metabolism and kinetics.

[3]Caution: For morphine, hydromorphone, and oxymorphone, rectal administration is an alternate route for patients unable to take oral medications. Equianalgesic doses may differ from oral and parenteral doses because of pharmacokinetic differences. **Note**: A short-acting opioid should normally be used for initial therapy of moderate to severe pain.

[4]Transdermal fentanyl (Duragesic) is an alternative option. Transdermal fentanyl dosage is not calculated as equianalgesic to a single morphine dosage. See the package insert for dosing calculations. Doses above 25 µg/h should not be used in opioid-naive patients.

[5]Not recommended. Doses listed are for brief therapy. Switch to another opioid for long-term therapy.

[6]Caution: Doses of aspirin and acetaminophen in combination opioid/NSAID preparations must also be adjusted to the patient's body weight.

[7]Caution: Codeine doses above 65 mg often are not appropriate because of diminishing incremental analgesia with increasing doses but continually increasing nausea, constipation, and other side effects.

Note: Published tables vary in the suggested doses that are equianalgesic to morphine. Clinical response is the criterion that must be applied for each patient; titration to clinical response is the criterion that must be applied for each patient; titration to clinical responses is necessary. Because there is not complete cross-tolerance among these drugs, it is usually necessary to use a lower than equianalgesic dose when changing drugs and to retitrate to response.

Codes: q=every. N/A=not available. N/R=not recommended. IM=intramuscular. SC=subcutaneous.

Jacox A, Carr DB, Payne R, et al. *Management of Cancer Pain. Clinical Practice Guideline* No. 9. AHCPR Publication No. 94-0592. Rockville, MD. Agency for Health Care Policy and Research, U.S. Department of Health and Human Services, Public Health Service, March 1994.

Table 28-3. Dose equivalents for opioid analgesics in opioid-naive adults < 50 kg

Drug	Approximate equianalgesic dose		Usual starting dose for moderate to severe pain	
	Oral	Parenteral	Oral	Parenteral
Opioid agonist[1]				
Morphine	30 mg q3–4h (repeat around-the-clock dosing) 60 mg q3–4h (single dose or intermittent dosing)	10 mg q3–4h	0.3 mg/kg q3–4h	0.1 mg/kg q3–4h
Morphine, controlled-release[3,4] (MS Contin, Oramorph)	90–120 mg q12h	N/A	N/A	N/A
Hydromorphone[3] (Dilaudid)	7.5 mg q3–4h	1.5 mg q3–4h q3–4h	0.06 mg/kg q3–4h	0.015 mg/kg q3–4h
Levorphanol (Levo-Dromoran)	4 mg q6–8h	2 mg q6–8h q6–8h	0.04 mg/kg q6–8h	0.02 mg/kg q6–8h
Meperidine[5] (Demerol)	300 mg q2–3h	100 mg q3h	N/R q2–3h	0.75 mg/kg q3–4h

Methadone (Dolophine, other)	20 mg q6-8h	10 mg q6-8h q6-8h	0.2 mg/kg q6-8h	0.1 mg/kg

Combination opioid/NSAID preparations[5]

Codeine[6] (with aspirin or acetaminophen)	180-200 mg q3-4h	130 mg q3-4h	0.5-1 mg/kg q3-4h	N/R
Hydrocodone (in Lorcet, Lortab, Vicodin, others)	30 mg q3-4h	N/A q3-4h	0.2 mg/kg	N/A
Oxycodone (Roxicodone, also in Percocet, Percodan, Tylox, others)	30 mg q3-4h	N/A q3-4h	0.2 mg/kg	N/A

[1]Caution: Recommended doses do not apply to patients with renal or hepatic insufficiency or other conditions affecting drug metabolism and kinetics.

[2]Caution: For morphine, hydromorphone, and oxymorphone, rectal administration is an alternate route for patients unable to take oral medications. Equianalgesic doses may differ from oral and parenteral doses because of pharmacokinetic differences. Note: A short-acting opioid should normally be used for initial therapy of moderate to severe pain.

[3]Transdermal fentanyl (Duragesic) is an alternative option. Transdermal fentanyl dosage is not calculated as equianalgesic to a single morphine dosage. See the package insert for dosing calculations. Doses above 25 ug/h should not be used in opioid-naive patients.

[4]Not recommended. Doses listed are for brief therapy. Switch to another opioid for long-term therapy.

[5]Doses of aspirin and acetaminophen in combination opioid/NSAID preparations must also be adjusted to the patient's body weight.

[6]Caution: Some clinicians recommend not exceeding 1.5 mg/kg of codeine because of an increased incidence of side effects with higher doses.

Note: Published tables vary in the suggested doses that are equianalgesic to morphine. Clinical response is the criterion that must be applied for each patient; titration to clinical response is the criterion that must be applied for each patient; titration to clinical responses is necessary. Because there is not complete cross-tolerance among these drugs, it is usually necessary to use a lower than equianalgesic dose when changing drugs and to retitrate to response.

Codes: q=every. N/A=not available. N/R=not recommended.

Jacox A, Carr DB, Payne R, et al. *Management of Cancer Pain. Clinical Practice Guideline* No. 9. AHCPR Publication No. 94-0592. Rockville, MD. Agency for Health Care Policy and Research, U.S. Department of Health and Human Services, Public Health Service, March 1994.

Table 28-4. Drugs and routes of administration not recommended for treatment of cancer pain

Class	Drug	Rationale for not recommending
Opioids	Meperidine	Short (2-3 hour) duration. Repeated administration may lead to CNS toxicity (tremor, confusion, or seizures). High oral doses required to relieve severe pain, and these increase the risk of CNS toxicity.
Miscellaneous	Cannabinoids	Side effects of dysphoria, drowsiness, hypotension, and bradycardia preclude its routine use as an analgesic.
	Cocaine	Has demonstrated no efficacy as an analgesic or coanalgesic in combination with opioids.
Opioid agonist-antagonists	Pentazocine Butorphanol Nalbuphine	Risk of precipitating withdrawal in opioid-dependent patients. Analgesic ceiling. Possible production of unpleasant psychomimetic effects (e.g., dysphoria, hallucinations).
Partial agonist	Buprenorphine	Analgesic ceiling. Can precipitate withdrawal.
Antagonist	Naloxone Naltrexone	May precipitate withdrawal. Limit use to treatment of life-threatening respiratory depression.
Combination preparations	Brompton's cocktail	No evidence of analgesic benefit to using Brompton's cocktail over single opioid analgesics.
	DPT (Meperidine, Promethazine, and Chlorpromazine)	Efficacy is poor compared with that of other analgesics. High incidence of adverse effects.

Anxiolytics alone	Benzodiazepine e.g., alprazolam	Analgesic properties not demonstrated except for some instances of neuropathic pain. Added sedation from anxiolytics may limit opioid dosing.
Sedative/ hypnotic drugs alone	Barbiturates Benzodiazepine	Analgesic properties not demonstrated. Added sedation from sedative/hypnotic drugs limits opioid dosing.

Routes of administration | **Rationale for not recommending**

Intramuscular (IM)	Painful. Absorption unreliable. Should not be used for children or patients prone to develop dependent edema or in patients with thrombocytopenia.
Transnasal	The only drug approved by the FDA for transnasal administration at this time is butorphanol, an agonist-antagonist drug, which generally is not recommended. (See opioid agonist-antagonists above.)

Jacox A, Carr DB, Payne R, et al. *Management of Cancer Pain. Clinical Practice Guideline* No. 9. AHCPR Publication No. 94-0592. Rockville, MD. Agency for Health Care Policy and Research, U.S. Department of Health and Human Services, Public Health Service, March 1994.

Box 28-1

Guidelines for Respiratory Depression

1. Always have a baseline respiratory rate
2. Respiratory depression is usually slow in onset and preceded by sedation
3. Respiratory depression usually occurs
   7 minutes after IV
   30 minutes after IM
   90 minutes after SC
4. Use a flow sheet to record respiratory rate and pain relief
5. Dilute Narcan 0.1 to 0.4 mg in 10 mL saline and administer intravenously over 2 to 4 minutes

From McGuire L: Pain. In Beare PG and Myers JL: *Principles and practice of adult health nursing*, St Louis, 1990, Mosby.

Opioid Side Effect Management

The expected side effects are:

- *Constipation.* All patients on opioids should be given stool softeners and agents to increase bowel motility to prevent constipation as opioids inhibit peristalsis in the GI tract. Preventing severe constipation requires treating consistently and prophylactically.[10]
- *Nausea/vomiting.* The intensity of nausea and/or vomiting in patients receiving opioids varies from patient to patient and from opioid to opioid. This side effect generally decreases after 2 to 3 days of repeated dosing.[13]
- *Sedation.* Opioids have a depressant effect on the central nervous system therefore some drowsiness can be anticipated. Do not confuse normal extended sleep patterns with sedation. Be aware that the person may have been exhausted from interrupted sleep patterns due to previous pain. If sedation persist for more than 3 to 5 days, possible added stimulation might be required.[9,18]
- *Confusion and/or hallucinations.* Impaired renal function and other possible causes of confusion to be ruled out: cerebral metastases, hypercalcemia, sepsis, and so on. Tolerance to these side effects usually develops within 48 to 72 hours.[18]

- *Pruritus.* This intense itching is more often observed with the administration of intraspinal narcotics, and is not frequently seen with the other routes of administration.
- *Respiratory depression.* Tolerance to this potential side effect develops rapidly (Box 28-1). Pain is a natural antagonist to the respiratory depressant effects of opiates and therefore pain provides a natural stimulant. When doses are escalated, respirations should be monitored.[9,18,29]

Table 28-5 Opioid Dosing Equivalence

Drug	Approximate Equianalgesic Dose	
	Oral	Parenteral
morphine[1,2]	30 mg q3-4hr	10 mg q3-4hr
hydromorphone (Dilaudid)	7.5 mg q3-4hr	1.5 mg q3-4hr
codeine[3]	130 mg q3-4hr	
hydrocodone[3] (Lorcet, Lortab, Vicodin, others)	30 mg q3-4hr	
oxycodone[3] (Roxicodone, also in Roxicet, Percocet Tylox and others)	30 mg q3-4hr	
methadone (Dolophine)	20 mg q6-8hr[4]	10 mg q6-8hr[4]
levorphanol (Levo-Dromoran)	4 mg q6-8hr[4]	2 mg q6-8hr[4]
meperidine (Demerol)	300 mg q2-3hr[4]	2 mg q3hr[4]
transdermal fentanyl[5] (Duragesic)		

[1]Short-acting oral products include MSIR, Rescudose, Roxanol, Roxanol 100 and others.
[2]Long-acting products with 8-12hr durations of action include MS-Contin and Oramorph SR.
[3]Codeine and oxycodone are often given as combination products with aspirin or acetaminophen. Hydrocodone is only available in such combination products. Propoxyphene is also marketed in combination with aspirin or acetaminophen; 65-130 mg of propoxyphene is equivalent to about 650 mg of aspirin.
[4]May be significantly longer in some patients.
[5]A 25 μg patch is approximately equivalent to 45-135 mg oral or 8-22 mg parenteral morphine sulfate per 24 hr.
Weissman DE and others: *Handbook of Cancer Pain Management,* ed 4, Wisconsin, 1994, Cancer Pain Institute, Wisconsin.

Box 28-2

ROUTES OF ADMINISTRATION

Oral

- Preferred route for analgesics; patients maintain control
- Allows greater mobility
- Drug levels peak in 1 to 2 hours
- Ease in administration
- Cost efficient

Rectal

- Good for patients who are NPO, nauseated, or unable to swallow
- May be more expensive than oral route and more difficult to obtain
- Most often a 1:1 ratio with oral

Transdermal

- Good for patients who are NPO, nauseated, or unable to swallow
- Takes 14-24 hours to peak initially; lasts approximately 17 hours after removal

IV continuous infusion

- Provides constant narcotic intravenous infusion to maintain constant blood levels
- No peaks and valleys in blood levels
- Recommended when unable to achieve pain control through oral or rectal routes with high dosages of narcotics or unable to use oral/rectal route
- Requires use of infusion pump with alarms

IV bolus

- Good for acute pain and/or procedures
- Provides most rapid onset but shortest duration
- Not recommended for constant pain due to peaks and valleys in bloodstream

IM injection

- Should be used mainly for acute short-term pain
- Painful administration; rotate sites
- Not recommended for chronic long-term pain especially cancer pain.

- Each patch lasts 2-3 days
- Ease in administration
- Difficult to titrate
- Not recommended for use with children, emaciated patients, or patients with a decrease in muscle mass

Subcutaneous infusion

- Provides prolonged parenteral administration of narcotics and/or intermittent bolus
- Avoids repetitive injections
- Avoids peaks and valleys in bloodstream
- Avoids need for intravenous access
- Readily managed at home
- Recommended for cancer patients who cannot take anything by mouth
- Requires use of infusion pump with alarms

Patient-controlled alagesia (PCA)

- Allows patient to receive a predetermined intravenous bolus of a narcotic by a pump mechanism.
- Gives patient sense of control, less anxiety
- Provides quick pain relief
- Patient may require less narcotic
- Eliminates the need for repeated injections

Spinal administration

Epidural
Dose: 5-10 mg morphine
Pain relief: 12-24 hours
Intrathecal (subarachnoid)
Dose 0.5-1.0 mg morphine
Pain relief: up to 36 hours

- Narcotic (usually morphine) administered through catheter into epidural or intrathecal space
- May be intermittent bolus or by continuous infusion pump
- Careful selection of the patient necessary as procedure is expensive and may be risky
- Side effects include nausea, vomiting, pruritus, sedation, urinary retention, respiratory depression
- Possible complication of infection and/or meningitis

Potentiators

General Principles of Analgesic Administration

- Choose the analgesic appropriate to the type and level of pain.
- Choose the easiest and most cost-effective route of administration.
- Schedule administration. Around the clock (ATC).
- Be prepared for breakthrough pain.
- Plan treatment of side effects.
- Never use placebos.

Routes of Administration

Routes of administration are detailed in Box 28-20.[2,3,6,12,18,19,28,29]

Nonpharmacologic Pain Relief Techniques[4,5,7,22]

Noninvasive Mechanical Interventions

Cutaneous Stimulation

- Activity that stimulates the skin for the purpose of relieving pain

Heat and Cold

- Decrease pain and muscle spasm
- Keep in mind whenever using heat or cold therapy: the age of the patient, medical history, condition of the skin, and any discomfort

Transcutaneous Electrical Nerve Stimulation (TENS)

- Consists of a pocket-sized battery-operated device that provides a continuous mild electrical current to the skin via electrodes

Behavioural Interventions

Relaxation

- State of relative freedom from both anxiety and skeletal tension

Distraction

- Focusing on stimuli (music, tapping, people, humor) other than the pain sensation
- Alters the patient's ability to tolerate pain

Imagery/Visualization

- Mentally creating a picture
- Focus on a close person, a place of enjoyment, a past event, or anything that is thought to bring pleasure
- Used to take the thoughts away from the painful sensation: very individual as to the person's preference

Humor

- Used as a distraction; can provide prolonged pain relief even up to 2 hours

Prayer

- Use of communication with a higher power

Play Therapy

- Use of games or toys
- Useful for children and adults

Biofeedback

- The ability to alter the body functions by intentional mental focusing; requires the skill of a professional person who is trained in the technique

Hypnosis

- The use of psychotherapy to alter the affective component as well as the sensory component of pain; the patient's perception of pain is modified

510 Pocket Guide to Oncology Nursing

Invasive Techniques

Nerve Blocks

- An injection of an anesthetic agent into or near to numb pain pathways can be performed with either a local temporary anesthetic agent or a permanent neurolytic agent

Neurosurgical Procedures

- Surgical or chemical (alcohol) interruption of pain pathways

Acupuncture

- The insertion of needles at various points into the body to relieve pain; stimulates large nerve fibers to close the gate in the spinal cord to pain impulses

Nursing Management

Nursing Diagnosis

- *Alteration in comfort, pain due to*

Interventions

- Assess: pain location, quality, duration, intensity, aggravating and relieving factors; loss of appetite, sleep disturbance, fatigue, behavioural changes and equianalgesic amount required per 24 hours
- Plan and intervene whether current treatment is adequate: Administer analgesics according to pain requirements Collaborate with other health care professionals Evaluate and document; provide patient instructions Conduct ongoing evaluation

Patient Teaching[1,13,25,26,30]

Some of the areas of patient education include:

- Cause of pain
- Anticipated outcome (pain relief)
- What to report to MD/RN

Unmanaged side effects
Uncontrolled pain
■ Medication information
■ Side effects of medications and what to do to prevent or treat them
■ Information to restructure attitudes and beliefs regarding addiction, medications, etc.
■ Plan for follow-up and who to call for emergency assistance
■ Client's and providers' responsibilities for pain management plan

Geriatric Pain Issues[1,22]

When working with an elderly population, analgesics are appropriate for pain management with the following considerations:

1. The dose may need to be *decreased.*
2. The interval between doses may need to be *lengthened.*
3. The frequency of assessment and evaluation is increased.
4. Other considerations
   ■ Distribution of drugs
     There are changes in the body composition (an increase of fat and decrease in heart, kidney, and muscle mass) as aging occurs, therefore, usual adult doses may need to be decreased to avoid toxic drug levels in the blood and tissue. Decreased circulating proteins due to serum proteins, malnutrition, or chronic disease potentially result in greater drug effect from higher concentration of unbound drug, with a greater risk of toxic effect
   ■ Metabolism of drugs
     There is limited research in the area of hepatic metabolic rates in relation to aging; allow for longer intervals between doses in the elderly
   ■ Excretion of drugs
     A decrease in renal mass, renal blood flow, glomerular filtration rate, and tubular secretion can all occur in the kidney due to aging. With reduced function, the drugs or their active metabolites may remain in the body longer

Bibliography

1. Agency for Health Care Policy and Research (AHCPR) "Acute Pain Management: Management of Cancer Pain. Clinical Practice Guideline." Rockville, MD: U.S. Department of Health and Human Services, Publication No. 94-0592, 1994.

2. *American Nurses' Association Position Statement on the Role of the Registered Nurse in the Management of Analgesia by Catheter Techniques*, Am Nurse, February:7, 1992.

3. Cole L and Hanning CD: *Review of the rectal use of opioids*, J Pain Sympt Manage 5(2):118, 1990.

4. Cushing M: *The legal side: Pain management on trial*, Am J Nurs 92(2):21, 1992.

5. Dalton JA: *Nurses' perceptions of their pain assessment skills, pain management practices, and attitudes toward pain*, Oncol Nurs Forum 16(2):225, 1989.

6. Enck RE: *Parenteral narcotics for pain control in the home care environment*, Caring 9(5):38, 1990.

7. Ferrell BR, and Ferrell BA: *Easing the pain*, Geriatr Nurs July/August:175, 1990.

8. Ferrell BR, McCaffery M, and Rhiner M: *Pain and addiction: an urgent need for change in nursing education*, J Pain Sympt Manage 7(2):117, 1992.

9. Foley KM and Arbit E: Management of cancer pain. In DeVita VT, Hellman S, and Rosenberg SA, editors: *Cancer: Principles & Practice of Oncology*, ed 4, Philadelphia, 1993, JB Lippincott.

10. Glare P and Lickiss JN: *Unrecognized constipation in patients with advanced cancer: a recipe for the therapeutic disaster*, J Pain Sympt Manage 7(6):369, 1992.

11. Gonzales GR: *Postherpes simplex type 1 neuralgia simulating postherpetic neuralgia*, J Pain Sympt Manag 7(2):320, 1992.

12. Johanson GA: *New routes of opiate administration*, Am Hospice Palliative Care, July/August:4, 1992.

13. Max MB: *Improving outcomes of analgesic treatment: is education enough?* Ann Intern Med 114(4):342, 1991.

14. McCaffery M and Beebe A: *Pain: A Clinical Manual for Nursing* Practice, St Louis, 1989, Mosby.

15. McCaffery M and Ferrell BR: *Opioid analgesics: nurses' knowledge of doses and psychological dependence,* J Nurs Staff Develop 8(2):77, 1992.

16. McGuire DB: *Cancer pain: pathophysiology of pain in cancer*, Cancer Nursing 12(5):310, 1989.

17. McGuire DB and Sheidler VR: Pain. In Groenwald SL and others, editors: *Cancer Nursing—Principles and Practice,* ed 3, Boston, 1993, Jones and Bartlett Publishers.

18. McGuire L: *Administering analgesics. Which drugs are right for your patients?* Nursing 90:34, 1990.

19. McLaughlin-Hagan M: *Continuous subcutaneous infusion of narcotics*, J Intrav Nurs 13(2):119, 1990.

20. Miaskowski C and Donovan M: *Implementation of the American Pain Society quality assurance standards for relief of acute pain and cancer pain in oncology nursing practice*, Oncol Nurs Forum 19(3):411, 1992.

21. Paice JA: *Unraveling the mystery of pain*, Oncol Nurs Forum 18(5):843, 1991.

22. Portenoy RK and Coyle N: *Controversies in the long-term management of analgesic therapy in patients with advanced cancer*, J Pain Sympt Manage 5(5):307, 1990.

23. Schug SA and others: *A long-term survey of morphine in cancer pain patients,* J Pain Sympt Manage 7(5):259, 1992.

24. Spross JA, McGuire DB, and Schmitt RM: *Oncology Nursing Society Position Paper on Cancer Pain — Part I (Scope of Nursing Practice Regarding Cancer Pain, Ethics and Practice),* Oncol Nurs Forum 17(4):595, 1990.

25. Spross JA, McGuir DB, and Schmitt RN: *Oncology Nursing Society Position Paper on Cancer Pain—Part II (Education, Research and list of cancer pain management resources)*, Oncol Nurs Forum 17(5):751, 1990.

26. Spross JA, McGuire DB, and Schmitt RN: *Oncology Nursing Society Position Paper on Cancer Pain—Part III (Nursing Administration, Pediatric Cancer Pain and Appendices)*, Oncol Nurs Forum 17(6):943, 1990.

27. Spross JA: *Pain management: issues in the hospital setting.* In Pain Management Issues in Research and Practice. American Cancer Society Publication, 1992.

28. Spross JA: *Cancer pain relief: an international perspective*, Oncol Nurs Forum 19(7 supplement):5, 1992.

29. Stanley TH and Ashburn MA: *Novel delivery systems: oral transmucosal and intranasal transmucosal*, J Pain Sympt Manage 7(13):163, 1992.

30. Walsh TD: *Prevention of opioid side effects*, J Pain Sympt Manage 5(6):362, 1990.

31. Weissman DE and others: *Handbook of cancer pain management*, ed 4, 1994, Wisconsin Pain Institute, Wisconsin.

32. World Health Organization (WHO). *Cancer pain relief and palliative care*, Geneva, Switzerland, 1990, World Health Organization.

Protective Mechanisms

29

Immunity

Immunity is a protective mechanism that serves to maintain the integrity of the body against foreign substances or agents. Three main functions of the immune system include: defense against invading organisms, homeostasis—removal of dead "self" cells, and surveillance—removal of mutant cells.[2,9,11,13]

Innate Immunity

Innate immunity is a nonspecific response to any breach of the skin and mucous membranes, present at birth, species specific, and provides initial protection against foreign substances and invading organisms. There are four mechanisms of innate immunity: mechanical barriers (skin and mucus membrane), chemical barriers (saliva, tears, sweat, gastric juices, cerumen), fever, and inflammation.

Acquired Immunity

Acquired immunity is the body's specific neutralizing response to foreign invaders and their products. This type of immunity is not fully functional at birth, and may take 6 to 7 years for the immune system to mature. As a person reaches late middle age, its level of functioning begins to decline. There are two main mechanisms of acquired immunity: cell-mediated immunity and humoral immunity.

Cell-mediated immunity—uses T cells as the primary effector cell, functions as immunoregulatory and cytotoxic cells, and provides defense against intracellular bacteria such as *Mycobacterium tuberculosis* and *Listeria monocytogenes,* fungi, viruses, and protozoa.

Humoral immunity—the part of acquired immunity that involves the production of antibodies. Antibodies are substances produced by plasma cells (sensitized B cells) in response to specific recognition of an antigen (foreign substance). They are serum proteins called immunoglobulins. There are five major categories of immunoglobulins: IgG, IgM, IgA, IgD, and IgE.

Skin

The skin is a multifunctional organ. Its recognized functions include the following:

- Distinguishes between pain, temperature, and touch
- Regulates loss of water and electrolytes
- Regulates body temperature by vasoconstriction and vasodilation
- Absorbs substances applied directly to the skin
- Excretes excess water and electrolytes
- Prevents entrance of external gases, liquids, and pathogens as long as intact and so protects the internal body
- Provides nutrition to underlying structures through abundant blood supply

Pathophysiology

A person with cancer may experience multiple disruptions of skin integrity.

Disease-Related Causes

Include malignant melanoma, basal cell carcinoma, squamous cell carcinoma, Kaposi's sarcoma, mycoses fungoides, metastatic tumors of the skin, acanthosis nigricans, acquired icthyosis, dermatomyositis, exfoliative dermatitis, and thrombocytopenia.

Treatment-Related Causes

Include drug extravasation, alopecia, hyperpigmentation, hyperkeratosis, photosensitivity, ulceration, radiation recall reactions, allergic skin eruptions, Stevens-Johnson reactions, erythema multiforme, radiation therapy, skin reactions, and surgical incisions.[16]

Complicating Factors

Include immobility, malnutrition, obstruction, infection, and pruritus.

Medical Management

Treatment of skin complications may include antibiotics, antifungals, and antivirals for infection, surgical procedures for incision and drainage, debridement, skin grafting, radiation therapy
for obstructive phenomena, chemotherapy to treat the underlying disease for relief of pruritus, and management of disfiguring, non-healing or ulcerating malignant skin lesions.[16,20]

Mucous Membranes

The oral mucosa provides a mechanical barrier to inhibit the
invasion of microorganisms.

Pathophysiology

The following conditions may occur as the result of disease or
treatment.

- *Stomatitis*—a general term referring to the inflammatory
  reaction and shallow ulcerative lesions occurring on the
  mucosal surfaces of the mouth and oropharynx 7 to 14
  days after the administration of certain chemotherapeutic agents and following radiation therapy to the head and
  neck.
- *Mucositis*—a general term referring to the inflammatory
  reaction and shallow ulcerative lesions occurring on mucosal surfaces, not limited to the mouth and oropharynx,
  frequently associated with the administration of certain
  chemotherapeutic agents and following radiation therapy
  to mucous membrane-bearing sites. Stomatitis, esophagitis, gastritis, enteritis, colitis, proctitis, and vaginitis
  are examples of treatment-related mucositis.

Disease-Related Causes

Include primary tumors of the head, neck, gastrointestinal tract,
respiratory tract, and genitourinary tract; agranulocytic oral ul-
cers; gingival hypertrophy and infiltration associated with acute
leukemia; non-Hodgkin's lymphoma or acute leukemia involving Waldeyer's ring; and Kaposi's sarcoma, among others.

Treatment-Related Causes

Include chemotherapy-induced mucositis, radiation-associated mucositis, xerostomia, parotitis, osteoradionecrosis of the bone, and surgical procedures.

Complicating Factors

Include infections, which may become systemic; bleeding from nonintact mucosal surfaces; poor nutritional status; and pain secondary to the lesions.

Medical Management

Treatment of complications involving nonintact mucous membranes includes antibiotics, antifungals, and antivirals for superinfections; platelet transfusion and antifibrinolytic agents for bleeding from mucous membranes; topical and systemic analgesics for pain; and dilation of strictures involving the esophagus and vagina.[6,10]

Bone Marrow Suppression

Anatomy and Physiology

The bone marrow is the production site for all formed blood elements: erythrocytes, granulocytes, monocytes, lymphocytes, and megakaryocytes. All blood cells arise from a common progenitor cell called the stem cell. The stem cell probably resembles and cannot be distinguished by sight from the small mature lymphocyte. The stem cell pool is self-renewing; for every stem cell that enters the differentiation and maturation pool, another cell returns to the stem cell pool. Conditions causing destruction of the stem cell pool lead to the development of marrow aplasia. Stem cells may be either pleuripontential (uncommitted) or unipotential (committed), see Figure 29-1.

Pathophysiology

The following terms are defined:

- *Leukopenia*—a condition said to occur when the total leukocyte complement is reduced. Leukopenia is a nonspecific finding and usually reflects a decrease in all WBCs.

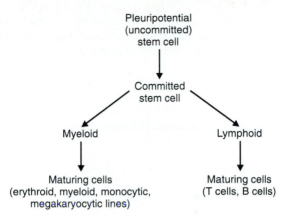

Figure 29-1. Stem cell differentiation and maturation.

- *Granulocytopenia*—a condition said to occur when the absolute granulocyte complement is reduced. When granulocytopenia occurs, there is a decrease in neutrophils, eosinophils, and basophils.
- *Neutropenia*—a condition that exists when there is an absolute decrease in the number of circulating neutrophils, usually less then 1,000/mm^3. The absolute neutrophil count (ANC) is calculated as follows:

Segs (%) + Bands (%) × White blood cell count = ANC
0.10   +   0.10   ×   2000   = 400/mm^3

Neutropenia is associated with a profound impairment in the inflammatory response, leading to lack or minimization of the usual signs and symptoms of infection such as erythema, swelling, heat, and pain. Purulence is not present.

ANC > 1,500/mm^3 = normal risk
ANC < 1,000/mm^3 = moderate risk
ANC < 500/mm^3 = severe risk
ANC < 100/mm^3 = extreme risk

- *Immunosuppression*—a condition that exists when lymphocyte function or interaction is suppressed. Immunosuppression may result from either disease process or treatment, may be primary or secondary, secondary immunosuppression being the most common.

- *Anemia*—a condition characterized by a decrease in circulating hemoglobin levels or circulating erythrocytes. Anemia occurs when loss or destruction exceeds production of RBCs.
- *Thrombocytopenia*—a condition characterized by decreased numbers of circulating platelets or thrombocytes,[7] and may result from decreased or ineffective production of platelets secondary to marrow replacement by tumor, exposure to marrow toxins or infectious agents, and ionizing radiation.
- *Pancytopenia*—a term used when there is a deficiency of all the cell elements of the blood (erythrocytes, platelets, and all the white blood cells [neutrophils, eosinophils, basophils, monocytes, macrophages, and lymphocytes]).

Complicating Factors

Complications associated with bone marrow suppression include increased susceptibility to infection secondary to neutropenia, fatigue associated with anemia, and increased risk of bleeding secondary to low platelet counts. Assessment should include identification of risk factors for the development of infection (Box 29-1). Sepsis, or blood-borne systemic infection, produces significant morbidity and mortality.

Box 29-1

Signs and Symptoms of Infection

Temperature > 38° C (100° F)
Flushed skin, diaphoresis
Shaking chills
White, cream-colored lesions in mouth
Erythema, swelling, or pain in skin, throat, eyes, joints, perineal or rectal areas
Cough, chest pain, tachypnea, or dyspnea
Changes in character or color of sputum, urine, or stools
Dysuria or frequency of urination
Malaise, lethargy, myalgias, or arthralgias
Skin rash
Confusion, mental status change

Medical Management

Infection

The medical management of suspected infection in the neutro-penic or otherwise immunocompromised patient includes its prompt recognition with a workup including cultures, radiologic studies, a thorough physical assessment, and the immediate in-stitution of broad-spectrum, empiric, intravenous antibiotics. Blood cultures should be obtained from both peripheral and cen-tral venous access sites, if present, for aerobic and anaerobic bacteria, fungi, and viruses if indicated. Cultures from body ori-fices, other body substances, and any suspicious lesions should be obtained before initiating antibiotic therapy. Sites of infec-tion in the neutropenic patient are the following:

- Lungs
- Skin
- Oral cavity
- Gastrointestinal tract
- Genitourinary tract
- Blood[12,14,17,18]

The choice of antibiotics will be based on the prevalence and sensitivities of organisms commonly cultured at the health care facility. The usual combination is that of an aminoglycoside and a semisynthetic penicillin with good antipseudomonal effect. Antibiotic therapy usually continues for a minimum of 10 to 14 days or until the patient's neutrophil count recovers to over 1,500/mm^3. If the patient continues febrile for greater than 72 hours it is advisable to reculture, and depending upon previous culture results, change antibiotic therapy.[14,20]

Bleeding

Workup should include a thorough physical examination, radio-logic examination as indicated by the clinical presentation, and laboratory evaluation, CBC, PT, PTT, and FDPs if indicated.[2] Treatment depends upon the cause of the bleeding. If the bleed-ing is secondary to thrombocytopenia or a qualitative platelet defect, platelet transfusions will be of value. If the bleeding re-sults from a coagulopathy such as DIC, platelets and coagula-tion factors may be replaced, using concentrates, cryoprecipitate, or fresh frozen plasma. Epsilon amnocaproic acid (Amicar) may be added to inhibit lysis of the clot by the fibrinolytic system.

Anemia

The workup should include a thorough physical assessment looking for the site of bleeding and the level of cardiorespiratory compensation. Laboratory examination should include complete blood count, reticulocyte count, lactic dehydrogenase, bilirubin, and a hemolysis screen if indicated. Transfusion of red blood cells is indicated if there is evidence of cardiac decompensation or if low hemoglobin levels are combined with low platelet counts. Transfusion of whole blood is not indicated unless there is massive bleeding and volume replacement cannot be accomplished by other means. Replacement of circulating red cell mass to improve oxygen carrying capacity should be accomplished by transfusion of packed red blood cells.

Nursing Management

Nursing Diagnoses for the Person with Cancer

- Potential disruption of skin integrity
- Potential disruption of oral mucous membrane
- Potential for vaginal/rectal mucositis
- Increased susceptibility to infection
- Fatigue associated with anemia

- Skin integrity; impaired
- Infection, potential
- Alteration in comfort
- Body image disturbance
- Body temperature altered
- Mobility impaired
- Gas exchange, impaired
- Communication, impaired
- Knowledge deficit
- Tissue integrity, impaired
- Sexuality patterns, altered
- Injury, potential
- Activity intolerance
- Anxiety, fear

Interventions: Disruption of skin integrity[4,7,16]

Assessment
- Inspect high risk skin areas for color, vascularity, edema, injuries, scars, lesions, nodules

Preventive measures to maintain intact skin
- Use draw sheet for turning and positioning

- Elevate head of bed to maximum of 30 degrees except for mealtimes
- Provide over-bed trapeze to assist in position change
- Use devices to provide protection and decrease pressure to sensitive areas
- Provide meticulous skin hygiene

Incontinence

- Offer bedpan and urinal every 2 hours
- Wash buttocks and perineum after each incontinence, pat or air dry
- Evaluate need for bowel and bladder retraining program

Immobility

- Use splints and braces to prevent contractures.
- Initiate referrals to rehabilitation medicine, social services, and vocational rehabilitation

Pruritus

- Maintain hydration of the skin by increasing fluid intake, apply water-soluble emollients to damp skin, and provide a humidified environment
- Use alternative methods of skin stimulation such as pressure, massage, vibration, and cold compresses

Interventions for Nonitact Skin

Assessment

- Inspect skin lesions and document: general character, location and distribution, configuration, size, morphologic structure, drainage, depth of lesion, presence of vital structure in lesion
- Monitor for signs and symptoms of infection

Nonulcerating lesions

- Use dry dressings to protect against irritation and trauma.
- Use occlusive dressings with topical medications for increased penetration

Ulcerating lesions

- Cleanse area with antibacterial soap using gentle motion. Rinse well. Prevent cross-contamination if local infection is present.
- Follow recommended protocol for debridement

Prevention and management of local infection
- Irrigate with antibacterial agent as prescribed
- Obtain specimens for culture as prescribed or if fever is present
- Apply dry, sterile, non-adherent dressing. Change and cleanse every eight hours or more often as needed

Hemostasis
- Use silver nitrate sticks or styptic pencils as prescribed for mild oozing.
- Apply 1:1000 epinephrine or topical thrombin to areas with moderate oozing as prescribed. Local radiation or application of hemostatic dressings may be used

Interventions: Disruption of oral mucous membranes[8,10]

Measures to decrease inflammation of mucous membranes
- Avoid exposure to chemical or physical irritants such as commercial mouthwashes, alcohol, tobacco, and hot and spicy or coarse foods
- Use a systematic oral care protocol, which includes oral hygiene measures before and after each meal and at bedtime as a minimum and every 2 hours around the clock when oral mucositis is present

Measures to increase comfort
- Use systemic analgesics when pain is uncontrolled by topical agents
- Safe, effective agents for oral care include normal saline (1 tsp/L of water) and sodium bicarbonate (1 tsp/L of water) alone or in combination (1:1)
- Brushing and flossing are the best defense against plaque build-up, but should be discontinued when the ANC is less than 1000 mm^3 and/or the platelet count is less than 50,000 mm^3 or mucositis is present. Toothettes or a gauze wrapped finger may be used instead
- Water soluble lubricants may be used for dry, cracked lips
- Dentures should be cleaned with a denture brush and an antimicrobial detergent such as chlorhexidine gluconate when oral care is done. Rinse with normal saline or water
- Modify dietary intake to include bland, soft or liquid foods (avoiding acidic foods and liquids) high in calories and protein, served at room temperature or cool, *not* hot or cold

Medical treatment
- Administer antibiotics, antifungals, analgesics, antivirals, dietary supplements, enteral, or parenteral nutrition as prescribed.
- For bleeding from oral mucosa, administer anti-fibrinolytics and platelets as prescribed, and/or apply topical thrombin and gelfoam.

Patient and Family Education
- Signs and symptoms of mucositis and infection
- Importance of fluids and adequate nutrition
- Necessity of dietary changes secondary to the presence or absence of oral and esophageal lesions
- Avoidance of trauma to mucous membranes secondary to smoking, alcohol, commercial mouthwash, poorly fitting dentures

Interventions: Vaginal/rectal mucositis[6,17]

Measures to decrease inflammation of mucous membranes
- Avoid exposure to chemical and physical irritants
- Encourage adequate fluid intake
- Wash perineum with soap and water following each urination and defecation; pat or air dry

Measures to minimize complications
- Modify dietary intake to minimize diarrhea and constipation
- Encourage frequent perineal hygiene measures
- Instruct female patients to wipe from front to back following urination and defecation
- Monitor patient for signs and symptoms of vaginal infection and/or rectal cellulitis/abcess.

Patient and Family Education
- Teach personal risk factors for development of mucositis —chemotherapy, radiation therapy.
- Teach signs and symptoms of mucositis, such as pain, itching, and discharge or drainage, which should be reported.

■ Identify situations that require professional interventions, such as fever, diarrhea, and uncontrolled pain.

Interventions: Increased susceptibility to infection[5,15]

General preventive measures
■ Wash hands with soap, water, and friction before and after all direct patient contact
■ Provide meticulous skin and oral hygiene for patient
■ Provide cooked diet only—no raw fruits or uncooked vegetables
■ Do not allow live plants or cut flowers in standing water in room
■ Avoid all sources of stagnant water in room such as water pitchers, denture cups, humidifiers, and respiratory therapy equipment. Change daily
■ Screen visitors for illnesses
■ Utilize Universal Precautions/OSHA requirements when caring for all patients

Interventions: Increased risk of bleeding[1,3,18]

General preventive measures
■ Limit invasive procedures
■ Avoid intramuscular injections
■ Avoid aspirin-containing medications or nonsteroidal anti-inflammatories
■ Suppress menses in premenopausal female patients by hormonal manipulation as ordered by the physician
■ Avoid hard toothbrushes or tooth flossing
■ Avoid use of rectal thermometers, suppositories, enemas, or rectal examinations
■ No alcohol-containing beverages

Assessment of bleeding
■ Apply pressure and/or pressure dressings to venipunctures, bone marrow aspiration and biopsy sites, and other sites of invasive procedures until hemostasis occurs
■ Observe sites of invasive procedures, such as vascular access device placement, for continued hemostasis and notify physician if bleeding is present or recurs

- Administer appropriate medications to prevent activities that raise intracranial pressure such as vomiting, coughing, sneezing, and straining in stool
- Report any complaints of headache with or without change in level of consciousness or vital signs
- Administer platelet transfusions and other blood component therapy as ordered

Patient and family education
- Assess for and report any evidence of frank bleeding including petechiae, purpura, and ecchymoses
- Avoid all aspirin-containing compounds. Read the label. Don't take any medications unless prescribed by your physician
- Report any feelings of increased weakness, change in stool color and consistency, emesis, headache, and change in level of consciousness

Intervention: Fatigue associated with anemia

Instructions include:
- Develop a progressive ambulation plan
- Seek assistance with such things as child care, meal planning and preparation, laundry, and house-cleaning
- Eat a nutritionally balanced diet
- Maintain usual patterns of sleep

Bibliography

1. Alexander EJ: Injury, potential for, related to thrombocytopenia. In McNally JC and others, editors: *Guidelines for oncology nursing practice,* ed 2, Philadelphia, 1991, WB Saunders.
2. Baird SB, McCorkle R, and Grant M: *Cancer nursing,* Philadelphia, 1991, WB Saunders.
3. Bavier AR: Alterations in hemostasis. In Johnson BL and Gross J, editors: *Handbook of oncology nursing,* New York, 1985, John Wiley & Sons.

4. Bord MA and others: Alteration in comfort, pruritus. In McNally JC and others, editors: *Guidelines for oncology nursing practice,* ed 2, Philadelphia, 1991, WB Saunders.

5. Brandt B: *Nursing protocol for the patient with neutropenia,* Oncol Nurs Forum 17(1s):9, 1990.

6. Clark JC: Mucous membrane integrity, impairment of, related to vaginal changes. In McNally JC and others, editors: *Guidelines for oncology nursing practice,* ed 2, Philadelphia, 1991, WB Saunders.

7. Couillard-Getreuer DL: Skin. In Johnson BL and Gross J, editors: *Handbook of oncology nursing,* New York, 1985, John Wiley & Sons.

8. Eilers J, Berger AM, and Peterson MC: *Development, testing and application of the oral assessment guide,* Oncol Nurs Forum 15:325, 1989.

9. Gallucci BB: *The immune system and cancer,* Oncol Nurs Forum 14(6s):3, 1987.

10. Goodman M and Stoner C: Mucous membrane integrity, impairment of, related to stomatitis. In McNally JC and others, editors: *Guidelines for oncology nursing practice,* ed 2, Philadelphia, 1991, WB Saunders.

11. Grady C: *Host defense mechanisms: an overview,* Semin Oncol Nurs 4(2):86, 1988.

12. Hughes WT: *Empiric antimicrobial therapy in the febrile granulocytopenic patient,* Infect Control Hosp Epidemiol 11:151, 1990.

13. Kluger MJ: *Fever: role of pyrogens and cryogens,* Physiol Rev 71:93, 1991.

14. Lieschke GJ and Burgess AW: *Granulocyte colony-stimulating factor and granulocyte-macrophage colony factor,* N Engl J Med 327:28, 1992.

15. McNally JC and Stair J: Potential for infection. In McNally JC and others, editors: *Guidelines for oncology nursing practice,* ed 2, Philadelphia, 1991, WB Saunders.

16. Owen P: Skin integrity, impairment of, related to malignant skin lesions. In McNally JC and others, editors: *Guidelines for oncology nursing practice,* ed 2, Philadelphia, 1991, WB Saunders.

17. Rostad M: *Current strategies for managing myelosuppression in patient with cancer,* Oncol Nurs Forum 18(2s):7, 1991.
18. Rostad M: Injury, potential for, related to anemia. In McNally JC and others, editors: *Guidelines for oncology nursing practice,* ed 2, Philadelphia, 1991, WB Saunders.
19. Styrt B: *Antipyresis and fever,* Arch Intern Med 150:1589, 1990.
20. Walsh TJ and others: *Empiric therapy with amphotericin B in febrile granulocytic patients,* Rev Infect Dis 13:496, 1991.

Psychosocial Issues

30

The Personal Meaning of Cancer

The meaning a cancer diagnosis holds for a particular individual is highly personal and is derived from numerous sources, including past experiences with cancer, cultural biases, the specific kind of cancer and necessary treatment and the potential responses from the treatments.[21]

Timing and Role Strain

Age and stage of life affect perceptions, understanding, and acceptance. The diagnosis of a malignancy in a child, young adult, or a person experiencing a productive middle age is often viewed as more devastating than in the elderly individual who has seemingly completed significant life events. Timing is significant not only in terms of development but also in relation to other stressors. Periods of life transitions, such as marriage, childbirth, retirement, or death in the family can intensify responses.[22]

Spiritual Distress

The person with cancer and those with whom significant relationships are shared may experience some degree of spiritual distress as they struggle with the effects of the diagnosis and its meaning. The perceived misfortune or tragedy uncovers concerns about the unfair distribution of suffering in the world. This often begs a confrontation with the concept of a kind and loving God. Attempts to explain or transform bad into good and pain into privilege are often used to defend God.[8]

Providing Support for Psychosocial Adjustment

Interdisciplinary Team Approach

Interdisciplinary team care is the standard in quality care delivery and may involve: nurse, physician, psychologist, psychiatrist, clergy, social worker, counselor, volunteer.

Structured Assessment

Structured assessment or data can determine the capacity of the patient and family to manage the situation. Symptom and well-being inventories can be used to measure anxiety, depression, hostility, general distress or well-being.[12,13,14]

As a result of nursing and other team members' assessments, numerous nursing diagnoses related to psychosocial care can be made (Box 30-1).

Adaptation Process

Adaptation to cancer can be addressed from several time frames: initial diagnosis, treatment, recurrence, advanced disease, and death, or long-term survival. The needs of the individual differ at each point on the continuum.

Initial Diagnosis and Treatment

The primary concern of the newly diagnosed person is life versus death. They experience an acute grief reaction to the diagnosis itself and the uncertainty of the outcome. During the initial diagnostic and treatment stage, the individual and family are often overwhelmed and have trouble comprehending all that is said.[9,10]

Recurrence

When cure is not feasible, the goal of therapy is control, or the longest possible disease-free period. This goal presents the patient and family with the double-edged sword of hope and fear. The psychosocial response to a recurrence is dependent on several variables: current symptoms, functional status, previous experience with cancer therapy, and ongoing expectations since initial diagnosis.[6]

Box 30-1

Nursing Diagnoses Related to Psychosocial Care*

Adjustment, impaired
Anxiety
Body image disturbance
Caregiver role strain
Coping, defensive
Coping, family: potential for growth
Coping, ineffective family: compromised
Coping, ineffective family: disabling
Coping, ineffective individual
Decisional conflict (specify)
Denial, ineffective
Family processes, altered
Fear
Grieving, anticipatory
Grieving, dysfunctional
High risk for caregiver role strain
Impaired communication (decreased attention and concentration)

Impaired problem-solving
Ineffective management of therapeutic regimen
Knowledge deficit (specify)
Noncompliance (specify)
Parenting, altered
Parenting, altered, potential
Powerlessness related to illness and hospitalization
Relocation stress syndrome
Self-esteem, disturbance
Self-esteem, chronic low
Self-esteem, situational low
Sleep disturbance related to anxiety and/or depression
Social interaction, impaired
Social isolation
Spiritual distress (distress of the human spirit)
Violence, potential for: self-directed or directed at others

*NANDA approved — 1992

Long-term Survival

When the individual's disease-free period ends, the fear of recurrence seems to decrease. A vital component of the care of people experiencing disease-free status is to provide them with current, appropriate information regarding the significance of the length of the disease-free interval in relation to their particular situation and the important role of follow-up.[4,11,23]

Patient and Family Coping Strategies

Alterations in Coping

Positive coping strategies have been characterized by several different types of behaviors. The following list provides examples of some strategies, identified by specific behaviors.[9,10,21]

- Avoidance behaviours are minimal: denial of the potential problem is minimized by gaining appropriate information, including referrals to appropriate health care providers.
- Problems are redefined into a solvable form such as: scheduling therapy to minimize disruptions in work and family activities.
- Realities are confronted: the possible outcomes of cancer therapies are realistically acknowledged and addressed.
- Alternatives are considered such as: having a backup plan for needed child care arrangements.
- Open and mutual communication with significant others is maintained: the feelings, concerns, and anxieties of the individual and significant others are addressed with honesty by both parties.
- Constructive help, including adequate medical care, is sought. The individual seeks a second opinion or actively searches for health care providers with whom he or she feels comfortable.
- Support is accepted when offered and assertive behaviors is used when necessary. The individual accepts support that is helpful and recognizes behaviours that are not helpful.
- Morale is enhanced through self-reliance or the use of available resources. The individual pursues activities that are personally meaningful and in addition recognizes that

compromises may need to be made, such as working part-time or reducing the amount of time spent in volunteer activities.

- Self-concept is as important as symptom relief and the individual who, while living with compromise, maintains a sense of control and does not behave as if powerless, continues to value self as a functioning being.
- Hope is self-pride, not self-deception. The ability to hope for a cure, increased life expectancy, or for an inevitable peaceful death does not indicate a lack of knowledge or understanding of the situation. Hope may include time-focused activities, such as the desire to witness the birth of a first grandchild. Ineffective coping strategies include: withdrawal, suppression, the excessive use of alcohol or other drugs, passive acceptance, and reckless impulsive behaviors. It is important to note that the individual or family may use an ineffective style in an isolated situation, usually in response to extreme stress.

Maladaptive coping may manifest itself as three or more of the following behaviors:[1,3,12]

- Poor eye contact and little facial expression, slow speech
- Nonfluctuating, generally negative mood
- Appetite significantly depressed, refusing adequate nutrition
- Sleep pattern characterized by early morning awakening, insomnia, or excessive daytime sleeping
- Lack of attention to hygiene and activities of daily living

Crisis Theory

Crisis is a state provoked when a person faces an important obstacle in relation to life goals and for a time finds it insurmountable through the use of customary problem-solving methods. Crisis theory describes three phases of response. In the precrisis phase the individual seeks to maintain equilibrium by adapting to physical and psychosocial changes within the context of normal life events. The crisis phase is characterized by disorganization. Attempts are made to solve the problem, which may or may not be successful.[14,16,17,19]

In the postcrisis phases, successful problem resolution reduces the crisis and can influence the individual's functioning in future crisis situations. If the postcrisis period is marked by deterioration in physical and emotional function, the individual may function at a level lower than in the precrisis state. If new skills are learned and personal growth occurs, future functioning may be at a higher level of coping.

Psychosocial Staging

As goals of therapy are adjusted to the stage of disease progression, likewise supportive care is adjusted to various psychosocial stages of response to the disease process that can be considered in conjunction with the physical stage of disease.[21,22]

- *Stage I: Existential Plight*—the first 100 days following diagnosis; as time progresses, the initial shock becomes focused on coping with treatment plans and therapy side effects.
- *Stage II: Mitigation and Accommodation*—this stage encompasses the issues faced during remission or the time after which cure is designated; adjustments are related to long-term side effects and the fear of recurrence; reinvestment in life occurs as plans for the future are again made.
- *Stage III: Decline and Deterioration*—recurrence signals a time-limited prognosis; realization of disease return may be related to the degree of symptoms experienced.
- *Stage IV: Preterminality and Terminality*—this stage acknowledges the beginning of the dying process; symptom control and personal choices should guide care.

Maximizing Quality of Life for Patient and Family

Survivorship

From the time of its discovery and for the balance of life, an individual diagnosed with cancer is considered a survivor. During the experience the individual first fights to beat the disease and then to sustain disease-free survival. Survivorship brings with it many aspects of rehabilitation. The physical, psychosocial, vocational, and financial effects of cancer are receiving more attention than ever.[3,4]

Cancer rehabilitation may be defined as the process of minimizing the physical, psychologic, social, and vocational dysfunction that may result from the disease or its treatment. Rehabilitation measures are aimed at restoration of function and prevention of further complications and include compensatory and supportive measures.[7,11,16]

Physical Rehabilitation

Physical rehabilitation should begin as soon as the likelihood of disability is recognized, such as the amputation of body part or limb, the loss of voice, the loss of bowel/bladder function. Functional restoration will be dependent on the degree of impairment, disability, or handicap experienced. Other physical changes, such as impaired fertility, may be the source of distress requiring psychosocial rehabilitation.[2,7]

Psychosocial Rehabilitation

Psychosocial needs are best assessed in a systematic manner that includes information about the family makeup and relationships, work history, religious and community involvements, educational status, financial resources, and, when possible, clues to prior coping mechanisms.[19,23]

Employment/Vocational Rehabilitation

The Americans with Disabilities Act (ADA) of 1990 requires equal opportunity in selection, testing, and hiring of qualified applicants with disabilities, including individuals with cancer or a history of cancer. This law prohibits discrimination against workers with disabilities and is similar to the Civil Rights Act of 1964 and Title V of the Rehabilitation Act of 1973.

Unless the effects of disease or treatment directly affect the individual's ability to perform the essential functions of a job there is no obligation to disclose information. The employee should be prepared to educate the employer and to stress specific job qualifications and abilities. The employer is required to provide reasonable accommodation. The Equal Employment Opportunity Commission (EEOC) assumes the federal government role of enforcing the standard. Local government offices can assist in investigations or claims.[2,7]

Finances, Insurance, and the Law

Currently no federal law guarantees a right to adequate health insurance. Cancer survivors do have the opportunity of keeping the health insurance obtained through their employer even after they are no longer employed. This opportunity is provided through The Comprehensive Omnibus Budget Reconciliation Act (COBRA) and The Employee Retirement and Income Security Act (ERISA). The COBRA plan can provide short-term coverage while seeking new employment or a new group plan. The ERISA law entitles the individual to file a claim when benefits are denied through discrimination. The ERISA law is enforced by the Pension and Welfare Benefits Administration of the United States Department of Labor.

Providing Comfort in Terminal Care

When cure or disease control are no longer attainable goals, there is a shift to palliative care. The transition into this phase may be gradual and the shifts in care needs are not always recognized and acknowledged. As caregiving needs change, role strain may increase. The distinct needs of the patient and the caregiver must be recognized.

Advanced Directives

A Supreme Court ruling has affirmed the constitutional right of liberty to refuse any medical treatment, including life-prolonging procedures and the right to name an agent to be a surrogate decision-maker for health care issues when the individual loses the personal capacity to do so. These rights are proclaimed by enacting an advance directive that is a signed, dated, and witnessed document. Some states require notarization of the document. The individual who signs such a document must provide copies to their family, physician, and other appropriate individuals and discuss the specific details with these individuals.

Hospice Care

Discussion of care goals will lead to planning for a method of care-delivery. The setting and use of available health care agencies are determined by the individual situation. Hospice involves physical care, counseling services, volunteer assistance, respite care, support at the time of death, and bereavement follow-up.

Bereavement

With long-term illness, there is an opportunity to prepare for the actual loss by anticipating it. The degree of emotional attachment and quality of communication within relationships influence the impact and outcome of grief. Constant pain, suffering, and a protracted death can increase the emotional pain. During the period of anticipation, the family may not only rehearse the impending death and feel depressed but also attempt to readjust their lives.[22]

The time necessary for grief resolution is highly variable. Behavioral adaptation may be a response to societal expectations and not a barometer of emotional healing. Clear evidence of grief resolution may be the ability to speak of the lost relationship comfortably and realistically, recounting pleasures and disappointments of the relationship. There are no timetables for grief and bereavement. The extent of follow-up must be individualized to the bereaved's needs and the constraints of the professional and institutional resources. Focus on high-risk needs and further referrals may be the priority.[14,15]

Support for the Caregiver

Priority-Setting

Priority-setting often parallels a hierarchy of needs. Physical needs must be met first. Emotional and social needs are more complex. The individual who successfully meets these needs may experience the personal growth that permits addressing spiritual needs. Care demands must be assessed in light of the priorities. The clarification of goals and priorities fosters shared responsibilities. The level of communication needed to establish priorities can also aid in minimizing demands, making problems manageable, and preventing burnout.[15,19]

Burnout is a syndrome of physical and personal exhaustion accompanied by negative attitudes and loss of concern for self and others. Family members and professional caregivers alike risk such a response when giving highly specialized care in emotionally charged situations. A cycle of frustration, helplessness, and cynicism can develop. The risk of burnout can be reduced by voicing frustration appropriately, developing a support system, setting priorities, and establishing reasonable expectations.

Life Enhancement Skills

Life enhancement begins with self-care. Attending to the needs of others must be balanced with attending to one's own needs. A nutritious diet, adequate sleep, and physical exercise aid in physical self-care. Psychic and social comfort can be achieved through a variety of activities that provide a form of decompression. Prodromal signs of distress or inappropriate coping must be recognized and confronted. Life enhancement skills are developed from a philosophy of being true to self, a personal spirituality, and commitment to caring for self and others. These skills can include such things as exercise, reading, writing, crafts, hobbies, music, dance, drama, and humor.

Nursing Management

Facilitate Positive Coping

1. Promote self-care
   - Nurse's role as coach, teacher, interpretor
   - Promote self-care
   - Assist patient/family with goal setting
   - Referrals-counseling, community programs
   - Behavioral techniques
     - relaxation
     - hypnosis
     - imagery
     - biofeedback
2. Patient's sense of maintaining control
3. Assist the patient with goal-setting
4. Refer for counseling

Bibliography

1. Doublsky J: Ineffective individual coping, In McNally JC and others, editors: *Guidelines for oncology nursing practice,* ed 2, Philadelphia, 1991, WB Saunders.
2. Dudas S and Carlson C: *Cancer rehabilitation,* Oncol Nurs Forum 15:183, 1988.

3. DuFault SK and others: Ineffective family coping, In McNally JC and others, editors: *Guidelines for oncology nursing practice,* ed 2, Philadelphia, 1991, WB Saunders.

4. Germino B: The impact of cancer on the patient, the family, and the nurse. In *Living with cancer: fifth national conference on cancer nursing,* New York, 1987, American Cancer Society.

5. Harvey CD and Heiney SP: Grieving, In McNally JC and others, editors: *Guidelines for oncology nursing practice,* ed 2, Philadelphia, 1991, WB Saunders.

6. Herth K: *The relationship between level of hope and level of coping, response and other variables in patients with cancer,* Oncol Nurs Forum 16(1):67, 1989.

7. Hoffman B: *Cancer survivors at work: job problems and illegal discrimination,* Oncol Nurs Forum 16(1):39, 1989.

8. Kubler-Ross E: *On death and dying,* New York, 1969, Macmillan.

9. Larson P: *Important nurse caring behaviors perceived by patients with cancer,* Oncol Nurs Forum 11(6):46, 1984.

10. Lind S and others: *Telling the diagnosis of cancer,* J Clin Oncol 7(5):583, 1989.

11. Loescher LJ and others: *Surviving adult cancers. Part 1. Physiologic effects,* Ann Intern Med 111(5):411, 1989.

12. Massie M and Holland J: *Assessment and management of the cancer patient with depression,* Advances in Psychosomatic Medicine 18:1, 1988.

13. Mor V and Masterson-Allen S: *The hospice model of care for the terminally ill,* Adv Psychosom Med 18:119, 1988.

14. North American Nursing Diagnoses Association: *Conference Proceedings,* St Louis, 1992, The Association.

15. Northouse L: *Family issues in cancer care,* Adv Psychosom Med 18:82, 1988.

16. Oberst M and others: *Caregivers demands and appraisal of stress among family caregivers,* Cancer Nurs 12(4):209, 1989.

17. Quigley K: *The adult cancer survivor: psychosocial consequences of cure,* Semin Oncol Nurs 5(1):63, 1989.

18. Rickel LM: *Making mountains manageable: maximizing quality of life through crisis intervention,* Oncol Nurs Forum 14(4):29, 1987.

19. Simko LO: Psychosocial dimensions of cancer. In Groenwald SL, editor: *Cancer nursing principles and practice,* ed 3, Boston, 1993, Jones & Bartlett.

20. Thorne SE: *Helpful and unhelpful communications in cancer care: the patient perspective,* Oncol Nurs Forum 15(2):167, 1988.

21. Wegman J: *Hospice home death, hospital death, and coping abilities of widows,* Cancer Nurs 10(3):153, 1987.

22. Weisman AD: *Coping with cancer,* New York, 1979, McGraw-Hill.

23. Weisman AD and Worden WJ: *The emotional plight of cancer: significance of the first 100 days,* Int J Psychiatry Med 7(1):145, 1976-77.

24. Welch-McCaffrey D and others: *Surviving adult cancers. Part 2. Psychological implications,* Ann Intern Med 11(6):517, 1989.

Impact of Cancer on Sexuality

31

Human beings are sexual from the time of birth until their death, and being sexual is a primary part of being human. If this factor is dismissed by the nurse or physician, the patient often perceives him- or herself as less than human. Until recently, health care professionals have been inclined to focus on the physical and emotional aspects of the human being while overlooking the psychosexual. This has been especially true with patients who are disabled, chronically ill, or over the age of 62.

Increased confidence in sexual assessment and intervention may be attained if specific information and "how-to's" are made available. The Oncology Nursing Society and American Nurses Association Outcome Standards for Cancer Nursing Practice have provided guidelines for the nurse, which include the area of sexuality.[8]

Psychosocial Development Through the Life Cycle

A person's sexual expression will vary throughout the life cycle. Although personal beliefs and values are influential, interference with the psychosexual stages of development by an event like disease may cause sexual dysfunction (Table 31-1). For the cancer patient, passage from one stage to the next may be precluded by the disease and its treatment or prognosis. Awareness of these stages will help the caregiver recognize patients at risk for possible sexual dysfunction.[1,15]

Table 31-1 Psychosexual Stages of Development

Stage	Basic Psychosocial Task	Sexual Tasks
Infancy (0-2 years)	Acquiring basic trust, learning to walk, talk	Gender identity
Childhood (2-12 years)	Acquiring sense of autonomy vs. shame and doubt; entering and adjusting to school	Pleasure-pain associated with sexual organs and eliminative functions; masturbation takes place with resulting shame and acceptance; secondary sex characteristics become evident
Adolescence (13-20) years)	Acquiring sense of identity vs. role confusion	Mastery over impulse control, acceptance of conflict between moral proscription and sexual urges, handling new physiologic functions (menses for girls and ejaculation for boys)
Young adulthood (20-45 years)	Acquiring sense of intimacy vs. isolation; vocational effectiveness; interpersonal security, "sexual adequacy"	Sexual adequacy and performance plus fertility concerns and questions related to parenting

Middle adulthood (50-70 years)	Acquiring sense of self-esteem vs. despair; adjusting to diminution of one's energy and competence; "empty nest syndrome" plus care of aging parents or their death; adjusting to change in physique and evidence of aging	For females, menopause and resulting vasomotor changes, atrophy of breasts, clitoral size, and vaginal lubrication; for males, delay on attaining an erection, a reduced compulsion to ejaculate, episodic impotence, possible prostatitis
Old age	Adjusting to loss of friends, family, confrontations with old age and dying, painful joint conditions, reduced hearing and visual acuity; adjustment to social stigmatization of being "old"	Reduced vitality, fear of incompetence or injury (coital coronary); fear of being viewed as "dirty old person," unavailability of a partner (widowhood); limited physical capacity and reduced options

Reprinted with permission from Schain W: Sexual problems of patients with cancer. In DeVita VT, Hellman S, and Rosenberg SA, editors: *Cancer: principles and practice of oncology,* 1985, JB Lippincott.

Anticipation of and Adaption to the Effects of Cancer

Sense of Adequacy

The *male sexual response* (desire, subjective arousal, erection, emission, ejaculation, and orgasm) has separate mechanisms of control and can therefore be affected independently. Although cancer therapy may destroy the capability for an erection, the pleasure of sexual arousal and orgasm often remains intact. This factor is important because men are often worried about whether they can function as they did before.

Female sexual response (desire, subjective arousal, vaginal expansion and lubrication, and orgasm) is not as well understood. Women with cancer may lose sexual desire during debilitating treatment, especially if the therapy affects the structure or innervation of the clitoris or vagina. This, along with painful intercourse, are factors that tend to interfere with orgasm. Emphasis here is on perceived damage resulting from therapy, which women feel will lead to rejection from their partner.[16,17,19]

Sense of Self-Esteem

Cancer patients are at much greater risk of having a negative body image because of mutilating surgery and devastating side effects of therapy. Cancer and its treatment can produce considerable loss of economic independence, alter role behavior and significant relationships, and reduce sexual responsiveness.[10]

Gratification and Performance

Cancer patients often feel undesirable and unattractive and, because they are now typecast as "ill," feel they are not supposed to be sexual. It has been reported that these patients desire touch more than overt sexual activity. The reason for this is unclear but may be related to side effects, fatigue, weakness, and pain, which all cause diminished libido.[11]

Site-Specific Issues Affecting Sexualtiy

The following nursing diagnoses apply to the nursing interventions that will be discussed in the Nursing Management section at the end of the chapter.

Principal Nursing Diagnoses

- Sexual dysfunction related to impotence, ineffective coping, lack of knowledge, change or loss of body part, and physiologic limitations
- Disturbance in self-esteem related to change in body image, self-concept, role performance, and personal identity

Secondary Nursing Diagnoses

- Activity intolerance related to fatigue
- Alteration in comfort related to acute/chronic pain, which decreases sexual desire
- Impaired verbal communication related to tracheostomy
- Social isolation related to cancer (incontinence, disfiguring surgery, superstitions of others)

Head and Neck Cancer

Many patients are more than 60 years of age at the time of diagnosis and may be entering a period of adjustment to a diminished sexual drive. The patient may also be an alcoholic, which will influence treatment and the rehabilitation process.[13,21] Patients with head and neck cancer often require rehabilitation, which may be accomplished with reconstructive surgery or prostheses or both. It is important to keep in mind that the expectations of the patient may differ from actual treatment results.

Sarcomas of Bone and Soft Tissue and Limb Amputation

Major limb amputation creates emotional hurdles for patients' perception of themselves, as well as acceptance by their partners. A decrease in self-esteem and a negative body image are common because of the presence of a gross defect that is obvious even when covered with clothes. The male may equate the loss of a limb to the loss of manhood. Some patients may view the surgery as a punishment for past transgressions.[7,19]

Hematologic Malignancies

Most men and women experience reduced desire for sexual intercourse during chemotherapy treatments, particularly during the first few days after receiving their drugs. This is usually due to increased weakness, fatigue, and intermittent nausea and vomiting.[25] Lack of sexual eagerness can also be induced by an effect on the testes or ovaries. Hormone levels can decrease resulting in difficulty with erections and vaginal dryness.

Myelosuppression and its consequences can cause fatigue and shortness of breath, which decrease sexual desire. Concern about bleeding and infection will be present due to low platelet and white blood cell/absolute neutrophil counts. A discussion may be needed to assess the feelings of the spouse or significant other. It is helpful to identify ways they can support the client's feelings of self-worth and masculinity or femininity.

Breast Cancer

Mastectomy makes an obvious change in the body's contour, which can lead to fears about loss of identity as a woman and a desirable sexual being. The partner's perceived importance of a breast can also impact the female's perspective should she choose mastectomy.[17,23]

A woman's response to treatment for breast cancer and its corresponding threat to sexuality will depend on several conditions:

- Her feelings about her femininity
- The value she bestows on her missing breast
- Her physical discomfort
- The response of her significant other
- The reinforcement she receives from the nurse regarding her sexual identity
- Her sense of self-worth

Female Pelvic and Genital Cancer

Surgical resection and/or radiation therapy for cancer of the cervix, uterus, ovary, vulva, diethylstilbestrol (DES) exposure, and bladder can be either simple or quite extensive. Women faced with this type of treatment have many apprehensions:[24]

- Threat to life
- Feelings of lost femininity
- Concern about what their external region will look like
- Ability to have intercourse and, if so, whether it will be painful
- Fear that along with loss of fertility will come loss of vitality and orgasmic potential
- Fear of physical aging, diminished libido, loss of vaginal lubrication, and dyspareunia

Male Pelvic Cancer

When the malignancy involves the prostate, testicle, or penis, there is a temporary or permanent disturbance in relation to erection, emission, and ejaculation. Orgasm is not as frequently affected and can actually be achieved even when genital function is lost. To promote adjustment and sexual rehabilitation, support and assistance for the patient and his partner are essential through knowledge and specific interventions.[26]

Colorectal Cancer

Regardless of the type of surgical diversion performed (colostomy, ileostomy, or urinary diversion), patients express many common reactions. These reactions may include: (1) greater-than-expected fatigue and weakness; (2) feelings of fragility and vulnerability to harm; (3) despair at the initial viewing of the stoma; (4) feelings of invalidism and depression; (5) fear of accidents, odor, leakage, and staining; (6) excessive emotional investment in the stoma; and (7) feelings of lost personal control.

Lung Cancer

Quality of life is always an important factor in relation to the person with cancer and should be especially important to those with a shortened life expectancy. Since treatment for these people is often palliative rather than curative, it is important to consider their feelings of masculinity, femininity, and self-esteem, along with the basic aspects of care such as pain control. Due to the often rapidly fatal nature of lung cancer, the patient and partner must make significant decisions and adjustments, which often affect the patient's sense of self-esteem and worthiness: (1) if the patient has been a smoker, he or she will probably have tremendous feelings of guilt to overcome or deal with; (2) if the patient's performance status is poor and remains so due to fatigue and weakness, he/she will be unable to continue as a productive member of the family; (3) if the patient/partner decides to take treatment (chemotherapy, radiation therapy), energy must be expended to cope with the side effects; and (4) if the patient/partner decides not to take treatment, there will be issues to resolve such as coping with an early death and caregiving. All these factors will affect the relationship the patient has with his or her partner, and it is no wonder there may be little time, energy, or desire for intimacy.[1,2,8]

Special Issues Influencing Sexuality

The Gerontologic Patient

When providing sexual counseling for the elderly, be aware that all couples will not be interested in sexual activity. Respect for this option is necessary. Various methods of sexual relating besides vaginal intercourse should be discussed with an elderly couple. For those patients who still have the desire for sexual involvement, the nurse may wish to suggest the following:

- For the partners to achieve lubrication and erection, longer precoital stimulation may be needed to compensate for slowed physical response.
- During prolonged hospitalization or nursing home confinement, privacy should be provided for couples to hold, touch, fondle, and have intercourse if desired. This applies to couples of any age.
- Warm baths, gentle massage, caressing and touching, masturbation, and fantasy all provide a sense of satisfaction and reassurance.

The Homosexual Patient

It must never be assumed that all patients have or wish to have a partner *or* that all partners are of the opposite sex. It is the nurse's responsibility to be knowledgeable about the entire patient population and not be judgmental. All patients are entitled to competence and a caring attitude.

Due to inexperience in the area of sensitivity to behavioral cues, obtaining information about sexual orientation may be missed because staff do not ask the right questions. Rather than asking about a spouse, husband, or wife, the nurse can ask the client if he or she is sexually active or whether they have a significant other.[16] Questions about sexual activity may deal with sexual preference such as "Do you prefer sexual activity with women, men, or both?"[5,10,12]

Sterility, Infertility, and Pregnancy

Generally speaking, male fertility is more susceptible to damage than the female's because of the constant mitotic cycles needed for spermatogenesis versus the relative inactivity of the female oocyte. Testes are more susceptible to injury than ovaries because rapidly dividing cells are most often affected by cancer therapies. Consequently, many chemotherapeutic agents alone, and especially in combination, can cause azospermia, oligospermia, or permanent sterility. Alkylating agents such as nitrogen mustard, cyclophosphamide, and chlorambucil cause sterility in the majority of treated males. However, depending on the drugs used, drug dose, and length of treatment, fertility may return, and the time frame can vary from 15 to 49 months after completion of therapy. Successful pregnancy is often limited due to abnormalities of the pretreatment sperm specimen. Frequently, the sperm have poor motility, and there is a growing number of patients who have attempted in vitro fertilization as treatment for male infertility with reported successes. Age is a factor for the female concerning possible ovarian dysfunction after treatment with chemotherapy because there are progressively fewer germ cells in the aging ovary.

Making a decision whether or not to treat the patient during pregnancy should take into consideration several factors: (1) gestation age of the fetus; (2) maternal and fetal health at the time of diagnosis; (3) mother's prognosis and likelihood of future pregnancies after treatment; and (4) the known teratogenic effects of the drugs to be used. Pregnancy after chemotherapy is not usually discouraged, although some oncologists are concerned about recurrence facilitated by hormonal and immunologic changes.[4,20,23,25]

Assessing and Preserving the Sexual Health of the Cancer Patient

Nursing Assessment Techniques

When performing a sexual health assessment, several elements can enhance both the nurse's and the patient's comfort during the discussion. Key elements that will promote optimal patient teaching can be found in Box 31-1.

Box 31-1

Sexual Health Assessment

- Privacy is essential when doing the assessment.
- Assure the patient of confidentiality.
- Try to obtain a sexual history early in your association with the patient. This implies that sexuality is an important and natural part of good health.
- Avoid overreaction in your verbal and nonverbal communication.
- Move from less sensitive to more sensitive issues.
- Determine the patient's goals for treatment.
- Realize when a problem is too complex to handle or when you do not know enough to be therapeutic and refer the problem.

VerSteeg describes an early assessment approach that is more comprehensive and addresses the following areas:[15]

- *Couple's relationship*
- *Understanding of cancer and its treatments*
- *Impact on sexuality*
- *Preparation for changes*
- *Planning and participation in care*
- *Control and optimism will help*
- *Expansion of sexuality*

The PLISSIT is a model frequently used for sexuality counseling or as a nursing intervention. Each step is taken depending on the nurse's knowledge and comfort level.[3]

- *P = permission*
- *LI = limited information*

- *SS = specific suggestions.*
- *IT = intensive therapy.*

A more complete model has been created by Schain.[19] Her model uses eight letters—PLEASURE—to cue the nurse to the topic area and to represent a good feeling.[3,15]

- *P = partner*
- *L = lovemaking*
- *E = emotions*
- *A = attitude*
- *S = symptoms*
- *U = understanding*
- *R = reproduction*
- *E = energy*

Nursing Management

Head and Neck Cancer

Interventions

- Sugarless mints and artificial saliva help freshen stale breath caused by a dry mouth.
- Candles, scented or not, can provide a relaxed ambience for both patient and partner.
- Tracheostomies should be cleaned of mucus and covered lightly during sexual activity.
- Partners should be made aware that the patient's heavy breathing may sound different..
- Various positions may need to be tried for sexual activity because the partner may be fearful of cutting off the patient's air supply.

Limb Amputation

Interventions

- If balance and movement are problems, pillows or other forms of cushions may be used to maintain a level pelvis.

- The female may need to assume the superior position during coitus.
- An upper extremity amputee may wish to use a side-lying position with the existing arm free to balance themselves.[7,8]

Hematologic Malignancies

Interventions

- The patient who is neutropenic should be advised against oral and anal sexual manipulation. The couple may bathe together.
- The importance of contraceptive measures during chemotherapy and radiation must be emphasized to all patients.
- Encourage sperm banking before initiation of chemotherapy.[8]

Breast Cancer

Interventions

- Until the woman is ready to disrobe or let her partner touch the wound area, she can wear a fancy camisole or short nightgown.
- The couple may make love by candlelight to decrease the impact of the change in body contour.
- Since many women derive great pleasure from stroking, sucking, and manipulation of the breast during foreplay, the remaining breast can continue to be stimulated if the woman so desires. Reassure the patient that manipulation will not cause another breast cancer.[14,19]

Female Pelvic and Genital Cancer

Interventions

Radical Hysterectomy

If a long-term indwelling catheter is present, vaginal sexual relations can be impeded. Partners may change positions, and rear entry intercourse can be practiced. Alternate ways of expressing physical love can also be fulfilling and can include oral, anal, and digital expressions.[13,18]

Pelvic Exenteration

To assure the most beneficial adjustment psychologically and sexually for the patient and her partner, it is necessary to provide specific alternatives and realistic information *before* surgery. After reconstruction there is usually decreased vaginal sensation. To promote total healing and the ability to detect early recurrence, a waiting period of 12 to 18 months is advised before resumption of sexual intercourse.[9,24]

Alternatives to sexual intercourse available to women who have had vaginal reconstruction and to those not interested in such surgery may include: nudity, cuddling, and general pleasuring; autoeroticism and mutual masturbation with a partner; oral-genital relations and anal love play; and fantasy.

Radical Vulvectomy and Cystectomy

It is imperative that the patient's partner be included in all education and counseling because of the radical nature of the treatment and long recuperative period after therapy.

Problems identified are vaginal tightness and dryness and self-conscious anxiety because of the ostomy. Scarring can develop as well as numbness and lost sensation due to impaired innervation of the perineum. Recommended remedies may include a vaginal estrogen cream and vaginal dilators to help decrease dyspareunia. Most women like to cover their ostomy appliance with a fabric cover, and feminine lingerie may also be worn during sexual activity. Kegel exercises are helpful to relieve tension and decrease dyspareunia.[24]

Radiation Therapy

The vagina will react to radiation by becoming shorter and narrower, having adhesions and problems with lubrication. The nurse may suggest the following:

- Continued sexual intercourse during treatment is usually encouraged to decrease possible adhesions and prevent shortening.
- A good water-soluble lubricating jelly is always needed to decrease vaginal discomfort.

- During sexual activity, the hips may be elevated or the adducted thighs lubricated to emulate a deeper vaginal barrel and improve sexual stimulation for a male partner.
- Vaginal dilators can be used if a woman does not have a sexual partner or is not sexually active.

Male Pelvic Cancer
Interventions
Prostate
One of the most important issues in the area of male pelvic cancers may be to help the patient and his partner develop a change in attitude toward sexual intercourse if erection is no longer possible or if it is impaired.[6,11,22]

- Many men become sexually aroused with erotic books, pictures, and/or movies.
- Long periods of foreplay, including romantic dinners, showering or bathing together, and using different rooms for lovemaking, may be stimulating.
- If full erections is not possible, mutual masturbation may allow the patient to reach orgasm and ejaculation.
- The risks and benefits of penile implants should be explained to the couple. Schover recommends waiting 6 months after surgery before installing a prosthesis.
- Intracavernous injections into the penis using papaverine to stimulate erections is becoming a common treatment.

Testicle
- Stress the fact that normal sexual desire and pleasurable sensations, erection, and orgasm will probably continue. If sexual desire is lost, serum testosterone should be checked; replacement therapy may be needed.
- Alpha-adrenergic stimulating drugs can increase ejaculation and occasionally the intensity of orgasm for some patients who have had retroperitoneal lymph node dissection.

Penis
- If partial penectomy has occurred, men report erections and orgasms of normal or near normal intensity with the phallic stump.

- Female partners must be advised to have a yearly Pap smear since they may be at risk for cervical cancer from exposure to the human papilloma virus.

Cystectomy

In addition to the interventions mentioned previously, the following are a few ways to decrease anxiety from a urostomy:[22]

- Before intercourse, the appliance should be emptied. Some patients secure the bag with a supportive belt.
- Like females, males may choose to wear a cover over their ostomy bag.
- To avoid friction on the stoma and pouch, other positions besides the missionary position may be tried.
- Some patients like to have their stomas touched during lovemaking, but they must be reminded that the stoma is fragile and too much rubbing may cause tearing. Objects should not be placed into the stoma.

Colorectal Cancer

Interventions

- Prepare the pouch before sexual activity by emptying and assuring the seal. If the ostomy is dry or controllable with irrigation, a small cover or patch may be sufficient cover.
- Deodorize the pouch (1 or 2 drops of Banish is helpful) and avoid foods that cause gas.
- Wear attractive camouflage like a cummerbund or cloth cover for the pouch.

Lung Cancer

Interventions

The nurse should encourage lung cancer patients and their partners to experience sexual closeness that does not necessarily lead to intercourse, which can exacerbate excessive fatigue and dyspnea. The following suggestions may be helpful:[1,2]

- When experiencing sexual closeness, the significant other should continue to treat the patient as a partner rather than an invalid.

- Being physically close, hand holding, sharing an intimate moment will enhance feelings of maleness and femaleness.
- Soft caressing or light massage with oils or creams is sensual and can help reduce pain/discomfort.

Bibliography

1. Bernhard J and Ganz P: *Psychosocial issues in lung cancer patients (Part 1),* Chest 99:1, 1991.
2. Bernhard J and Ganz P: *Psychosocial issues in lung cancer patients* (Part 2), Chest 99:2, 1991.
3. Cooley M, Yeomans A, Cobb S: *Sexual and reproductive issues for women with Hodgkin's disease: application of PLISSIT model,* Cancer Nurs 9:248, 1986.
4. Doll D, Ringenberg Q, and Yarbro Y: *Management of cancer during pregnancy,* Arch Intern Med 148, 1988.
5. Ducharma S and Gill K: *Sexual values, training and professional roles,* J Head Trauma Rehab 5:2, 1990.
6. Gritz E and others: *Long term effects of testicular cancer on sexual functioning in married couples,* Cancer 64:1989.
7. Heiney S: *Adolescents with cancer: sexual and reproductive issues,* Cancer Nursing 12:2, 1989.
8. Hogan CM: Sexuality dysfunction related to disease process and treatment, In McNally JC and others, editors: *Guidelines for oncology nursing practice,* ed 2, Philadelphia, 1991, WB Saunders.
9. Hoskins WJ, Perez CA, and Young RC: Gynecologic tumors. In DeVita VT, Hellman S, and Rosenberg SA, editors: *Cancer: principles and practice of oncology,* ed 4, Philadelphia, 1993, JB Lippincott.
10. Lefebure K: *Sexual assessment planning,* J Head Trauma Rehabil 5:2, 1990.
11. Levison V: *The effect on fertility, libido, and sexual function of post-operative radiotherapy and chemotherapy for cancer of the testicle,* Clin Radiol 37:161, 1986.
12. MacElveen-Hoehn P: *Sexual assessment and counseling,* Semin Oncol Nurs 1:69, 1985.
13. McDonald T and others: *Impact of cervical intraepithelial neoplasia diagnosis and treatment on self-esteem and body image,* Gynecol Oncol 34, 1989.

14. Renshaw D: *Sexual and emotional needs of cancer patients,* Clin Ther 8:242, 1986.

15. Schain W: *A sexual interview is a sexual intervention,* Innovations Oncol Nurs 4:2, 1988.

16. Schover L: *Sexuality and cancer: for the man who has cancer, and his partner,* New York, 1988, American Cancer Society.

17. Schover L: *Sexuality and cancer: for the woman who has cancer, and her partner,* New York, 1988, American Cancer Society.

18. Schover L and Fife M: *Sexual counseling of patients undergoing radical surgery for pelvic or genital cancer,* J Psychosocial Oncol 3:15, 1986.

19. Schover L, Schain W, and Montague D: Sexual problems. In DeVita V, Hellman S, and Rosenberg S, editors. *Cancer principles and practices of oncology,* ed 4, Philadelphia, 1993, JB Lippincott.

20. Shell J: Sexuality for patients with gynecologic cancer. In Lowdermilk D, editors: *NAACOGs clinical issues in perinatal and women's health nursing,* Philadelphia, 1990, JB Lippincott.

21. Shell J: The psychosexual impact of ostomy surgery. In *Progressions: developments in ostomy and wound care,* St Louis, 1992, Mosby.

22. Shell J: Sexual function and activity in the person with genitourinary cancer. In Berry D, editor: *Urologic oncology nursing manual,* Philadelphia, 1993, CoMed Communications.

23. Stair J: Sexual dysfunction: infertility, In McNally JC and others, editors: *Guidelines for oncology nursing practice,* ed 2, Philadelphia, 1991, WB Saunders.

24. Wallace L: *Sexual adjustment after radical genital surgery.* Nurs Times 83:51, 1987.

25. Weeks D: Acute leukemia and pregnancy. In Lowdermilk D, editor. *NAACOGs clinical issues in perinatal and women's health nursing.* Philadelphia, 1990, JB Lippincott.

26. Zinreich E and others: *Pre- and post-treatment evaluation of sexual function in patients with adenocarcinoma of the prostate,* Int J Radia Oncol Biol Phys 19:3, 1990.

Infusion
Therapies

Table A-1 Common Antibiotics, Antifungals and Antivirals

Medication	Route/Dose	Indications/Precautions
ANTIBIOTICS		
Amikacin	IV 15 mg/kg every 8 hours	Severe systemic infection of CNS, respiratory, GI, urinary tract Monitor renal function carefully Monitor for signs of hearing loss, tinnitus, and vertigo Observe for signs of superinfection. Infuse over 30-60 minutes
Aztreonam	IV/IM 500-1,000 mg every 8-12 hours	Gram-negative infections Elicit history of allergies Monitor liver function Monitor renal function Monitor coagulation. Monitor neurotoxicity Observe for signs of superinfection

Carbapenem Imipenem/cilastin	IV 250-500 mg every 6 hours	Gram-positive infections (anaphylaxis) Elicit allergy history Monitor renal function Monitor liver function Monitor CBC and Coombs' test Observe for signs of superinfection
Cefoperazone	IV 2 gms every 8 hours	Suspected gram-negative sepsis Infuse over 30 minutes Not approved for pediatric patients Monitor prothrombin time and for diarrhea Administer vitamin K as ordered

Ceftazidine	IV 150 mg/kg/day every 8 hours	Suspected gram-negative sepsis
		Infuse over 30 minutes
		Maximum dose 2 gms every 8 hours
		Monotherapy for pediatric patients, second line
		  therapy for adults
		Monitor for diarrhea and development of drug
		  resistance

Continued.

Table A-1 Cont'd.

Medication	Route/Dose	Indications/Precautions
Gentamicin	IV 3-5 mg/kg every 8 hours	Severe systemic infection of CNS, respiratory, GI, urinary tract Monitor renal function carefully Monitor for signs of hearing loss, tinnitus, and vertigo Observe for signs of superinfection Infuse over 30-60 minutes
Norfloxicin	PO 400 mg bid	Reduction of bowel flora, anaerobes Administer on empty stomach Do not administer with antacids or carafate Discontinue when granulocyte recovery is maintained
Penicillin VK	PO 250 mg bid	Prophylaxis of gram-positive infections post BMT. Check for allergy to penicillin Monitor for rash
Piperacillin	IV/IM 100-300 mg/kg every 4-6 hours	Gram-positive infection Monitor renal function carefully Elicit allergy history

Tobramycin	IV 5 mg/kg/day	Be prepared for possible allergic reaction (anaphylaxis) Monitor CBC and liver function tests carefully Monitor serum electrolytes (K^+ and Na^+) (hypokalemia) Suspected gram-negative sepsis Infuse over 20 to 30 minutes Do not administer at same time as ceftazidine, or cefoperozone Monitor peak and trough blood levels. Monitor for nephrotoxicity (elevated BUN and creatinine) and ototoxicity (ataxia, diminished hearing)
Trimethoprim-sulfamethoxazole	PO 1 DS tablet bid IV 15-20 mg/kg/day	Prophylaxis of *Pneumocystis carinii* pneumonia post BMT Avoid with sulfa allergy. Administer per transplant center protocol. Monitor for rash, decreasing WBC, and increasing BUN and creatinine.

Continued.

Table A-1 Cont'd.

Medication	Route/Dose	Indications/Precautions
Vancomycin	IV 1 gm every 12 hours (adult) IV 40 mg/kg/day (pediatrics) PO 125 mg every 6 hours	Suspected or proven gram-positive infections Infuse over 60 minutes PO is used for *C. difficile* enterocolitis only (not absorbed orally) Monitor peak and trough blood levels Monitor for nephrotoxicity (elevated BUN and creatinine) and ototoxicity (ataxia, diminished hearing)
ANITFUNGALS Amphotericin B	IV 0.5-1 mg/kg/day	Treatment of fungal infections resistant to fluconazole Infuse through D5W only over 3 to 6 hours. Administer test dose at initiation of therapy (1 mg in 100 mL D5W) Monitor for increased temperature and chilling rigor during infusion Premedicate with diphenhydramine, actetaminophen, or hydrocortisone as ordered Monitor electrolytes and for nephrotoxicity

Fluconazole	PO 500 mg bid IV 100-200 mg/day	PO for reduction of bowel flora (used with norfloxacin) IV for treatment of fungemia Monitor for overgrowth of resistant strains of fungus—surveillance cultures Monitor for elevated liver function tests and nephrotoxicity Discontinue PO when granulocyte recovery is maintained
Ketoconazole	Oral	Treatment of fungal infections. Monitor GI symptoms (nausea, vomiting, diarrhea), liver function, and food and drug interaction
ANTIVIRALS Acyclovir	PO or IV 250-500 mg/m^2 every 8 hours	Prophylaxis and treatment of herpes simplex or cytomegalovirus Infuse over 2 hours (doses >500 mg must be diluted in 500 mL of fluid) Monitor for increased BUN and creatinine
Ganciclovir	IV 2.5 mg/kg every 8 hours IV 5 mg/kg every 12 hours	Prophylaxis and treatment of cytomegalovirus (CMV) Infuse over 1 hour, handle administration and disposal using chemotherapy precautions

Continued.

Table A-1 Cont'd.

Medication	Route/Dose	Indications/Precautions
		Administer with immunoglobulin for cases of CMV pneumonitis
		Monitor for decreased WBC and increased BUN and creatinine
		Colony stimulating factors may be given to maintain WBC
Foscarnet	IV 40-60 mg/kg every 8 hours	Second line therapy for herpes simplex or cytomegalovirus infections
		Monitor for electrolyte disturbances, nephrotoxicity and decreased WBC
		Monitor for seizure activity
Immunesuppressant Immunoglobulin	500 mg/1gm as indicated IV 0.4 mg/kg every week × 6 PO 50 mg/kg/day every 6 hours	IV prophylaxis for herpes simplex and cytomegalovirus
		IV treatment for CMV pneumonitis in conjunction with ganciclovir
		PO treatment of rotavirus
		Administer IV slowly 20 to 30 mL/hr
		Monitor for chills, hypotension, and increased temperature during infusion

Table A-2 Biotherapy Drugs

Drug Class	Route/Dose (mg/in²)	Major Side Effects/Toxicities	Nursing Guidelines
Bacillus Calmette-Guerin (BCG)	Intradermal Intralesion, Intravesical as directed	Depends on route of administration; may cause burning sensation to skin; bladder mucosa, inflammatory reactions	This drug aids immune system in killing tumor cells. This is a live virus, other compromised patients should not be in close contact with this patient. Assess for skin reaction and signs of infection
Epogen (recombinant Human Erythropoietin)	50 to 500 IU/kg maintenance, 25 to 100 IU/kg SC./IV	Flulike syndrome; potential for DVT, thrombus of fistula and hypertension	Increases transferrin and ferritin levels, anemia of chronic diseases, and chemotherapy related to myelo-suppression; refrigerate; reconstitute with accompanying diluent; *do not shake* when reconstituted
GCSF-Granulocyte Colony Stimulating Factor (Neupogen)	5 mcg/kg IV SC,	Myalgias, arthralgia, chills, fever, bone pain, fatigue, anorexia, weight gain, headache, rash, confusion	Follow reconstitution guidelines; *do not mix with normal saline or flush lines with normal saline*; do not shake medication after reconstitution; final concentration ideally 15 mcg/mL; drug

Continued.

Table A-2 Cont'd.

Drug Class	Route/Dose	Major Side Effects/Toxicities	Nursing Guidelines
			stability is 6 hours after mixing; *use nonfiltered tubing; infuse in more than 30 minutes; do not IV bolus/push;* designate a specific IV line to prevent side effects and drug incompatibilities **Do not give until 24 hours after chemotherapy has been given*
GMCSF-Granulocyte Macrophage Colony Stimulating Factor (Leukine, Prokine)	250 mcg/m² for 7-14 days as indicated SC/IV	Urticaria, bone pain, fever, arthralgia, nausea, dyspnea, acute respiratory distress syndrome (ARDS), pleuritis, angioedema, broncho constriction, anaphylaxis Capillary leak syndrome with edema and pleural effusion with doses greater than 16 to 32 mcg/kg	Follow reconstitution guidelines; *mix only with normal saline,* final concentration ideally to be 10 mcg/mL; *do not shake after mixing;* drug stability is 6 hours after mixing; *use nonfiltered tubing, infuse over 2 hours,* designate a specific IV line to prevent drug incompatibilities **Do not give until 24 hours after chemotherapy has been given*

Interferon (Alpha) (Roferon, Intron A)	3 million units day or 3 times weekly to 50 million units m² for 5 days every 3 weeks SC/IV	Fever, chills, myalgia, arthralgia, headache, fatigue, leukopenia, thrombocytopenia, and anemia	Intravenous administration results in a rapid clearance with a half-life of 4 to 8 hours; dosage: million units/m². Dose may be given daily × 3 days; daily; or three times in a week
Interleukin-2 (Proleukin)	10,000 to 600,000 u/kg for 8 hours for a total of 14 doses IV,SC, IA, IP	Chills, fever, headache, malaise, myalgia, fatigue, hypotension, tachycardia, edema, weight gain, ascites, decreased vascular resistance, dyspnea, pulmonary edema, oliguria, proteinuria,	Follow guidelines for reconstitution, filtration, and evaluation of compatibility with concomitant medications such as antiemetics and vasopressors; *monitor side effects.*

Continued.

Table A-2 Cont'd.

Drug Class	Route/Dose	Major Side Effects/Toxicities	Nursing Guidelines
		azotemia, increased BUN and creatinine, nausea, vomiting, diarrhea, mucositis, erythema, dry skin rash, confusion, lethargy, anxiety, depression, psychoses, anemia, thrombocytopenia, eosinophilia, lymphopenia	
Interleukin-3 Multi-CSF (IL-3)	SC/IV 1,000 mcg/m^2	Low grade fever, headache, flushing, erythema, bone pain, lethargy, N&V	Targets multi-potential committed progenitor cells. Increases leukocytes. Monitor WBC count
Tumor Necrosis Factor (TNF)	50 to 100 mcg/kg bolus continuous infusion IM, sub.q./IV	Flulike syndrome, fever, chills, hypotension, myalgias, headaches, anorexia	TNF selectively targets transformed cells and is produced by lymphocytes, NK cells, astrocytes and microglial cells; it is pivotal in pathogenesis of infection, inflammation, and injury; it participates in beneficial processes of host defense and tissue homeostasis

Table A-3 Most Commonly Used Chemotherapeutic Drugs

Class	Route	Dose	Infusion Solution/Duration	Major Side Effects/ Toxicities	Nursing Action
ALKYLATING AGENTS					
Busulfan (Myleran)	PO	2-6 mg/m^2	NA	Myelosuppression, nausea, vomiting, pulmonary fibrosis	Promote compliance Increase toxicity with high dosage
Carboplatin (CBDCA)	IV IP	250-500 mg/m^2	D5W>30 min D5W	Myelosuppression, nausea, vomiting, mild nephrotoxicity and neurotoxicity	Hydration; premedicate with antiemetics Drug decomposes if mixed in NS
Chlorambucil (Leukeran)	PO	0.1-0.3 mg/kg	NA	Myelosuppression, sterility, stomatitis	Promote compliance
Cisplatin	IV IV IP, IA	50-120 mg/m^2 15-20 mg/m^2	150/1,000 mL >6 hr 1 hr	Nausea, vomiting, renal neurotoxic damage, ototoxicity, electrolyte imbalance	Hydration, I&O; obtain 12-24 hr creatinine clearance, Premedicate with antiemetics
Cyclophosphamide (Cytoxan)	IV High-dose IV PO	400 mg/m^2 1-1.5 g 50-200 mg/m^2	20 mg/mL SW	Nausea, vomiting, alopecia, myelosuppression, hemorrhagic cystitis, cardiotoxic pneumonitis	Hydration, I&O; obtain 12-24 hr creatinine clearance, force fluids, void frequently

Continued.

Table A-3 Cont'd.

Class	Route	Dose	Infusion Solution/Duration	Major Side Effects/ Toxicities	Nursing Action
Estramustine	PO	600 mg/m²	NA	Toxicity, nausea, vomiting, gynecomastia; cardiac toxicity	Educate patient about side effects; drug may be given in divided doses
Hexamethyl-melamine (HMM, HXM)	PO	150 mg/m²	NA	Myelosuppression, neurotoxicity, anorexia, nausea, vomiting	Premedicate with antiemetics
Ifosfamide (Isophosphamide Naxamide)	IV	700–2,000 mg/m²	50–100 mg/mL D5W Bolus or continuous infusion	Myelosuppression, nephrotoxicity, nausea, vomiting, phlebitis, neurotoxicity, alopecia, hemorrhagic cystitits	Provide hydration, monitor I&O; administer MESNA concomitantly
Mechlore-thamine (Nitrogen mustard)	IV Topical	1–6 mg/m² 10 mg dissolve in 50 mL H₂O; apply daily to weekly	10 mg/10 mL NS/SW 1 mL/min	Severe nausea, vomiting, extravasation, myelosuppression	Vesicant; use in < 60 min after reconstitution

	Route	Dose	Administration	Side effects	Nursing considerations
Melphalan (Alkeran)	PO	Dose will vary according to protocol		Nausea, vomiting may occur with high-dose, myelosuppression	Promote compliance
Thiotepa	PO	6-10 mg/m^2		Myelosuppression, headache, fever, occasional nausea	Observe for reactions
	IV	8 mg/m^2	60 mg/60 mL D5W		
	Instill bladder		Bolus >30 min; weekly		
ANTIBIOTICS					
Bleomycin	IV	10-20 u/m^2	5/15u/mins	Fever, chills, pulmonary toxicity, hyperpigmentation, alopecia, stomatitis, hypotension	Use glass bottle for infusion
	IM	10	IM test dose; then 1 u/min		Auscultate breath sounds at least bid
	SC	10	q wk		Test dose prior to initial dosing
			q wk		

Continued.

Table A-3 Cont'd.

Class	Route	Dose	Infusion Solution/Duration	Major Side Effects/ Toxicities	Nursing Action
Dactinomycin (Actinomycin D)	IV	1-2 mg/m^2	1-5 min	Potentiates effects of radiation therapy, myelosuppression, alopecia	Vesicant; administer free-flowing IV
Daunorubicin (Cerubidine, Daunomycin)	IV	30-60 mg/m^2	1 mL/min	Myelosuppression, alopecia, nausea, vomiting, stomatitis, red urine, cardiotoxic	Vesicant; cumulative dose 500-600 mg/m^2
Doxorubicin (Adriamycin)	IV	50-75 mg/m^2	5 mg/mL/SW 1mL/min	Myelosuppression, alopecia, nausea, vomiting, diarrhea, red urine	Vesicant; cumulative dose 550 mg/m^2; incompatible with many drugs (e.g., heparin)
Idarubicin (Idamycin)	IV	18-25 mg	1 mg/mL/NS Bolus: 1 mL/min	Myelosuppression, alopecia, nausea, vomiting, mucositis	Vesicant; administer free-flowing IV

Drug	Route	Dosage	Dilution/Rate	Side Effects	Special Considerations
Mitomycin C (Mutamycin)	IV	10-20 mg/m^2	0.5 mg/mL D5W/NS 1 mL/min	Myelosuppression, alopecia, nausea, vomiting, fever, stomatitis, urine color change	Vesicant
Mithramycin (Plicamycin, Mithracin)	IV	25-50 µg/kg	150 mL D5W >30 min.	Thrombocytopenia, hepatotoxicity, nausea, vomiting, phlebitis	Vesicant; monitor liver and kidney function tests
ANTIMETABOLITES					
Cytarabine (Ara-C, Cytosar)	IV	100-200 mg/m^2	1-20 mg/mL Bolus >60-min or 24-hr continuous infusion; infuse over 60 min; <60 min increases toxicity	Potent myelosuppressant, anorexia, alopecia, nausea, vomiting, hepatotoxicity, neurotoxicity with increased dosage and intrathecal administration; conjunctivitis	Monitor for neurotoxicity with high dose; force fluids; administer antiemetics; use decadron eye drops as prophylactic measure
	High dose IV	3 g Variable			

Continued.

Table A-3 Cont'd.

Class	Route	Dose	Infusion Solution/Duration	Major Side Effects/ Toxicities	Nursing Action
	IT	20/30 mg	Use preservative-free solution slowly NA		
Floxuridine (FUDR)	SC IA	10 mg 0.1-0.6 mg/kg	24-hr continuous infusion	Myelosuppression, oral and gastrointestinal ulceration, nausea, vomiting	Observe and patient teaching for arterial catheterization
Fluorouracil (5-FU)	IV	400-600 mg/m^2	1,000 mL/NS 24-hr continuous infusion Bolus	Myelosuppression, alopecia, skin rash, nausea, vomiting, ataxia, diarrhea, stomatitis	Observe; incompatible with anthracyclines; observe and patient teaching for arterial catheterization
	IV IA	500 mg/m^2 20-30 mg/kg	24-hr continuous infusion		

Drug	Route	Dose	Diluent/Rate	Side Effects	Comments
Fludarabine (Fludara)	IV	30 mg/m^2 × 5 days	30 mL D5W/NS 15–30 min	Myelosuppression, flu-like syndrome, nausea, vomiting, dyspnea	Decreases Cd-4 lymphocytes
Hydroxyurea	IV PO	500–3,000 mg/m^2; 1,000 mg/qd	100 mL D5W/NS Over 30 min	Myelosuppression, stomatitis, alopecia, dysuria, nausea, vomiting, allergic reactions	Observe; oral daily dose may be given in divided doses with meals
Methotrexate (Mexate)	IV	25–40 mg/m^2	10/100 mL/NS Bolus >10 min	Oral and gastrointestinal ulceration, myelosuppression, stomatitis, renal toxicity, nausea, vomiting, diarrhea	Dosage 1 g/m^2 or > require hydration, alkylinization of urine and folinic acid rescue
	IV	7,500 with rescue			
	IM	25 mg/m^2	NA		
	IT	12 mg/m^2	10 mL preservative-free D5W 1–5 min		
6-Mercaptopurine(6-MP)	PO	100 mg/m^2	NA	Myelosuppression, hepatotoxicity, stomatitis, anorexia	Promote compliance

Continued.

Table A-3 Cont'd.

Class	Route	Dose	Infusion Solution/Duration	Major Side Effects/ Toxicities	Nursing Action
6-Thioguanine (6-TG)	PO	100 mg/m²	NA	Myelosuppression, nausea, vomiting	Promote compliance
HORMONES **Androgens**					
Fluoxymesterone (Halotestin)	PO	10-30 mg qd	NA	Nausea, vomiting, edema, liver function abnormalities, virilization in the female	Educate the patient about virilization
Testosterone	PO IM	Variable 100 mg 3 × /wk breast	NA	Mild fluid retention, monitor FBS with diabetes mellitus	Educate the patient: female—masculinization and menstrual irregularity; male—gynecomastis, impotence
Progestins Megestrol acetate (Megace)	PO	40-80 mg qd	NA	Mild fluid retention, hypercalcemia with breast cancer	Teach patient to recognize and report side effects

Medroxyprogesterone acetate (Provera)	PO	400-800 mg/ 2 ×/wk	NA	Mild fluid retention, hypercalcemia with breast cancer	Teach patient to recognize and report side effects
Medroxyprogesterone acetate (Depo-Provera)	IM	400-800 mg/ 2 ×/wk	NA	Acute local hypersensitivity, possible IM injections	Teach patient to recognize and report side effects
Estrogens					
Diethylstilbestrol (DES)	PO	10/breast 0.5-1.5/prostate	NA	Breakthrough bleeding, spotting, premenstrual-like syndrome, feminization in males	Instruct patient about changes
Conjugated estrogen (Premarin)	PO	10 mg tid breast 1.25-2.5 mg tid prostate	NA	Breakthrough bleeding, premenstrual-like syndrome	Educate patient about changes
Chlorotrianisene (TACE)	PO	12-25 mg qd prostate	NA	Increase or decrease in weight, breakthrough bleeding	Educate patient about changes

Continued.

Table A-3 Cont'd.

Class	Route	Dose	Infusion Solution/Duration	Major Side Effects/ Toxicities	Nursing Action
ANTIHORMONAL AGENTS		Dosage not administered by m² and may be given in divided dosages			
Aminoglutethi-mide (Cytadren)	PO	500/1,000 mg qid	NA	Myelosuppression, dermatitis, masculin-ization, drowsiness, lethargy, weakness	Monitor for neurotoxicity
Flutamide (Eulexin)	PO	250-750 mg tid	NA	Gynecomastia, hepa-totoxicity, libido effect	Educate patient about changes
Leuprolide (Leupron)	SC/IM	Variable	NA	Impotence, amenor-rhea, hot flashes	Educate patient about changes
Milotane	PO	2-16 g/day	NA	Nausea, vomiting	Administer in divided doses
Tamoxifen (Nolvadex)	PO	10-20 mg bid	NA	Hot flashes, nausea, vomiting, transient bone or tumor pain	Educate patient regarding changes
Zoladex (Goserelin)	IM	3.6 mg monthly	NA	May increase bone pain, hot flashes, decreased libido, impo-tence, gynecomastia	Educate patient about changes

NITROSUREAS

Drug	Route	Dose	Concentration/Diluent/Time	Toxicities	Administration
Carmustine (BCNU)	IV	25-125 mg/m^2	100 mg/mL D5W > 30 min	Myelosuppression, stomatitis, nausea, vomiting, hepatotoxic pneumonitis, pulmonary fibrosis	Administer slowly: vein irritant Contains alcohol; patient may feel inebriated
Lomustine (CCNU)	PO	70-150 mg/m^2	NA	Nausea, vomiting, thrombocytopenia, myelosuppression	Administer at bedtime with antiemetics
Semustine (MeCCNU)	PO	150-200 mg/m^2	NA	Myelosuppression, nausea, vomiting, renal and hepatic toxicities	Administer on empty stomach with antiemetics
Streptozocin (Zanosar)	IV	0.5-1.5 g	100 mg/mL DW >15 min	Mild myelosuppression, diarrhea, nausea, vomiting, chills, acute hypoglycemia	Administer slowly: vein irritant

Continued.

Table A-3 Cont'd.

Class	Route	Dose	Infusion Solution/Duration	Major Side Effects/ Toxicities	Nursing Action
CORTICOSTEROIDS					
Dexamethasone (Decadron)	IV IM PO	Dose varies with reason for drug	Bolus NA	Gastrointestinal fluid and electrolyte disturbances, possible neuromuscoloskeletal imbalances	Teach patient about side effects; IV rapid bolus may cause rectal itching
Hydrocortisone (Solu-Cortef)	IV	Dose varies with reason for drug	Bolus	Fluid and electrolyte disturbance	Teach patient about side effects
Prednisone (Deltasone)	PO	40-100 mg/day	NA	Fluid and electrolyte disturbance, manifestations of latent diabetes mellitus	Instruct patient to take medications after meals with gradual tapering after long-term use; teach side effects of drug
Prednisolone	PO	40 mg	NA	Similar in action to prednisone	Same as prednisone

VINCA PLANT ALKALOIDS

Drug	Route	Dose	Fluid/Rate	Side effects	Comments
Vinblastine (Velban)	IV	4-20 mg/m²	mg/mL NS 1 mL/min	Myelosuppression, stomatitis, neurotoxicity, alopecia	Vesicant; monitor for neurotoxicity
Vincristine (Oncovin)	IV	0.5-2 mg/m²	mg/mL NS 1 mL/min	Neurotoxicity, constipation, alopecia, stomatitis	Vesicant; monitor bowel function and neurotoxicity Administer stool softeners
Vindesine (Eldisine)	IV	2-4 mg/m²	mg/mL NS 1 mL/min	Myelosuppression, constipation, alopecia, neuropathy	Vesicant; monitor bowel function and neurotoxicity
Podophyllin alkaloids					
Etoposide (VP-16)	IV	50-100 mg/m²	50 mL NS Over 30-60 min	Nausea, vomiting, leukopenia, anemia, alopecia, hypotension	Administer drug slowly; may test dose before infusion
	PO	400 mg	NA		
Teniposide (VM-26)	IV	50-130 mg/m²	100-250 mL NS Never give IV push; slow IV infusion only	Anaphylaxis, myelosuppression, severe hypotension, alopecia	Vesicant; slow infusion only; may test dose before infusion

Continued.

Table A-3 Cont'd.

Class	Route	Dose	Infusion Solution/Duration	Major Side Effects/ Toxicities	Nursing Action
					High dose VP-16: use glass container for solution (solution will melt tubing) and give in nonfiltered tubing (e.g., albumin tubing)
MISCELLANEOUS AGENTS					
Asparaginase (Elspar)	IV	1,000 IU kg/ day 2–20 days	2,000 U/mL NS 1 mL/min	Anaphylactic shock, nausea, vomiting, hyperglycemia, hepatotoxic	Monitor closely Follow anaphylaxis protocol; test dose prior to initial dosing
	IM, Subq	6,000 IU kg 3 ×/wk	5,000 U/mL NA		
Dacarbazine (DTIC-Dome)	IV	75–1,450	10 mg/mL D5W 10–15 min or 24-hr continuous infusion	Myelosuppression, venous spasm, flu-like syndrome, paresthesia, pruritus	Vesicant; premedicate with antiemetics

Levamisole	PO	1-5 mg/kg	NA	Mild gastrointestinal complaints	Observe
Leucovorin	PO IV	200-500 mg/m² × 3 days/ 1 week	500 mg/m²; 250 mL/NS	Allergic reaction, irritant, myelosuppression, diarrhea, stomatitis, dehydration	Increased toxicity with increased dosage
Leustatin (cladribine, 2-CdA)	IV	0.09 mg/kg/ day	10 mg vial/ 1 mg/mL; prepare 24 hr continuous 7 day infusion in 100 mL NS 100 mL via continuous infusion × 7 days	Myelosuppression, fever, nausea, rash, injection site reaction	Incompatible with D5W; calculate dose by multiplying patient's weight in kg by 0.09 mg (120 lb ÷ 2.2 lb/kg = 54.5 kg; 54.5 kg × 0.09 mg = 4.9 mg/ day); prepare central venous access ambulatory pump

Continued.

Table A-3 Cont'd.

Class	Route	Dose	Infusion Solution/Duration	Major Side Effects/ Toxicities	Nursing Action
Mitoxantrone (DHAD)	IV	15	10 mL NS or D5W >30 min	Myelosuppression, diarrhea, nausea, vomiting, phlebitis, bluish discoloration of urine, alopecia	Irritant; monitor laboratory values, teach side effects
Pentostatin (2'-deoxycoformycin)	IV	4 mg/m^2 q14 days	1 mg/mL 5 min or more	Myelosuppression, rash, nausea, vomiting, diarrhea, stomatitis, elevated liver enzymes, *neurotoxic*, cough, shortness of breath	Monitor laboratory values; assess neurologic toxicities and other side effects

Procarbazine (Matulane)	PO	100-150 mg/m² NA		Myelosuppression; avoid use of narcotics, epinephrine, antihistamines	Incompatible with ethanol, antidepressants, food rich in tyramine will get hypertensive crisis
Paclitaxel (Taxol)	IV	200 mg/m²	500 mL NS 4-24 hr	Alopecia, nausea and vomiting, neutropenia, skin rash, *allergic reaction*, cardiac arrhythmias	Ensure recommended pre-medications are given prior to taxol infusion; follow anaphylaxis protocol; monitor vital signs and cardiac dysrhythmias; prepare Taxol solution in a glass bottle and infuse via non-PVC tubing

NA, not applicable; *SW*, sterile water; *D5W*, dextrose water 5%; *NS*, normal saline; *PO*, by mouth; *SC*, subcutaneous; *IM*, intramuscular; *IV*, intravenous; *IP*, intraperitoneal; *IT*, intrathecal; *qd*, daily; *qid*, four times a day; *bid*, twice a day; *tid*, three times a day. Nadir usually occurs 7-21 days after drugs are given. Adapted from Chabner BA and Myers CE: Clinical pharmacology of cancer chemotherapy. In DeVita VT, Hellman S, Rosenberg SA, editors: *Cancer: principles and practice of oncology*, ed 4, Philadelphia, 1993, JB Lippincott.

Table A-4 Investigational Chemotherapy Drugs: Phase II Drugs

Drug	Disease Evaluation	Toxicities
Amonafide	Acute myelocytic leukemia, esophagus, ovarian, sarcoma	Myelosuppression, alopecia, diarrhea, nausea and vomiting, seizure, dyspnea, rash, temporary orange tint in urine
Didemnin B	Brain, prostate, melanoma, non-small cell lung	Anaphylaxis, myalgia, myopathy Anorexia, nausea and vomiting, diarrhea, transient hepatotoxicity; may induce insulin-dependent diabetes
Diaziquone (AZQ)	Brain	Myelosuppression, alopecia, gastrointestinal distress
Dihydroxyazacytidine (DHAC)	Mesothelioma	Myelosuppression, chest pain, nausea and vomiting, diarrhea, stomatitis, pleural effusion
Edatrexate (10-EdAM)	Head and neck, bladder, non-small cell lung	Leukopenia, nausea and vomiting, diarrhea, mucositis, stomatitis, respiratory infection, pulmonary fibrosis, fatigue, alopecia
Fazarabine	Brain, lung	Myelosuppression, pulmonary emboli, nausea and vomiting
Merberone	Gastrointestinal, hepatic, melanoma, renal	Myelosuppression, myalgia, nausea and vomiting, hypouricemia, diarrhea, stomatitis, alopecia, phlebitis

Pala	Colon (synergetic with 5-FU)	Nausea and vomiting, diarrhea, stomatitis, skin rash
Piroxantrone (Oxantrazale)	Breast, gastric, head and neck, melanoma, pancreas, renal, sarcoma	Myelosuppression, alopecia, nausea and vomiting, hyponatremia, stomatitis, fatigue, diarrhea, vesicant, cardiotoxic
Topotecan	Lung, ovary, hepatic, gastric, ovary, renal, skin	Neutropenia, thrombocytopenia, alopecia, nausea and vomiting, rash, fever, microscopic hematuria, myelosuppression, nephrotoxicity, dermatitis
Trimetrexate (TMXT, TMQ)	*Pneumocystitis carinii*	Myelosuppression etc.

From Southwest Oncology Group Research Protocols, Southwest Oncology Group; National Cancer Institute, 1994.

Table A-5 Investigational Chemotherapy Drugs: Phase I Drugs

Drug	Disease Evaluation	Toxicities
Adozelesin	Preclinical: leukemia, lung, melanoma, colon, pancreas, ovary	Undetermined
Biantrazole	Breast	Myelosuppression, alopecia, nausea and vomiting, phlebitis
Crisnatol mesylate	Glioma	Somnolence, dizziness, blurred vision, unsteady gait, confusion, vertigo, nystagmus
Camptothecan (CPT-11)	Colon, lung, cervix, ovary	Myelosuppression, gastrointestinal toxicities, alopecia, anorexia
Gemcitabine	Breast, colon, lung, head and neck, pancreas	Myelosuppression, dermatitis, fever, flu-like syndrome, hypotension, alopecia, mucositis, elevated liver enzymes
Ilmofosine	Renal, colon, breast, lung	Intravascular hemolysis, nausea and vomiting, diarrhea, phlebitis, fever
Suramin	HIV, Kaposi sarcoma, ovary, hormone resistant prostate, refractory lymphoma	Adrenocortical insufficiency, transient paresthesia, muscle weakness, rash, coagulopathy, myelosuppression, liver function test abnormality

Drug	Indication	Toxicity
Taxotere	Breast, lung, ovary, pancreas	Neutropenia, alopecia, dermatitis, mucositis, phlebitis, mild anaphylactic reaction
Terephthalamidine	Hodgkin's seminoma	Anorexia, nausea and vomiting, weight loss, weakness
Tetraplatin (Ormaplatin)	Esophagus, gastric	Myelosuppression, nausea and vomiting, mild parathesia
Toremifene	Breast	Vaginal discharge, hot flashes, mild sweating
Vinorelbine (Navelbine)	Hodgkin's, ovary, breast	Leukopenia, nausea and vomiting, alopecia, constipation, decrease deep tendon reflexes, phlebitis

From Fields SM and Von Hoff DD: *New anticancer agents*, Highlights on Antineoplastic Drugs 10(2):16, 1993.

Table A-6 Anaphylaxis Chemotherapeutic Drugs with Anaphylactic Potential

Drugs	Signs and Symptoms	Precautions
Asparginase (Elspar)	Respiratory distress, increased pulse, respirations, hypotension, facial edema, anxiety, flushed appearance, hives, itching. Risk for anaphylaxis increases with each dose	Test dose prior to initial IV/IM dosing. Monitor 30 min/IM; 60 min/IV post drug administration. Keep vein open with IV normal saline prior, during, and 30/60 min post IV administration of Asparginase. Initiate drug infusion slowly (mg/m^2/titrate infusion). Code cart, O$_2$, suction equipment, drugs for anaphylaxis at or near patient's bedside
Test Dose Procedure: Prepare 10,000 IU Asparginase with 5 mL NS. Inject 0.1 mL of solution (200 IU) into 9.9 mL NS. Inject intradermally 0.1 mL of concentration (20 IU) to make a wheal in inner aspect of arm. Observe wheal for 60 min for erythema, swelling, and itching prior to infusion.		
Bleomycin	Dyspnea, hypotension, increased pulse and respiration, rash	Test dose prior to initial IV dosing. Initiate drug infusion slowly (10–20 mL/15 min). Monitor vital signs and auscultate breath sounds q4hr during and for 24 hours postinfusion and/or on scheduled basis in outpatient setting
Test Dose Procedure: Inject 2 U Bleomycin intradermal to make a wheal in inner aspect of arm. Observe for erythema, edema, and itching prior to first 2 doses of Bleomycin infusion.		

Etoposide (VP-16)	Hypotension, bronchospasm, chest pain, increased pulse, respirations, facial flush, fever, chills, diaphoresis.	Initiate drug infusion slowly (10-20 mL/15 min). Infuse total volume over at least 60 minutes. Monitor vital signs q15 min × 4; q30 min × 2 and q4hr, during and 24 hours postinfusion
Taxol	Hypotension, dyspnea with bronchospasm, urticaria, abdominal and extremity pain, angioedema and diaphoresis. Incidence is increased with shorter infusions.	Ensure recommended premedications are given prior to taxol infusion. Dexamethasone 20 mg PO 12 and 6 hr; diphenhydramine 50 mg IV bolus 30 to 60 min; cimetidine 300 mg IV infusion 30 to 60 min; antiemetic (e.g., Zofran) 10 mg in 50 mL IV infusion over 15 min.

Continued.

Table A-6 Cont'd.

Drugs	Signs and Symptoms	Precautions
		Obtain baseline vital signs; then monitor q15 min × 4; q1 hr × 4; then q4 hr during infusion. Code cart, O$_2$, suction equipment, and drugs for anaphylaxis at or near bedside
Teniposide (VM-26)	Severe hypotension, anxiety, increased pulse, respirations, fever	Initiate drug infusion slowly (10-20 mL/30 min). Total infusion time 60-120 min. Monitor vital signs q15 min × 4; q30 min × 2, during and postinfusion; then monitor q4hr × 24 hr

Data from American Hospital Formulary Service, American Society of Hospital Pharmacists, Inc., Bethesda 1992, *Physicians Desk Reference*, Medical Economics Data, New Jersey, 1994, Medical Economics Data.

Table A-7 Extravasation: Chemotherapeutic Vesicant Drugs with
Recommended Antidotes

Drug	Antidote

ALKYLATING AGENT
Mechlorethamine
  (nitrogen mustard)
	Isotonic
	Sodium thiosulfate
	Dilute 1.6 mL sodium thio-
	  sulfate 25% with 8.4 mL
	  of sterile water; inject 1
	  to 4 mL through existing
	  IV access; inject subq if
	  IV access is removed
	Apply ice pack and/or
	  cold compresses

ANTIBIOTICS
Actinomycin D
Dacarbazine
Daunorubicin
Doxorubicin
Epirubicin*
Esorubicin*
Idarubicin
Mithramycin
Mitomycin C
Piroxanthrone*
	Hydrocortisone 100 mg/mL
	Inject 0.5 mL IV through
	  existing IV line and 0.5
	  mL subcutaneously into
	  extravasated site; apply
	  cold compresses
	Dexamethasone 4 mg/mL
	Inject 0.5 mL IV through
	  existing IV line and 0.5
	  mL subcutaneously into
	  extravasated site; apply
	  cold compresses/ice
	  packs immediately, *do*
	  not apply pressure
	Alternative protocol
	Topical DMSO 1 to 2 mL
	  of 1 mmol DMSO 50% to
	  100%
	Apply topically one time
	  at the site; apply cold
	  compresses

BISANTRENE	Sodium bicarbonate 1
	  mEq/mL
	Mix equal parts of sodium
	  bicarbonate with sterile

Continued.

Table A-7 Cont'd.

Drug	Antidote
	normal saline (1:1 solution); resulting solution is 0.5 mEq/mL Inject 2 to 6 mL (1 to 3.0 mEq) IV through existing IV line and subcutaneously into extravasated site; apply cold compresses
VINCA ALKALOIDS Vinblastine Vincristine	Hyaluronidase (Wydase) 150 U/mL Add 1 mL sterile sodium chloride Inject 1 to 6 mL (150 to 900 U) subcutaneously into extravasated site with multiple injections; apply warm compresses
LOCAL ANTIDOTE (may be used for daunorubicin, doxorubicin, and mitomycin)	Topical cooling may be achieved using: Ice packs Cooling pad with ice water circulating Cryogel packs changed frequently Cooling of site to patient tolerance for 24 hr. Elevate and rest extremity 24-48 hr.†

*Investigational Drugs

Table A-8 Blood Component Therapy

Component	Indications	Special Considerations
PACKED RED BLOOD CELLS (PRBC)	Hemoglobin <8.0 gm Patient is symptomatic Active bleeding	Must be ABO and Rh compatible Infuse over 2 to 4 hours Monitor for transfusion reaction (liver, chills, urticaria)
• Leukocyte poor PRBC Leukocytes are removed during transfusion	Patient has experienced febrile transfusion reactions Patient is at risk for alloimmunization	Infuse through a high-efficiency leukocyte depletion filter
• Washed PRBC Blood is washed with 1,000 mL normal saline and repacked prior to transfusion	Patient has known severe allergic reaction to plasma and leukocytes	Infuse at 20-30 gtts/min until completion of unit Unit expires within 24 hours of washing

Continued.

Table A-8 Cont'd.

Component	Indications	Special Considerations
PLATELET CONCENTRATES		
	Platelet count <20,000 Active bleeding Prior to minor procedures or surgery	ABO compatibility preferred but not necessary One hour or 24 hour posttransfusion increments are monitored to determine effectiveness Splenomegaly, DIC, fever, sepsis may increase demand Monitor for transfusion reactions Prophylaxis with diphenhydramine, acetaminophen, hydrocortisone (Administer IV as rapidly as patient can tolerate; recommend 150-200 mL/hr)
• Random donor (RDP) Several units (6-10) harvested from whole blood are pooled into one bag	Patient has had no prior transfusions Patient has had no reactions or alloimmunization	Units expire about 4 hours after pooling

• Leukocyte poor RDP Leukocytes are removed prior to or during transfusion	Patient is at risk for alloimmunization Patient has experienced febrile transfusion reactions	Unit is either centrifuged and leukocytes mechanically trapped (Leukotrap) or a special high-efficiency leukocyte depletion filter is used for infusion
• Single donor (SDP) Platelets are collected by pheresis from one donor	Patient is refractory to RDP Patient is at risk for alloimmunization	Try to match ABO/Rh of patient Usually transfuse with special high-efficiency leukocyte depletion filter Unit expires within 24 hours of collection
• HLA matched Platelets are collected by pheresis from a donor whose HLA typing closely matches patient	Patient is refractory to RDP and SDP Patient is at risk for alloimmunization	Patient must have been HLA typed Unit expires within 24 hours of collection

Continued.

Table A-8 Cont'd.

Component	Indications	Special Considerations
• Resuspended platelets Plasma is removed from pooled units and an equivalent amount of normal saline is added	Patient has experienced severe reaction to platelet concentrates despite prophylaxis	Prophylaxis is usually needed
FRESH FROZEN PLASMA	Patient has had multiple PRBC transfusions Abnormal coagulation factors	Provide ABO compatible component Transfuse immediately after thawing
IRRADIATED COMPONENTS Gamma radiation delivered to blood components inactivates lymphocytes within product	Severely immunocompromised patients at risk for GVHD	Component is not radioactive Component should be labeled as being irradiated. Red blood cells and platelets are not affected.

Table A-9 Miscellaneous Blood Products Infusion Guidelines

Product	Infusion Guidelines
Cryoprecipitate *Volume* 10 to 20 mL/unit; total of 10 mL normal saline is added in blood bank; usual order 8 to 10 units *Filter* Special component filter	Rapid infusion: recommend 30 minutes to 1 hour *Comments:* Crossmatch not required; need not be ABO of Rh specific; each unit contains approximately 150 grams of fibrinogen and 80 units of Factor VIII; blood bank does not thaw and pool until requested; required preparation time: 20 minutes
Albumin—25% salt poor *Volume* 12.5 g/50 mL *Filter* Special tubing comes with product	Infuse within 1 hour at 1 mL/min; average pediatric dose and rate: 1 g/kg, infuse 4 mL/kg *Comments:* Dosage based on BSA requirements (estimating blood and plasma volume): refer to manufacturer's package insert; very hypertonic
Albumin—5% *Volume* 12.5 g/250 mL	Infuse within 1 hour at 2 to 4 mL/min; average pediatric dose and rate: 1 g/kg, infuse 10 mL/kg

Continued.

Table A-9 Cont'd.

Product	Infusion Guidelines
Filter Special tubing comes with product	*Comments:* Dosage based on BSA requirements (estimating blood and plasma volume): refer to manufacturer's package insert
Plasma Protein Fraction (PPF) *Volume* Varies according to scheduled dose *Filter* Special tubing comes with product	Infuse no more than 1 to 10 mL/min *Comments:* No typing or crossmatching required; used for volume expansion
Rh$_o$ Immune Globulin (RhoGam) *Volume* 1 mL *Filter* None	Given intramuscularly (IM) *Comments:* Usually ordered from blood bank; to achieve optimal effect, must be administered within 72 hours to Rh negative patients who have been exposed to Rh(D) antigens through transfusion or pregnancy
Immune Serum Globulin (ISG)	
Immune Serum Globulin	May be given IV or IM

Table A-10 Blood Transfusion Reactions

Type of Reaction	Signs and Symptoms	Interventions
Hemolytic	Fever, chills, back pain, substernal tightness, dyspnea, circulatory collapse, urticaria, vomiting, diarrhea, hemoglobinuria, renal shutdown, bleeding diathesis	Prevent by proper identification of patient and blood for transfusion Discontinue transfusion. Send to blood bank and obtain urine and blood specimens per hospital policy for transfusion reaction workup Administer saline diuresis, furosemide, and mannitol to prevent acute tubular necrosis
Allergic	Urticaria, itching, bronchospasm, anaphylactoid reactions	Elicit history of prior allergic reactions. Premedicate with diphenhydramine and/or corticosteroids If reaction occurs, stop transfusion. Follow hospital policy for suspected transfusion reaction. For anaphylactoid reaction, administer epinephrine, maintain airway and perfusion. Administer additional emergency measures as needed.

Continued.

Table A-10 Cont'd.

Type of Reaction	Signs and Symptoms	Interventions
Febrile (leukocyte antigens)	Fever with or without rigors, tachycardia, tachypnea, hypotension, cyanosis, fibrinolysis, leukopenia	Elicit history of febrile reactions. Premedicate with acetaminophen If reaction occurs, stop transfusion and follow hospital policy for suspected febrile reaction Administer saline washed or leukocyte-poor red blood cells
Bacterial (gram-negative organisms and endotoxin release)	Fever, rigors, circulatory collapse, mental confusion, septic shock	Maintain proper blood storage and administration conditions. Stop transfusion immediately Obtain blood for cultures, return blood to lab for culturing. Administer emergency treatment as needed Administer antibiotics as ordered

Table A-11 Adult Central Venous Catheters: Recommended Nursing Management

Type	Heparinization	Dressing	Blood Sampling
CENTRAL VENOUS CATHETERS			
Short-term Use (2-8 weeks)			
Subclavian Single, Dual, and Triple Lumen	After each use, flash *each* lumen with 5 mL Normal Saline (NS), then heparinized saline 2 mL (100 μ/mL). For catheter *not* in use, flush *each* lumen with heparinized saline 2 mL (100 μ/mL) *every 12 hours.*	Daily sterile dressing change at site for duration of catheter placement. Gauze dressing change *every 24 hours;* bio-occlusive change *every 72 hrs.* Change Luer-Lok injection caps *every 72 hours.*	Shut off all IVs for *one (1) full minute.* Withdraw 5 mL blood. Discard. Withdraw blood sample. Flush lumen with 5 mL NS, then heparinize or resume IV. TPN–SHUT OFF IV 10 MINUTES.
PERIPHERAL INSERTED CATHETER			
Longline PICC§ (Use gentle pressure on syringe plunger for PIC catheters)	After each use, flush *each* lumen with 2 mL NS, then heparinized saline 1 mL (100 μ/mL)	Sterile dressings at the site for duration of the catheter placement; Change dressing after first 24 hours, then *every 72 hours.*	Shut off all IVs for *one (1) full minute.* Withdraw 1.5mL blood. Discard. Withdraw blood sample. Flush lumen with 2.5 mL NS then heparinize or resume IV.

Continued.

Table A-11 Cont'd.

Type	Heparinization	Dressing	Blood Sampling
	For catheter *not* in use, flush *each* lumen with heparinized saline 1 mL (100 μ/mL) *every 12 hours*	Change Luer-Lok injection caps *every 12 hours*	TPN-SHUT OFF IV 10 MIN ONLY blood sample from PIC catheter 4.0 Fr (18 gauge) or larger
TUNNELED CATHETERS *Long-Term Use (1-3 years)* Broviac Hickman Quinton-Raaf *(single, dual, triple, and quad lumens)*	After each use, flush *each* lumen with 5 mL NS, then heparinized saline 2 mL (100 μ/mL) For catheter *not* in use, flush *each* lumen with heparinized saline 2 to 5 mL (100 μ/mL) *daily/ biweekly*	Daily sterile dressing change at exit site for at least 14 days. Gauze dressing change *every 24 hrs;* bio-occlusive change *every 72 hrs.* Thereafter, cleanse exit site daily (Betadine/alcohol). Optional daily clean dressing. Change Luer-Lok injection caps *weekly*	Shut off all IVs for one (1) *full minute.* Withdraw 5 mL blood. Discard. Withdraw blood sample. Flush lumen with 5mL NS, then heparinize or resume IV. TPN-SHUT OFF IV 10 MINUTES.

GROSHONG

Single, Dual and Triple lumen

Does not require heparin to maintain catheter patency. *Use force when flushing.* Flush *each* lumen with 5 mL NS after each use, except for TPN, then flush with 30 mL NS. For catheter *not* in use, flush with 5 mL NS weekly*

Daily sterile dressing change at exit site for at least 14 days. Gauze dressing change *every 24 hrs;* bio-occlusive change every 72 hrs. Thereafter, cleanse exit site daily (Betadine/alcohol). Optional daily clean dressing. Change Luer-Lok injection caps *weekly*

Shut off all IVs for *one (1) full minute.* Withdraw 5 mL blood. Discard. Withdraw blood sample. Flush lumen with 30 mL NS *vigorously,* then resume IV or apply injection cap*. TPN-SHUT OFF IV 10 MINUTES

IMPLANTABLE VASCULAR ACCESS DEVICES

- Davol Port
- Infuse-A-Port
- Life Port
- Omega Port
- Port-A-Cath

After each use, flush *each* port with huber needle—10 mL NS, followed by heparinized saline (100 μ/mL).† For port *not* in use, flush each port with 3 to 10 mL

Sterile bio-occlusive dressing when port accessed. Steri-strips at new incision site for 3 days. When incision site healed and port not accessed, no dressing

Shut off all IVs for *one (1) full minute.* Withdraw 5 mL blood. Discard. Withdraw blood sample. Flush with 20 mL NS followed by 3 to 10 mL

Continued.

Table A-11 Cont'd.

Type	Heparinization	Dressing	Blood Sampling
	heparinized saline (100 μ/mL) *every 30 days* (venous placement). Intermittent flush > 1 day/use NS and/or low dose/ volume heparin‡	required. When port is accessed for continuous infusion, change needle and extension tubing every 5-7 days	heparinized saline (100 μ/mL)* or resume IV. TPN-SHUT OFF IV 10 MINUTES
Tunneled catheters heparinization varies process	10-1,000 μ/mL concentration; frequency daily, biweekly, weekly and amount 2-5 mL		

* Selected oncologists use 2 to 5 mL heparinized saline (100 μ/mL).
† Check manufacturer's specific recommendations regarding volume. Oncologists use heparin 10 mL (100 μ/mL).
‡ Assess patient, disease, platelet count with frequency/volume/concentration of heparinization schedule.
§ Use 5 mL or larger syringes when flushing and/or blood sampling from PIC catheter.

Bibliography

Infusion Therapies

1. LaRocca JL and Otto SE: *Pocket guide to intravenous therapy,* ed 2, St Louis, 1993, Mosby.

2. Skidmore-Roth, L: *Mosby's 1994 Nursing Drug Reference,* St Louis, 1994, Mosby Year Book.

3. Walker, RH: Editor-in-chief, *Technical Manual,* American Association of Blood Banks, Arlington, VA, 1994.

Index

Drug	Zofran	Vincristine*	Vinblastine*	Vancomycin	Tobramycin	Sodium Bicarbonate	Ranitidine	Potassium Chloride	Morphine Sulfate	Mitoxantrone	Metoclopromide	Methotrexate	Mesna	Meperidine	Magnesium Sulfate
Aminophylline	I				C		C	C	I		C			I	
Amphotericin B	I				C		I	I							
Bleomycin	C										CY	I			
Carmustine	C														
Cisplatin	C										CY	CY	I		C
Cyclophosphamide	C										CY	CY			
Cyclosporin	C			CY⁴	CY⁴	CY⁴					CY	CY			
Cytarabine	C										C				
Dacarabazine															
Daunorubicin															
Dopamine						I	CY⁴	C							
Doxorubicin												I			
5-Flurouracil	?										CY	CY			
Furosemide	I	I	I								I	I			
Heparin	C	I	I	I	I	CY		C	CY⁴	I	C			CY	CY
Magnesium Sulfate	C			CY⁴	CY⁴	I		C			C				
Meperidine															
Mesna															
Methotrexate	C														
Metoclopromide						I	C	C	C					CY	C
Mitoxantrone															
Morphine Sulfate	C					I	C				C				
Potassium Chloride	C			C		C			CY		C			CY⁴	C
Ranitidine	C										C	I			
Sodium Bicarbonate				I				C	I		I	C		I	I
Tobramycin															
Vancomycin	C					I	C	C	CY⁴					CY⁴	CY⁴
Vinblastine															
Vincristine															
Zofran				C			C	C	C		C				C

? - Call your pharmacist about drug stability
C - Compatible: documented physically
CY - compatible for 24 hours
CY⁴ - Compatible via Y-site infusion
CY⁴ - Compatible via Y-site infusion, 4 hours
CY⁸ - Compatible via Y-site infusion, 8 hours
I - Incompatible: physical instability has been documented
* - Incompatible with other drugs in solution or syringe
- no information available; DO NOT assume compatibility